Prevention and Treatment of Diabetic Late Complications

This publication is sponsored by Bayer AG, Leverkusen, W.-Germany.

Diabetes Forum Series, Volume 2

Prevention and Treatment of Diabetic Late Complications

Editors: C. E. Mogensen, E. Standl

Walter de Gruyter
Berlin · New York 1989

Deutsche Bibliothek Cataloging-in-Publication-Data

Prevention and treatment of diabetic late complications / ed.: C. E. Mogensen ; E. Standl. – Berlin ; New York : de Gruyter, 1989
ISBN 3-11-012297-9
NE: Mogensen, Carl E. [Hrsg.]

Library of Congress Cataloging-in-Publication Data

Prevention and treatment of diabetic late complications / editors, C.E. Mogensen, E. Standl.
p. cm. –
Includes bibliographical references.
ISBN 0-89925-637-6 (U.S.)
1. Diabetes—Complications and sequelae. I. Mogensen, Carl Erik. II. Standl, E. (Eberhard)
[DNLM: 1. Diabetes Mellitus—complications. WK 835 P9438]
RC660.P744 1989
616.4′62—dc20
DNLM/DLC
for Library of Congress 89-17135
CIP

Medical science is constantly developing. Research and clinical experience expand our knowledge, especially with regard to treatment and medication.

For dosages and applications mentioned in this work, the reader may rely on the authors, editors and publisher having taken great pains to ensure that these indications reflect the standard of knowledge at the time this work was completed.

Nevertheless, all users are requested to check the package leaflet of the medication, in order to determine for themselves whether the recommendations given for the dosages or the likely contraindications differ from those given in this book. This is especially true for medication which is seldom used or has recently been put on the market and for medication whose application has been restricted by the German Ministry of Health.

The quotation of registered names, trade names, trade marks, etc. in this copy does not imply, even in the absence of a specific statement that such names are exempt from laws and regulations protecting trade marks, etc. and therefore free for general use.

Typesetting: Arthur Collignon GmbH, Berlin. – Printing: Gerike GmbH, Berlin. – Binding: Lüderitz & Bauer GmbH, Berlin. – Printed in Germany.

Editors

Prof. Dr. C. E. Mogensen
Medical Department M
Second University Clinic
of Internal Medicine
(Diabetes and Endocrinology)
Kommunehospitalet
DK-8000 Aarhus C
Denmark

Prof. Dr. E. Standl
Third Med. Department
City Hospital Schwabing
and Diabetes Research Unit
Kölner Platz 1
D-8000 Munich 40
FRG

List of First-mentioned Contributors

Prof. Dr. D. A. Greene
Room 5510 C, MSRB-I, Box 068
1150 W. Medical Center Drive
University of Michigan,
Medical Center
Ann Arbor, Michigan 48 109
USA

Prof. Dr. Ava Grenfell
52 Talfourd Road
GB-London SE 15 5 NY
Great Britain

Priv.-Doz. Dr. H. U. Janka
Third Med. Department
City Hospital Schwabing
and Diabetes Research Unit
Kölner Platz 1
D-8000 Munich 40
FRG

Dr. T. Jensen
Steno Memorial Hospital
Niels Steensensvej 2
DK-2820 Gentofte
Denmark

Dr. Eva M. Kohner
Hammersmith Hospital
Du Cane Road
GB-London W12 OH5
Great Britain

Dr. Lori M. B. Laffel
Joslin Diabetes Center
Harvard Medical School
1 Joslin Place
Boston, Massachusetts 02 215
USA

Prof. Dr. K. Pyörälä
Department of Medicine
University of Kuopio
SF-70 210 Kuopio
Finland

Preface

Diabetes mellitus is a very common disorder characterized by hyperglycemia. There are several syndromes associated with diabetes mellitus, but the major disease entities are type I or insulin dependent diabetes, and type II or non-insulin dependent diabetes. Diabetes is very common throughout the world, especially type II diabetes, whereas insulin dependent diabetes has a considerably higher frequency in certain countries, for instance Scandinavian countries, and also in North America. This type of diabetes is rare in Japan, where type II diabetes is much more common.

Type I diabetes is believed to be a chronic autoimmune disease associated with selective islet beta-cell destruction, leading to a deficient insulin secretion and subsequently to the clinical disease diabetes mellitus. The exact etiology of type II diabetes has remained a mystery until today. It is clearly genetically influenced and often associated with obesity. Still uncertain is how heterogeneous this syndrome may be, and it is equally uncertain whether the primary lesion or lesions are in the pancreas or in the peripheral tissue, with insulin resistance as a major pathogenetic mechanism.

However, both types or, in fact, all types of diabetes are quite often complicated by vascular and neurological disorders, occurring in the context of the disordered metabolism. Longstanding hyperglycemia is, indeed, the major factor associated with diabetic complications.

There has been considerable progress with respect to the study of diabetic complications over the last years, and the editors, therefore, believe that it is now time to sum up this recent extension of our knowledge within the field of diabetic complications. Today we have a much clearer understanding of the long-term complications of diabetes. The frequency in relation to diabetes duration has been greatly clarified over the recent years, in particular with respect to diabetic eye disease and diabetic kidney disease. Also great progress has been achieved regarding the understanding of the etiology and pathogenesis of long-term diabetic complications, although much further work needs to be done. This is probably because a number of factors are involved in the disease process, e. g. metabolic, hormonal, and hemodynamic aberrations. Therefore, it is also difficult to formulate a single pathogenetic process to explain the broad spectrum of diabetic complications, in the eyes as well as in the nerves, the vasculature, the heart and the kidney. Each organ seems specifically to be modified in its response to hyperglycemia and other aberrations associated with diabetes mellitus. Although we do not understand exactly the disease process, much progress has taken place within the field of the treatment of complications. Of course, a major issue is treatment of hyperglycemia and associated metabolic abnormalities. Apparently, if all blood glucose values were normalized right from the beginning of diabetes we believe that there would be no diabetic complications. Therefore, optimising antidiabetic treatment is a major issue for the diabetologists, and obviously diet intervention, treatment with insulin, and classical oral agents are the major treatment modality, although new perspectives are emerging. Unfortunately, it is difficult to normalize blood glucose values, which is evidenced from mean values of glycated hemoglobin in our diabetic clinics. Quite often mean values are around 8 per cent, provided a normal reference value of 5.5%, suggesting that many patients experience long-term hyperglycemia. A number of non-glycemic intervention modalities are important in all organ systems. In general, the modality is easily understood on the basis of the pathogenesis of the disease, e. g. antihypertensive treatment in patients with diabetic nephropathy and associated elevated blood pressure. In other instances we do not know the exact way in which a certain treatment modality acts. E. g., the exact mechanisms in the development of diabetic eye disease are not clarified, nor is it fully understood through which mechanisms laser treatment exerts its effects, although this treatment modality certainly is effective and is now standard treatment in the Western World. This volume will provide a fairly broad review of the major diabetic complications, even if not all aspects are included, e. g. diabetic skin disease. The reader of this volume is presented with a summary of our present knowledge on important pathogenetic mechanisms and classification systems with respect to the various entities of complications, and also an update of our treatment procedures. In addition, this volume will provide the reader with key references to the wide-ranging literature on diabetic complications.

Finally, the editors would like to express their sincere thanks to Bayer AG for a very fine and effective cooperation. We are also pleased to acknowledge the excellent and kind cooperation with the publisher, Walter de Gruyter & Co. in Berlin.

Aarhus and Munich
July 1989

Carl-Erik Mogensen and *Eberhard Standl*

Contents

History of diabetic complications

A. Grenfell

Introduction

The introduction of insulin in 1922 was one of the great achievements of modern 20th century medicine. It provided a lifesaving remedy for many diabetic patients and led to a new era for diabetes. However, although most of the features of diabetic complications had been described well before the introduction of insulin it was not until patients survived for longer periods that the full extent and often fatal nature of diabetic complications was realised. Lundbaek in 1954 [1] introduced the concept of diabetic angiopathy – a specific widespread diabetic small vessel disease – as the common mechanism leading to diabetic complications. Considerable advances have been made since then in our understanding of diabetic complications yet we still do not sufficiently understand the underlying pathogenesis of these complications to allow for effective preventive measures.

In this chapter I intend to trace the history of those small vessel complications specific to diabetes as described by Lundbaek, namely retinopathy, neuropathy, and nephropathy. Despite the importance of large vessel disease in diabetes in terms of mortality and morbidity I shall not cover these complications since they are non-specific and very similar in nature, if not frequency, in the non-diabetic, and well described elsewhere.

Retinopathy

Eye changes in diabetes were first noted almost 200 years ago. Rollo in 1798 [2] in the first detailed monograph on diabetic eye complications described an association between diabetes and cataract that was given much prominence over the next 100 years. However by the early 1900s it was being suggested that the incidence of cataract in diabetic patients was no greater than in non-diabetic patients. It was suggested that the only truly 'diabetic cataract' was that found in juvenile diabetics as bilateral fine subcapsular dots first described by Schnyder in 1923 and called snowflake opacities [3]. Interest however, had been directed towards more specific diabetic eye disease by the introduction of the ophthalmoscope in 1850 by Helmholtz.

One of the earliest descriptions of diabetic retinitis was by Jaeger in 1855 [4] who suggested that the fine deep retinal haemorrhages and waxy exudates he saw might be specific to diabetes. However, it was noted that such changes were also found in patients with vascular disease and hypertension and it was suggested that similar factors were operating in diabetic patients. Capillary microaneurysms were described by MacKenzie in 1877 [5] from post-mortem studies and were thought to be specific for diabetes. He also described retinal and vitreous haemorrhage characteristic of diabetic retinopathy. Thus by the turn of the century most of the features of diabetic retinopathy had been described. These observations were further extended by two large surveys of diabetic patients [3, 6]. Waite and Beetham (1935) in a survey of 2002 diabetic patients described deep retinal haemorrhages and waxy exudates. They also noted that in the 31 patients with vessel proliferation and vitreous haemorrhage over 90% had severe renal and/or vascular disease.

A classic description of diabetic retinopathy was given by Ballantyne and Lowenstein in 1944 [6] who focussed attention once again on the importance of microaneurysms as the earliest lesion in diabetic retinopathy. They described retinopathy as occurring in 5 stages: – 1) microaneurysms plus or minus punctate haemorrhages and small exudates, 2) dot and blot haemorrhages plus waxy exudates, 3) large haemorrhages, vascular abnormalities, new vessels in the vitreous body and early proliferation of vessels, 4) advanced stages of 3), 5) retinal detachment and end stage features. Yet even as late as 1952 it was stated by Warren and LeCompte [7] that "the question as to whether the diabetic eye shows any characteristic or pathognomonic changes is still disputed".

Many histological studies of diabetic retinopathy have been performed. Friedenwald (1953) [8] using periodic acid-Schiff staining of whole mounts of the retina clearly demonstrated that capillary microaneurysms were a true entity. This was confirmed by the injection studies of the retina by Ashton (1959) [9]. Both Friedenwald and Ashton commented on the association of microaneurysms with intercapillary glomerulosclerosis and speculated as to whether there may be any pathogenetic relationship. Friedenwald suggested that both may represent disturbances in the metabolism of muccopolysaccharides.

Considerable uncertainty remained however as to the aetiology of retinopathy as the coexistence of hypertension, arteriosclerosis and renal disease confused the picture. Waite and Beetham [3] suggested that these factors were of aetiological importance yet following this time there were many reports of retinopathy occuring in the absence of hypertension, arterial and renal disease. It was postulated that small haemorrhages resulted from capillary dilatation with slowing of blood flow and suggested that this was related to hyperglycaemia rather than other factors. Ballantyne in 1945 [10] emphasised the possible role of venous stasis in the production of capillary dilatation and haemorrhage. An alternative suggestion was that increased capillary fragility accounted for retinal haemorrhage and this led to a vogue in treatment with a variety of agents such as vitamin C, citrin, hesperidin and rutin [11].

By the mid 1960s proliferative retinopathy was established as pathognomonic of diabetes and the association with diabetic nephropathy, neuropathy and vascular disease firmly established. Root and colleagues from the Joslin clinic had already coined the term "triopathy" to describe the clinical association of retinopathy with nephropathy and neuropathy [12]. In the Joslin clinic series retinopathy almost always preceded proteinuria and usually occurred in patients under the age of 40 years with previously poor diabetic control. They also showed that the commonest causes of death in patients with proliferative retinopathy were nephropathy and coronary heart disease.

The treatment of diabetic retinopathy has a long and interesting history. Dietary manipulations were used in an attempt to reduce circulating lipids and decrease capillary fragility as these were thought to have a beneficial effect. Reduction of dietary lipids led to a decrease in hard exudates but had no effect on proliferative retinopathy or vision. Various vitamins and flavanoids were used in the late 1950s in an attempt to reduce capillary fragility but there was no real clinical evidence of benefit.

A large variety of drugs (iodides, salicylates, Vitamin K, heparin, clofibrate) have been used in the treatment of diabetic retinopathy but to date no medical therapy has proved to be effective. Two deserve mention. Heparin was used in an attempt to reduce chylomicrons and triglycerides from the blood but apart from reducing hard exudates had little effect. Clofibrate has also been used and reduces the number of waxy exudates but appears to have little influence on the development of maculopathy or visual acuity. Whether aldose reductase inhibitors have a role to play in the future remains to be seen.

Adrenalectomy was used for some time in the treatment of diabetic retinopathy, the rationale being that it would stabilize brittle diabetes and control hypertension. Overall benefit was small and complicated by the need for replacement therapy.

Pituitary ablation survived for a much longer time as a treatment for diabetic retinopathy. Two observations provided the basis for such treatment. Firstly that of Houssay and Biasotti in 1931 [13] who showed that hypophysectomy ameliorated the metabolic effects of pancreatomised animals and secondly that of Poulsen in 1953 [14] who reported significant improvement of severe retinopathy in a woman with post-partum pituitary failure. Early attempts at hypophysectomy met with little success mainly due to the fact that the patients selected had such severe retinopathy that improvement was unlikely to occur. By 1962 pituitary ablation was still an investigational form of therapy despite reports of a reduction in retinal and vitreous haemorrhage following pituitary ablation [15]. However, following this time until the early 1970s increasing numbers of patients were treated with pituitary ablation by a variety of methods. The overall results showed an improvement or stabilisation in about 50% of cases. However, there was a substantial morbidity and some mortality and no really convincing evidence that pituitary ablation altered the course of proliferative retinopathy. The only randomised trial was reported by Lundbaek in 1968 [16] who showed that in a matched series of patients and controls hypophysectomy resulted in better preservation of visual acuity with slower development of new vessels.

The present day laser treatment of diabetic retinopathy originated with the use of light photocoagulation by Meyer-Schwickerath in the 1950s in Germany for the treatment of a variety of retinal conditions. In 1963 he published details on 139 diabetic patients treated with a xenon arc to photocoagulate microaneurysms and new vessels [17]. The treated patients showed better preservation of vision than controls. Further encouraging reports were published during the 1960s but by 1971 it still remained a relatively new procedure with most of the relevant chapter in the 11th edition of Joslin's diabetes devoted to pituitary ablation [11]. However, it was stated in this chapter that 'the possible role of photocoagulation in altering the course of retinitis proliferans has been sufficiently established to warrant further investigation of potential long term benefits'. By this time many patients were declining to have pituitary ablation due to the unpleasant side effects and increasing numbers began to be treated with photocoagulation.

Neuropathy

Some of the earliest descriptions of diabetic neuropathy were given by Rollo [2] who described pain and paraesthesia in the legs of diabetic patients although during his time diabetes was commonly considered to result from disease of the nervous system. It was Marchal de Calvi [18] who first suggested that diabetes might be the cause rather than the result of neurological disease. He described pain in the sciatic distribution, peripheral anaesthesia, and frequent absence of the tendon jerks in diabetic patients. This was followed by several clear descriptions of diabetic neuropathy with notable contributions. Bouchard (1884) described the frequent absence of tendon reflexes in the legs [19]. Pavy (1885) gave a classic description of neuropathy – "they cannot feel properly in their legs, ... their feet are numb, ... their legs seem heavy ... darting or lightening pains are often complained of. Or there may be hyperaesthesia ... not unfrequently there is deep-seated pain". He noted that pain was especially prominent at night and that there was usually loss of patellar tendon reflex [20]. Althaus (1885) noted the close similarity of diabetic neuropathy to tabes-dorsalis [21] and this led to the introduction of the term pseudo-tabes. Motor manifestations in the legs were described by Charcot (1890) who compared the neuropathy of alcohol with that of diabetes [22].

Auche (1890) reviewed the literature, added new cases of his own, and attempted experimentally to reproduce the nerve lesions by injecting them with concentrated sugar solutions [23]. He stated that the nervous system complications of diabetes may involve all nerve functions including motor, sensory, special sensory, intellectual, and nutritional. He described the following symptoms: pain especially at night, paraesthesia, hyperaesthesia and anaesthesia, paralysis, vasomotor and trophic changes and depression of reflexes. He did not think there was bladder or rectal involvement. Thus, by the turn of the century the clinical picture of diabetic neuropathy was almost complete and, apart from the description of autonomic neuropathy, little was to be added in the next 50 years.

The first real description of autonomic neuropathy was not until 1945 yet references to clinical symptoms such as peripheral oedema, abnormal sweating, and bladder problems had been made before this time [24]. Rundles (1945) gave the first clear description of autonomic neuropathy in his survey of 125 diabetic patients with neuropathy [25]. He stated: "The unusual tendency of diabetic neuropathy to involve autonomic nerves results in such extraordinary diverse clinical manifestations of the neuritic disease as neuropathic (Charcot) joints, grossly disturbed gastrointestinal and genito-urinary function, abnormal orthostatic blood pressure regulation etc". He also described abnormal sweating patterns, peripheral oedema and abnormal pupillary reactions and noted that these features tended to occur together.

Despite further clinical features during the 1950s and 1960s tests to assess autonomic function were invasive and complex and autonomic neuropathy was considered a rare complication of diabetes. The introduction of simple non-invasive autonomic function tests during the 1970s led to a realisation that autonomic neuropathy was much more common in diabetes than previously realised. During the last decade there has been a much better understanding of the natural history of diabetic neuropathy and better definition of the various syndromes [26].

The highly variable nature of diabetic neuropathy has led to numerous attempts at classification. Pryce (1893) suggested that diabetic neuropathy be divided into two types: a patchy motor variety, and a sensory or ataxic variety [27]. Whereas Von Leyden (1893) suggested classification into 3 groups: a hyperaesthetic or neuralgic form, a paralytic or motor form and an ataxic or pseudo-tabetic form [28]. More recently Sullivan (1958) suggested division into an asymmetrical painful, mainly motor variety and a symmetrical distal and predominantly sensory neuropathy [29]. Pirart (1978) in his careful documentation of over 4000 patients between 1947 and 1973 failed to detect any regular pattern of clinical manifestations and suggested that no really satisfactory classification was possible [30]. However, the occurrence of certain groups of clinical features with sufficient frequency has led to continued attempts at classification.

Despite extensive study in recent years the pathogenesis of diabetic neuropathy remains almost as uncertain and controversial as in 1945 [25]. Debate still continues over the relative contribution of metabolic and vascular factors to the pathogenesis of diabetic neuropathy [31].

The importance of hyperglycaemia in the development of diabetic neuropathy was for many years of considerable uncertainty. Was diabetic neuropathy a complication or concomitant of diabetes? It was pointed out that symptoms may be present at the time of diagnosis of diabetes or appear when diabetes is first brought under control. Also there often seemed to be no relationship between the duration and/or severity of diabetes and the presence of neuropathy and several cases of apparent diabetic neuropathy were described without manifest diabetes. It was suggested by Ellenberg that neuropathy was a separate manifestation of diabetes and largely independent of carbohydrate metabolism [32]. Yet many workers provided evidence to the contrary. Rundles pointed out that he had not "seen a patient where 'diabetic' neuropathy actually preceded the appearance of diabetes mellitus" and that there was a striking correlation between diabetic control and the development of neuritic complications. He stated "the conclusion is inescapable that diabetic neuropathy is not only truly 'diabetic' in etiology but results from the abnormal metabolism of chronically unregulated diabetes" [25]. Pirart clearly showed that there was a relationship between the degree of hyperglycaemia and the occurrence of neuropathy [30]. He showed that the annual incidence of neuropathy was related to the duration of diabetes. Neuropathy was rare at the time of diagnosis in young patients but was much more frequent in those diagnosed as diabetic over the age of 40 years. This was due to the presence of un-diagnosed diabetes in the older subjects rather than a greater propensity to neuropathy.

The metabolic abnormalities of hyperglycaemia in diabetic nerves and their role in diabetic neuropathy have received much attention in recent years. It has been suggested that persistent hyperglycaemia activates the polyol pathway in nerves via the enzyme aldose reductase which results in the accumulation of sorbitol in nerve. Myo-inositol uptake by nerve is also thought to be inhibited leading to altered phosphoinositide metabolism and a reduction in axolemmal sodium-potassium ATPase with consequent alteration in nerve conduction and finally structural damage. However, not all workers agree on these findings and such ideas remain controversial.

Arteriosclerosis has long been recognised as a complication of diabetes and its widespread presence in amputated and autopsy specimens of lower limbs from diabetics led to the suggestion for an aetiological role in diabetic neuropathy. Both Charcot [22] and Pryce [27] suggested this possibility which was re-emphasised by Dry and Hines in 1941 [33]. Large vessel disease has since been discarded as a cause for diabetic neuropathy but a role for small vessel disease has been suggested by many workers. Lundbaek (1954) was one of the first to suggest a generalised specific small vessel disease to account for diabetic complications [1]. Fagerberg (1959) suggested that diabetic microangiopathy might account for most of the manifestations of diabetic neuropathy [34]. He described stenosis and hyalinisation of the intraneural vessels with subendothelial deposits together with thickening of the capillary basement membrane. These ideas assumed less importance as theories for the role of metabolic abnormalities in diabetic neuropathy were developed. More recently, however there has been renewed interest in the role of vascular lesions in the pathogenesis of diabetic neuropathy.

Microvascular abnormalities have been clearly demonstrated in both endoneurial and perineurial vessels in patients with neuropathy [35] and the severity of neuropathy shown to relate to the number of 'closed' capillaries. Recent autopsy studies of nerve trunks from diabetic patients have concluded that ischaemia of the nerve trunk is important in the pathogenesis of diabetic neuropathy [36]. Endoneurial hypoxia has been demonstrated in the nerves of patients with sensorimotor neuropathy [37]. Both metabolic and vascular factors may have a role since hyperglycaemia may act through the non-enzymatic glycosylation of vasa nervorum and the endoneurial matrix to cause ischaemia. Further work is required to unravel the relative contribution of theses various factors to the pathogenesis of diabetic neuropathy and provide clues for treatment and preventive measures.

Nephropathy

Proteinuria in association with diabetes has been recognised since at least 1770 [38, 2], but its significance was not realised until 1936 when Kimmelstiel and Wilson described the specific renal histology associated with the clinical features of hypertension, the nephrotic syndrome and renal failure in diabetic patients [39]. The glomerular and renovascular lesions characteristic of diabetes had already been described but their significance overlooked.

The first description of proteinuria in diabetics is attributed to Cotunnius in 1770 [38] but it was not until Bright's famous studies associating proteinuria with renal disease [40] that interest in proteinuria and diabetes was really stimulated. During the 19th century the association of proteinuria with diabetes was established and in some cases it was noted to occur with oedema and renal failure, poor vision and cardiac disease. It was gradually realised that proteinuria, especially if persistent, meant a poor prognosis for the diabetic patient although even as recently as 1941 it was stated that proteinuria in diabetes was of little importance [41].

Glomerular lesions in the diabetic kidney received little attention before 1900. Characteristic lesions were described but the significance of these lesions and their relationship to the clinical syndrome of diabetic nephropathy was not appreciated [42].

Kimmelstiel and Wilson described the renal histology at autopsy in eight patients of whom 7 had diabetes, together with hypertension, albuminuria, oedema, and renal failure [39]. The glomeruli showed a striking nodular accumulation of hyaline material in the central lobules with decrease in the number of capillaries so that "in many cases there remains only a ring of open capillaries surrounding the central hyaline mass". The capillary walls were thickened and when collapsed merged with the central hyaline mass. There was marked arteriosclerosis with hyalinisation of the afferent arterioles. They considered that the glomerular lesion was a thickening of the intercapillary connective tissue and so called it intercapillary glomerulosclerosis.

These findings were extended by other workers who confirmed the existence of a specific histology of the kidney in diabetes. 'Diffuse glomerulosclerosis' was described and distinguished from the 'nodular' form of Kimmelstiel and Wilson [43]. Destruction of glomeruli was more closely associated with the diffuse disease which also correlated more closely with the clinical course. Dispute however continued over the histogenesis of the lesion. That is whether it was truly 'intercapillary' and due to expansion of the intercapillary tissue or rather derived from a thickening of the capillary walls themselves i.e. 'intracapillary' or 'intramural'.

Arteriolar lesions were also shown to be of some importance in the pathology of diabetic nephropathy. Both afferent and efferent arterioles were shown to be involved in hyaline arteriosclerosis [43] often sufficiently characteristic of diabetes to be of aid in the diagnosis of diabetic nephropathy by light microscope.

The clinical features originally described by Kimmelstiel and Wilson were subsequently shown to vary, and many cases of intercapillary glomerulosclerosis were found to be asymptomatic [44, 7]. However, patients with the most severe lesions generally had the most severe clinical features [44]. Intercapillary glomerulosclerosis was shown to be more closely related to the duration of diabetes than the age of the patients and was found particularly in young diabetics of long duration [7].

The introduction of percutaneous renal biopsies in 1951 rapidly led to a greater understanding of the disease. Early electron microscopy demonstrated two primary changes – a thickening of the capillary basement membrane and an extracellular accumulation of hyaline or basement membrane-like material. The presence and nature of the mesangium was established and it was suggested that some of the earliest changes in the kidney in diabetes consisted of the accumulation of basement membrane-like material in the mesangium together with basement membrane thickening. As the mesangial deposits enlarged they were thought to compress and distort adjacent endothelial cells and so lead to capillary closure and destruction of the glomerulus.

Electron microscopy with its greater resolution and magnification made possible the detection of changes at the onset of diabetes and so presented an entirely new concept of diabetic complications. The observation by Siperstein in 1968 that basement membrane thickening of quadriceps muscle capillaries could be seen in 'pre-diabetics' precipitated a controversy on the pathogenesis of microangiopathy that was to continue for the next ten years [45]. Siperstein proposed that microangiopathy was not due to the metabolic derangements of diabetes but was due to genetic predisposition. This was not confirmed by other workers for either muscle or glomerular capillaries [46, 47] and fuelled much dispute especially over techniques for fixing and analysing specimens. Osterby in careful morphometric studies showed that there was no glomerular basement membrane thickening at diagnosis of diabetes and that this was not detectable until at least two years of diabetes [46]. More recently comparison of muscle and glomerular capillary basement membrane widths from identical twins discordant for insulin-dependent diabetes has confirmed that the non-diabetics do not show any thickening of the basement membrane [48]. Further evidence for the argument that the abnormal metabolic state of diabetes is necessary for the development of these lesions comes from the work of Mauer and colleagues in Minneapolis which showed the development of characteristic lesions in normal kidneys transplanted into diabetic patients [49].

Interest in factors underlying the rate of progression of the renal lesion in diabetic nephropathy was stimulated by an autopsy report describing a patient with diabetes and unilateral renal artery stenosis [50]. The kidney with the stenotic artery showed ischaemic changes only, whereas the other kidney showed marked glomerulosclerosis. It was suggested that this was due to exposure of the kidney to hypertension as well as diabetes. This observation was confirmed and extended by a study of rats with experimentally induced renal artery stenosis and diabetes [51]. It was shown that in the kidney exposed to diabetes and hypertension the development of diabetic glomerular lesions was accelerated whereas in the kidney protected from hypertension these lesions did not occur. Such changes were not seen in non-diabetic rats. Thus it was suggested that haemodynamic factors, namely increased glomerular capillary blood flow and increased capillary pressure may influence the rate at which diabetic nephropathy progresses.

Similar factors appear to be important in man. A genetic predisposition to hypertension may be important in determining those at high risk of developing diabetic nephropathy although these observations were not confirmed in large Danish studies (T. Deckert, personal communication) [52]. Treatment of hypertension in insulin-dependent diabetic patients has been shown to reduce the decline in glomerular filtration rate [53, 54]. In addition it has been suggested that those diabetic patients with the highest GFR early in the course of their disease may be the most likely to subsequently develop diabetic nephropathy [55].

Summary

Diabetic nephropathy is an important cause of morbidity and mortality and may account for up to one quarter of patients on renal replacement programmes. Retinopathy still causes significant morbidity and diabetes remains this single most common cause of blindness in the working population. Neuropathy is of importance especially in terms of foot lesions which account for a significant proportion of hospital bed occupancy. The last 50 years have seen a great increase in our understanding of the basic pathology and physiology of these diabetic complications. However, much remains to be done especially in understanding the basic pathogenetic mechanisms and how to recognize those at risk, if these devastating complications are to be prevented.

References

[1] Lundbaek K. Diabetic angiopathy. A specific vascular disease. Lancet 1954; 1: 377.
[2] Rollo J. Cases of the Diabetes Mellitus, 2nd edn. London: Dilly, 1798.
[3] Waite JH, Beetham WP. Visual mechanism in diabetes mellitus; comparative study of 2002 diabetics and 457 non-diabetics for control. N. Engl J Med 1935; 212: 367, 429.
[4] Jaeger E. Beiträge zur Pathologie des Auges. Wien, 1855; 33.
[5] MacKenzie, Roy London Opthal Hosp Report 1877; 9: part 2: 152.
[6] Ballantyne AJ, Lowenstein A. Pathology of diabetic retinopathy. Trans Opthal Soc UK 1944; 63: 95.
[7] Warren S, Le Compte PM. The pathology of diabetes mellitus. London: Henry Kimpton, 1952.
[8] Friedenwald JS. Diabetic retinitis; the opthalmologists view. (Soc Proc) Arch Opthal 1953; 50: 124.
[9] Ashton N. Diabetic retinopathy; a new approach. Lancet 1959; 2: 625.
[10] Ballantyne AJ. The state of the retina in diabetes mellitus. Trans Opthal Soc UK 1946; 66: 503.
[11] Bradley RF, Ramos E. The eyes and diabetes. In: Marble A, White P, Bradley RF et al, eds. Joslin's Diabetes Mellitus 11th edn. Philadelphia: Lea and Febiger, 1971; 478.
[12] Root HF, Pote WH, Frehner H. Triopathy of diabetes; sequence of neuropathy, retinopathy, and nephropathy in 155 patients. Arch Intern Med 1954; 94: 931.
[13] Houssay BA, Biasotti A. Pankresdiabetes und Hypophyse beim Hund. Arch ges Physiol 1931; 227: 664.
[14] Poulsen, JE. Houssay phenomenon in man; recovery from retinopathy in a case of diabetes with Simmond's disease. Diabetes 1953; 2: 7.
[15] Luft R, Olivecrona H, Iknos D et al. Hypophysectomy in man. Further experience in severe diabetes mellitus. Brit Med J 1955; 2: 752.
[16] Lundbaek K, Malmos R, Andersen HC et al. Hypophysectomy for diabetic angiopathy. A controlled clinical trial. In: Goldberg MF, Fine SL, eds. Symposium on treatment of diabetic retinopathy. Washington DC: US Government Printing Office, 1968; 291.
[17] Meyer-Schwickerath G. Treatment of vascular disease of the retina with light coagulation. Trans Canad Opthal Soc 1963; 26: 137.
[18] Marchal de Calvi. Recherches sur les accidents diabetiques. Paris: P. Asselin, 1864.
[19] Bouchard M. Loss of the knee-phenomenon in diabetes. Br Med J 1884; 237.
[20] Pavy FW. Introductory address to the discussion on the clinical aspects of glycosuria. Lancet 1885; 2: 1085.
[21] Althaus J. On sclerosis of the spinal cord. London: Longman, 1885.
[22] Charcot M. Sur un cas paraplegie diabetique. Arch Neurol (Paris) 1890; 19: 318.
[23] Auche B. Des alteration des nerfs peripheriques chez les diabetiques. Arch de Med exper et d'anet path 1890; 2: 635.
[24] Jordan WR. Neuritic manifestations in diabetes mellitus. Arch Intern Med 1936; 57: 307.
[25] Rundles RW. Diabetic neuropathy: general review with report of 125 cases. Medicine (Balt) 1945; 24: 11.
[26] Clarke BF, Ewing DJ, Cambell IW. Diabetic autonomic neuropathy. Diabetologia 1979; 12: 195.
[27] Pryce TD. On diabetic neuritis with a clinical and pathological description of three cases of pseudo-tabes. Brain 1893; 16: 416.
[28] Von Leyden E. Beiträge zur Klinik des Diabetes mellitus. Wien med Wchnschr 1893; 43: 926.
[29] Sullivan JF. The neuropathies of diabetes mellitus. Neurology (Minneap) 1958; 8: 243.
[30] Pirart J. Diabetes mellitus and its degenerative complications: a prospective study of 4,400 patients observed between 1947–1973. Diabetes Care 1978; 1: 168, 252.

[31] Asbury AK. Understanding diabetic neuropathy (editorial). N Engl J Med 1988; 319: 577.
[32] Ellenberg M. Diabetic complications without manifest diabetes: complications as presenting clinical symptoms. JAMA 1963; 183: 926.
[33] Dry TJ, Hines EA. The role of diabetes in the development of degenerative vascular disease, with special reference to the incidence of retinitis and peripheral neuritis. Ann Intern Med 1944; 14: 1893.
[34] Fagerberg S-E. Diabetic neuropathy: a clinical and histological study on the significance of vascular affections. Acta Med Scand 1959; 164 (suppl 345): 1.
[35] Timperley WR, Boulton AJM, Davies-Jones GAB et al. Small vessel disease in progressive diabetic neuropathy with good metabolic control. J Clin Pathol 1985; 38: 1030.
[36] Dyck PJ, Karnes JL, O'Brien P et al. The spatial distribution of fiber loss in diabetic polyneuropathy suggests ischaemia. Ann Neurol 1986; 19: 440.
[37] Newrick PG, Wilson AJ, Jakubowski J. Sural nerve oxygen tension in human diabetes. Br Med J 1986; 293: 1053.
[38] Cotunnius D. De Ischiade Nervosa. Vienna, 1770.
[39] Kimmelstiel P, WilsonHier ist Memory Taste 1Hier ist Memory Taste 1 C. Intercapillary lesions in the glomeruli of the kidney. Am J Pathol 1936; 12: 83.
[40] Bright R. Cases and observations illustrative of renal disease accompanied with the secretion of albuminous urine. Guy's Hospital Rep 1836; 1: 338.
[41] Iversen P, Bjering T, Bing J. De Medicinske nyrelidelser. Munksgaard, Copenhagen, 1941.
[42] Bell ET, Clawson BJ. Primary (essential) hypertension. A study of four hundred and twenty cases. Arch Path (Chicago) 1928; 5: 939.
[43] Bell ET. Renal lesions in diabetes mellitus. Am J Pathol 1942; 18: 744.
[44] Rogers J, Robbins SL. Intercapillary glomerulosclerosis: a clinical and pathological study. Am J Med 1952; 12: 688.
[45] Siperstein MD, Unger RH, Madison LL. Studies of muscle capillary basement membranes in normal subject, diabetic and pre-diabetic patients. J Clin Invest 1968; 47: 1973.
[46] Osterby R. Morphometric studies on the peripheral glomerular basement membrane in early juvenile diabetes 1. Development of initial basement membrane thickening. Diabetologia 1972; 8: 84.
[47] Williamson JR, Kilo C. Current status of capillary basement membrane disease in diabetes mellitus. Diabetes 1977; 26: 65.
[48] Steffes MW, Sutherland DER, Goetz FC et al. Studies of kidney and muscle biopsy specimens from identical twins discordant for type 1 diabetes mellitus. N Engl J Med 1985; 312: 1282.
[49] Mauer SM, Steffes MW, Connett J et al. The development of lesions in the glomerular basement membrane and mesangium after transplantation of normal kidneys to diabetic patients. Diabetes 1983; 32: 948.
[50] Berkman J, Rifkin H. Unilateral nodular diabetic glomerulosclerosis (Kimmelstiel–Wilson): Report of a case. Metabolism 1973; 22: 715.
[51] Mauer SM, Steffes MW, Azar S et al. The effect of Goldblatt hypertension on development of the glomerular lesions of diabetes mellitus in the rat. Diabetes 1978; 27: 738.
[52] Krolewski AS, Canessa M, Warram JH et al. Predisposition to hypertension and susceptability to renal disease in insulin dependent diabetes mellitus. N Engl J Med 1988; 318: 140.
[53] Mogensen CE. Long-term antihypertensive treatment inhibiting progression of diabetic nephropathy. Br Med J 1982; 285: 685–688.
[54] Parving H-H, Andersen AR, Smidt UM et al. Early aggressive antihypertensive treatment reduces the rate of decline in kidney function in diabetic nephropathy. Lancet 1983; 1: 1175.
[55] Mogensen CE, Christensen CK. Predicting diabetic nephropathy in insulin-dependent patients. N Engl J Med 1984; 311: 89.

Epidemiology and clinical impact of diabetic late complications in IDDM

L.M.B. Laffel, A.S. Krolewski

Introduction

An individual has a 1% lifetime risk of developing Type I Insulin-dependent diabetes (IDDM) accompanied by complications involving the large and small blood vessels [1]. This chapter will review specifically the epidemiology of the eye, kidney, and cardiac problems in IDDM patients. This should enhance the understanding of the clinical impact of late diabetes complications and assist in the development of efficient programs designed to prevent or postpone their late occurrence in IDDM patients. The discussion will focus mainly on individuals whose diabetes was diagnosed before the age of thirty years. Data regarding the natural history of the late complications in IDDM patients diagnosed after 30 years of age are discussed in the next chapter.

Two indices of disease frequency are generally used to describe the epidemiology of disease: the incidence rate and the prevalence rate [2]. Prevalence describes the number or proportion of cases of disease in a population at a given point in time, for example, the per cent of diabetic patients with proliferative retinopathy among all diabetic patients studied. This cross-sectional measure is often useful in planning health care needs. However, it may be an unreliable index of disease occurrence in a population, and, therefore, will not be used in this review. On the other hand, the incidence rate assists in study of disease etiology. The incidence rate describes the number of new cases, for example, of proliferative retinopathy, that develop in a diabetic population during a given time interval, usually one year, among individuals free of this complication at the start of the interval. This rate can be summarized into an individual's lifetime risk in a measure called cumulative incidence (Figs. 1B, 2B, 3B, 4A, 4B).

Diabetic retinopathy

The most frequent complications of insulin-dependent diabetes are eye complications. After a delay of about four years, the incidence rate of background

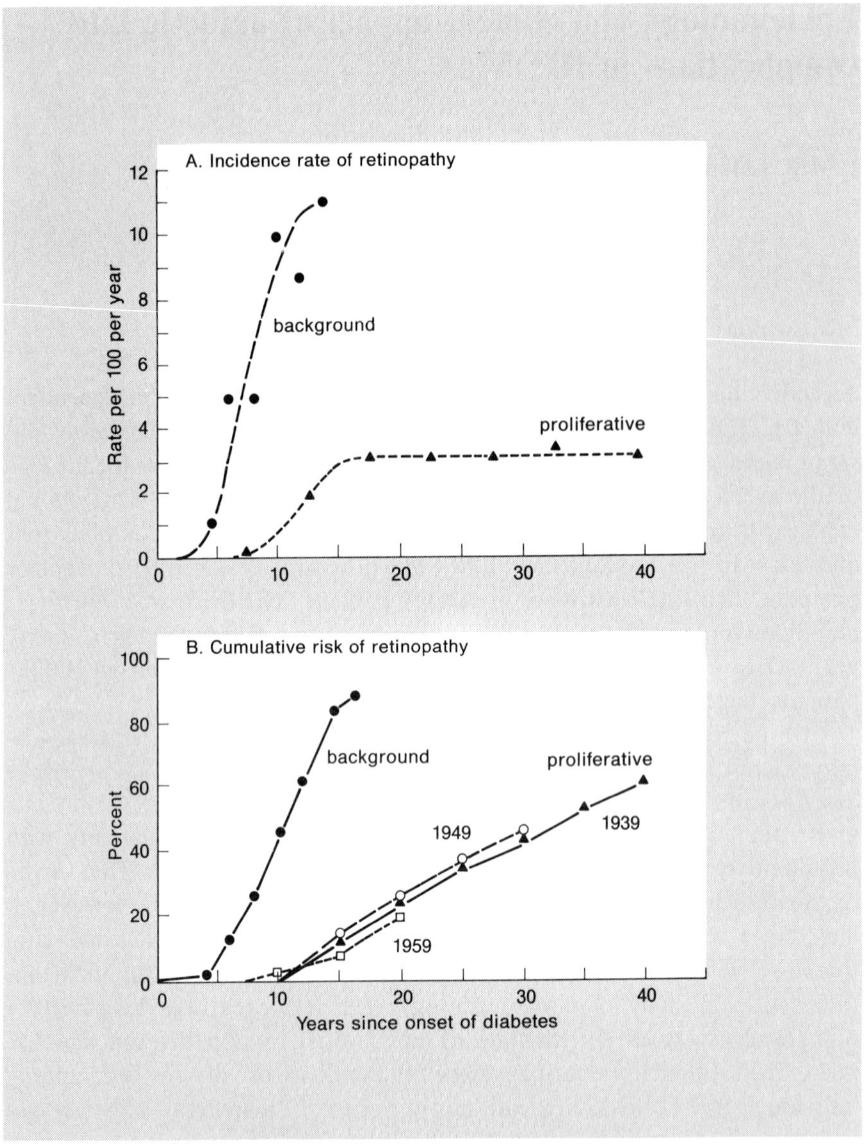

Fig. 1 Incidence rate and cumulative risk of background and proliferative retinopathy, according to diabetes duration in IDDM patients.
Panel A. Incidence rate of background retinopathy [4] and proliferative retinopathy [6], according to diabetes duration.
Panel B: Cumulative incidence of background retinopathy [4] and proliferative retinopathy [6], according to diabetes duration.
(Printed with permission of the authors and publishers [1].)

retinopathy, manifested as microaneurysms and hemorrhages in the retina, increases rapidly with the duration of diabetes [3, 4]. During the fifth year of diabetes, background retinopathy develops in only 1 of 100 patients, whereas in the fourteenth year, it develops in 11 of 100 patients who have remained free of eye changes up to that time (Fig. 1A). After fifteen years, almost all patients with type I diabetes have some retinopathic lesions (Fig. 1B). One can infer that these eye lesions are an outcome of the diabetic condition since they are almost ubiquitous with diabetes and extremely rare in persons without diabetes.

The development of background retinopathy appears to be necessary (but not sufficient) for the development of proliferative changes, the leading cause of blindness in patients with Type I diabetes [5]. The emergence of vulnerability to proliferative retinopathy is reflected in its incidence rate (Fig. 1A), which increases rapidly between the 10th and 15th year of diabetes, the time by which background retinopathy has developed in nearly all patients. After the initial fifteen year lag period, proliferative retinopathy develops at the constant rate of 3 per 100 previously unaffected patients yearly, regardless of whether they have had diabetes for 20 or 40 years. This constant incidence rate yields a cumulative risk of 62% after 40 years [6].

The incidence rate of proliferative retinopathy relates directly to the level of uncontrolled diabetes during the several years immediately preceding the onset of this complication but not during the first 5 years of diabetes [6, 7]. For example, long duration IDDM patients with background retinopathy were followed prospectively for 4 years [8]. Individuals in the highest quartile of glycohemoglobin at the start of the study were more than 20 times as likely to develop preproliferative or proliferative retinopathy as those in the lowest quartile of glycohemoglobin. In the Wisconsin Epidemiologic Study of Diabetic Retinopathy, the glycosylated hemoglobin level during the preceding several years was also a significant predictor of the development of retinopathy and progression to proliferative retinopathy [9]. The group in the highest quartile of glycosylated hemoglobin displayed a risk of developing proliferative retinopathy that was 22 times greater than that in the lowest quartile group of glycosylated hemoglobin level. Of note, the risk of developing severe retinopathy appeared to be reduced with increasing age, independent of the age of diabetes onset or its duration. For example, IDDM patients 45 years of age or older were half as likely to develop preproliferative or proliferative retinopathy as those under 35 years of age [8].

In summary, diabetic eye disease appears to be a multi-stage process determined by multiple factors. The pattern of occurrence of severe eye complications suggests two separate stages: the development of background retinopathy followed by neovascularization. In addition, the pattern of constant risk of proliferative retinopathy after the fifteenth year suggests universal vulnerability to the eye lesions. The factors governing the emergence of background changes may differ from those governing the onset of proliferative retinopathy although they may both be dependent upon uncontrolled diabetes. It remains to be established what specific metabolic and/or hemodynamic factors related to uncontrolled diabetes impact upon the development and progression of each stage.

Diabetic nephropathy

The most devastating late complication of insulin-dependent diabetes is diabetic nephropathy. The clinical syndrome of diabetic nephropathy is characterized by persistent proteinuria and rising arterial blood pressure culminating in renal failure or premature death due to coronary artery disease. A stage of incipient diabetic nephropathy with subclinical increases in urinary albumin excretion termed microalbuminuria has been shown to predict the occurrence of diabetic nephropathy. Three separate studies involving IDDM patients have examined the progression of microalbuminuria to persistent proteinuria [10, 11, 12]. Diabetic individuals with urinary albumin excretion values ranging from 15 to 200 mcg/min had a significantly increased risk of developing clinical diabetic nephropathy compared to patients with lower albumin excretion rates. However, the natural history of microalbuminuria remains ill-defined as longitudinal studies involving various ages of IDDM patients with different diabetes durations are presently lacking. Further, the interpretation of urinary albumin excretion in the range termed microalbuminuria remains unclear as many factors have been shown to impact upon its determination including glycemic control and exercise [13, 14, 15]. Therefore, this review will focus on the occurrence and determinants of the more clearly defined stages of persistent proteinuria and its inevitable progression either to renal failure or death due to coronary artery disease.

The incidence rate of diabetic nephropathy heralded by the onset of persistent proteinuria is shown according to diabetes duration in Figure 2A. The risk of persistent proteinuria has been shown repeatedly to increase with duration of diabetes during the first 15 years and then to decline [16, 17]. After a five year lag period, it rises to its peak of 2.5 per 100 annually during the second decade of diabetes and then declines to an annual rate of about 1 per 100 among the previously unaffected individuals. This pattern of occurrence does not support the generally held belief that diabetes duration is the main determinant of all late complications. Rather, the declining

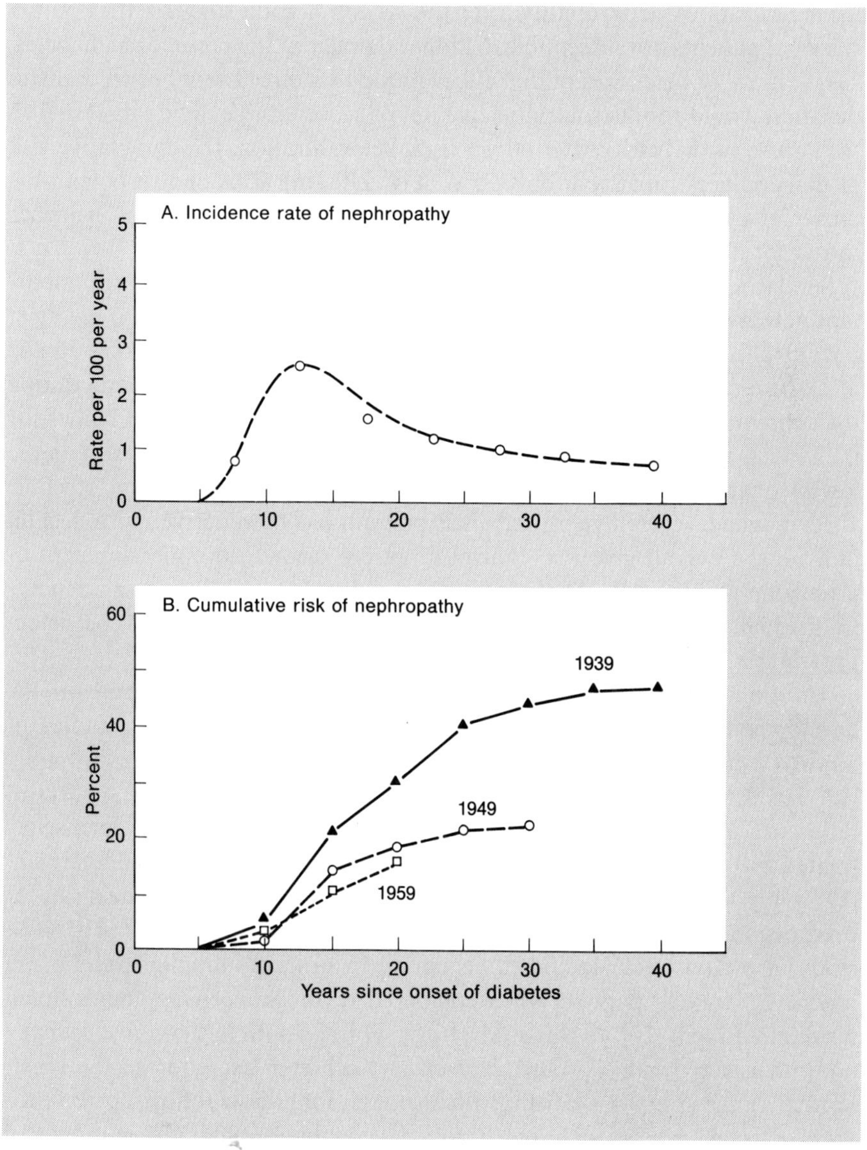

Fig. 2 Incidence rate and cumulative risk of nephropathy according to diabetes duration in IDDM patients.
Panel A: Incidence rate of nephropathy as measured by the incidence rate of persistent proteinuria [16], according to diabetes duration.
Panel B: Cumulative incidence of nephropathy as measured by the cumulative incidence of persistent proteinuria [16], according to diabetes duration.
(Printed with permission of the authors and publishers [1].)

incidence rate of nephropathy after the second decade suggests that only a subset of patients are susceptible to kidney damage in the presence of diabetes. The scarcity of new cases of diabetic nephropathy after twenty years diabetes duration would result from the depletion of susceptible individuals earlier in the course of diabetes. After 40 years diabetes duration, the cumulative risk of diabetic nephropathy is only 35% (Fig. 2B) [16]. This contrasts with the universal vulnerability to eye lesions noted above by the constant incidence rate from the second decade.

Similar to retinopathy, uncontrolled diabetes also appears to be an important determinant of diabetic kidney disease. Those individuals with the most uncontrolled diabetes, as measured, by glycemic index during the first decade of diabetes, have the greatest risk of developing persistent proteinuria during the subsequent decade (Fig. 3), a risk that is four and a half fold higher for individuals in the highest quartile of glycemic index compared to those in the lowest quartile [16]. The glycemic index, which is the proportion of clinic visits in which severe hyperglycemia is present, has been derived to reflect an individual's overall glycemic control in an era prior to the measurement of glycohemoglobin levels. As can be seen in the figure, clinic non-attenders (individuals with fewer than 9 visits) have the highest risk of persistent proteinuria. Similar findings have been reported by others [18].

Additional indirect support for the influence of hyperglycemia on the development of persistent proteinuria comes from preliminary studies of improved glycemic control during the stage of incipient diabetic nephropathy [19, 20]. Investigators from the Steno Hospital have shown a significant difference in progression of microalbuminuria between patients intensively treated with insulin pump therapy and those receiving conventional treatment [19]. Only the latter patients developed persistent proteinuria; their rate of progression correlated directly with the degree of hyperglycemia. The Oslo study also showed a significant reduction in urinary albumin excretion in intensively treated patients when compared to those receiving conventional insulin treatment [20]. In this study, most subjects, both in the conventionally and intensively treated groups, had urinary albumin excretion in the upper normal range for non-diabetics. Further, the long-term follow-up for progression is lacking. Nonetheless, it does appear that optimal glycemic control may be able to normalize urinary albumin excretion if it is instituted prior to the onset of persistent proteinuria [21].

Uncontrolled diabetes, while fundamental, does not appear sufficient to cause diabetic nephropathy. Other genetic and/or environmental factors must influence its pathogenesis. The association between elevated systemic blood pressure and kidney disease is well recognized [22]. The usual interpretation

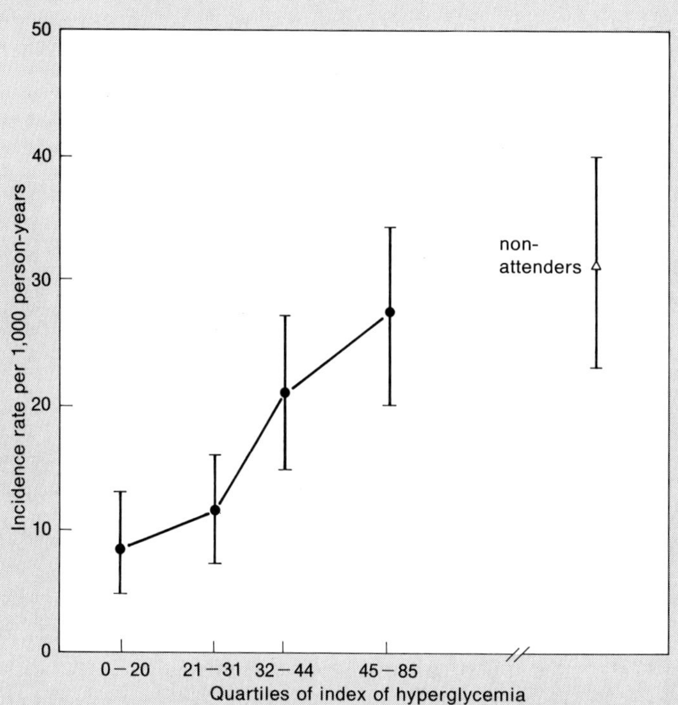

Fig. 3 Incidence rates of persistent proteinuria during the second and third decades of diabetes according to quartiles of the index of hyperglycemia during the first 15 years of diabetes and among patients who were non-attenders (patients having less than 9 visits during this period) [16]. The index of hyperglycemia is the percentage of the total number of blood glucose values (in mg/dl) recorded during visits to the Joslin Clinic that exceeded the following criteria: 180 fasting; 240 less than 1.5 hours after eating; 220 1.5 to 2.4 hours after eating; 200 2.5 to 3.4 hours after eating; and 180 3.5 or more hours after eating. Clinic visits that occurred subsequent to the onset of persistent proteinuria were excluded from the computation.
(Printed with permission of the authors and publishers [16].)

has been that this association, including the hypertension associated with diabetic nephropathy, is secondary to the renal disease. However, elevated systemic pressure has been noted to accompany microalbuminuria, preceding the onset of persistent proteinuria by many years [15, 23, 24]. Further, individuals who survive forty years of diabetes without nephropathy are remarkably free of hypertension despite their advancing age [18, 25, 26]. These observations suggest that susceptibility to renal complications in Type I diabetes might arise through a genetic predisposition to hypertension, a finding recently supported in separate studies [27, 28]. We have found that patients in whom nephropathy develops within the first twenty years of diabetes frequently have parents with hypertension (a familial predisposition to hypertension) and also have high red blood cell sodium-lithium counter-transport (a putative marker of hypertension risk) [29] when compared to a matched group of diabetics without renal complications [27]. Parents of proteinuric diabetic patients have also been shown to have higher arterial blood pressures than parents of non-proteinuric patients [30]. Thus, in the diabetic individual, an underlying predisposition to hypertension may be one mechanism by which renal damage ensues. Poor glycemic control and a predisposition to hypertension appear to act synergistically upon the development of diabetic nephropathy; i. e. diabetic nephropathy develops mainly among those individuals with a predisposition to hypertension *and* poor glycemic control [27]. The exact mechanisms underlying this interaction are unclear at present.

In addition to poor glycemic control and genetically determined susceptibilities, some environmental factors may also influence the risk of diabetic nephropathy. The cumulative risk of diabetic nephropathy in patients with Type I diabetes diagnosed in 1949 and 1959 is only half that in patients with the disease diagnosed in 1939 (Fig. B3) [16]. This contrasts with the similarity in risk for proliferative retinopathy in the same three cohorts of patients (Fig. 2B) [6]. Similar findings of declining incidence of persistent proteinuria in the more recent decades have also been reported from the Steno Hospital [31]. Environmental influences, either dietary, infectious, or pharmacologic (i. e. insulin type or purity) in nature, present earlier in this century appear to have changed favorably to diminish the risk of diabetic nephropathy. However, the exact mechanisms by which environment influences interact in the susceptible individual with uncontrolled diabetes remain unknown.

Once persistent proteinuria develops, there is inexorable progression to chronic renal failure unless death supervenes due to coronary artery disease [32] (see below). Progression to renal failure occurs within 3 to 20 years (median 10 years) after the onset of persisent proteinuria [16]. However, the rate of decline in renal function differs significantly among individuals and appears to vary directly with the level of diastolic blood pressure [33, 34]. The level of glycemic control does not appear to determine the decrement in renal function once the stage of persistent proteinuria is reached [16, 21, 33]. However, attained age appears to effect the decline in renal function [33]; individuals over 45 years of age appear to progress more slowly.

In summary, diabetic nephropathy consists of at least two separate stages. The first, the onset of persistent proteinuria, is determined by the level of diabetes control and an underlying susceptibility, which may be a predisposition to essential hypertension. The second stage consists of two separate outcomes: the decline in renal function to end-stage renal disease and an acceleration of atherosclerosis leading to coronary artery disease. The progression of persistent proteinuria to renal failure does not appear to be affected by hyperglycemia but seems to be influenced by other factors such as blood pressure, aging, and perhaps, certain dietary factors, such as protein intake [35, 36]. Modifications of these factors do not prevent the appearance of renal failure but they may delay its appearance. The ability to modify the acceleration of atherosclerosis is unclear.

Premature coronary artery disease

Coronary artery disease (CAD) is the leading cause of death in the diabetic population. Its occurrence and contribution to mortality are particularly increased among Type I insulin-dependent patients. The cumulative mortality for both men and women by age 55 years in a cohort of IDDM patients followed for 20 to 40 years was 35% (Fig. 4A) [37]. This was far higher than the corresponding risk for non-diabetic persons in the Framingham Heart Study of 8% for men and 4% for women [38]. In addition to excess mortality in the diabetic cohort, there was an excess of symptomatic and asymptomatic coronary artery disease as well; the cumulative risk for all forms of CAD (angina, acute non-fatal myocardial infarction, and asymptomatic CAD assessed by stress testing) was nearly 50% by age 55 [37]. This risk was similar in both men and women.

The enormous excess of morbidity and mortality due to CAD in Type I diabetes is mainly attributable to the premature development and acceleration of atherosclerosis in the coronary arteries [39, 40]. The mechanisms responsible for this are unclear. However, certain features of CAD occurrence provide insight into its pathogenesis. For example, CAD occurs only after the age of 30 years regardless of whether the onset of IDDM was in early childhood or late adolescence (Fig. 4B) [37]. In the general population, the

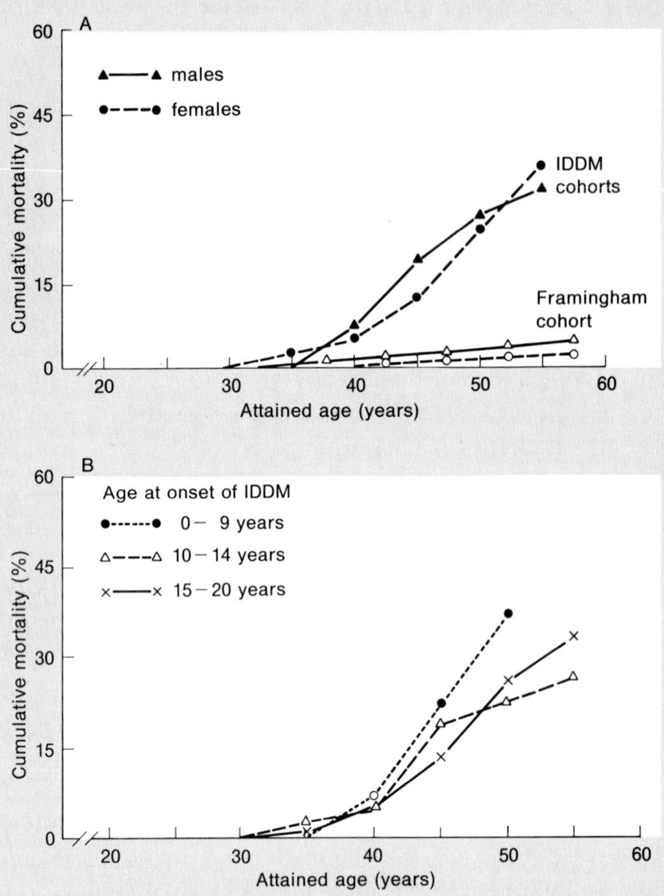

Fig. 4 Cumulative mortality due to coronary artery disease.
Panel A: Cumulative mortality due to coronary artery disease up to age 55 years in IDDM patients [37] compared to the population of the Framingham Heart Study [38, 44].
Panel B: Cumulative mortality due to coronary artery disease up to age 55 years in IDDM patients according to age of diabetes onset, at 0–9 years, 10–14 years, or 15–20 years [37].
(Printed with permission of the authors and publishers [16].)

first atherosclerotic lesions in the coronary arteries occur in the second and third decades of life [41]. Autopsy studies of U.S. casualities of the Korean and Vietnam wars have shown partial occlusion of coronary arteries due to fibrous plaques in half of the victims in their third decade [42, 43]. However, progression of these lesions to the point that they are clinically manifest as CAD requires several more decades [41, 44]. On the other hand, individuals with IDDM often develop severe, clinically significant coronary atherosclerotic lesions as early as their third decade, regardless of whether diabetes developed at 5 or 20 years of age [37]. Therefore, the appearance of CAD would seem to be determined by the natural history of atherosclerosis rather than by diabetes duration. This suggests that diabetes exposure does not impact upon the initiation of atherosclerotic lesions but rather it influences their progression during the third and fourth decades of life [45].

Relative to non-diabetic individuals, patients with IDDM have significantly more severe lesions, involving all three coronary arteries in the distal as well as proximal segments [40]. Thirty-two IDDM patients were compared with a group of 31 age-matched and symptom-matched non-diabetic patients undergoing CAD evaluation with cardiac catheterization [40]. Multi-vessel coronary disease occurred in 80% of the diabetic group compared with 22% of the non-diabetic group. Reduced ejection fraction and abnormal wall motion were detected in 60% and 71%, respectively, of the diabetic subjects compared with the significantly lower rates of 26% and 32%, respectively, in the non-diabetic subjects [40]. Diabetic women and men displayed the same degree of angiographic abnormalities. Presently, the diabetes-related factors responsible for this severe atherosclerosis are unclear.

Concomitant kidney disease is one well recognized factor leading to CAD, in part due to associated hypertension and hyperlipidemia [46]. Our previous study found a risk for CAD that was 15 times higher among patients with persistent proteinuria than among those without this renal complication [37]. Investigators from the Steno Memorial Hospital reported an eight-fold increased risk of CAD during the six year period following the onset of persistent proteinuria, and related it possibly to elevations in serum cholesterol and blood pressure [47]. Proteinuria, however, remained an independent risk factor for increased cardiovascular mortality after controlling for hypertension and hyperlipidemia in another study [32]. In contrast, the risk for CAD appears to be independent of proliferative retinopathy, the other major microvascular complication [37].

Diabetes appears to increase the risk for atherosclerosis independently of nephropathy [37, 48]. Indeed, uncontrolled diabetes is associated with platelet and coagulation disturbances, as well as lipid abnormalities [49–56]. These abnormalities, together with endothelial dysfunction or damage that has been demonstrated *in vitro* in studies mimicking diabetes [57], may play a role in advancing the early atherosclerotic lesions to raised plaques and premature CAD [58]. This constellation of abnormalities may gain particular importance among patients with nephropathy where there is clustering of many risk factors associated with CAD.

The effect of diabetes on CAD risk may not be the same among IDDM patients in all countries. The large impact of IDDM on the development of premature CAD parallels the frequent occurrence of the initial atherosclerotic lesion in the general population. Thus, in countries with a low risk of CAD in the general population, CAD may be an infrequent outcome of IDDM. Such a finding would support the notion that diabetes exposure modifies the progression of atherosclerotic lesions rather than their initiation. Thus, coronary artery disease, too, appears to be a multi-stage, multi-factorial process where diabetes seems to be modifying its natural history in concert with genetic and environmental factors.

Summary and implications

The pattern of occurrence of the late diabetic complications suggests that they are outcomes of distinct processes with specific constellations of determining factors. However, there may be some overlap in pathogenesis involving various functional and morphologic changes induced by uncontrolled diabetes. Knowledge of the determinants for each complication is important in order to develop preventive programs designed to reduce the associated morbidity and mortality.

Our present knowledge suggests that primary prevention of eye lesions may not be feasible as background changes appear to be a ubiquitous outcome of the diabetic state with the current means of insulin replacement therapy. However, secondary prevention of blindness appears possible with the early recognition and treatment of preproliferative and proliferative lesions. Primary prevention of diabetic nephropathy involves the recognition of susceptible individuals and institution of various treatment interventions prior to the onset of irreversible proteinuria. Such treatment modalities, as intensive insulin therapy, pharmacologic treatment to reduce systemic and intrarenal blood pressure, and, perhaps, dietary modifications, remain in the research arena at this time. Secondary prevention following the onset of persistent proteinuria involves interventions known to slow the inexorable decline in renal function such as normalization of systemic blood pressure and protein restriction. Prevention of atherosclerosis involves the recognition of individuals with conventional risk factors such as hyperlipidemia, hypertension, and a positive family history for premature CAD. Such individuals could be targeted to special risk factor reduction programs.Alternatively, individuals at risk for diabetic nephropathy could be identified and receive interventions designed to reduce their risk of renal disease and, consequently, their risk of CAD as well.

References

[1] Krolewski AS, Warram JH, Rand LI et al. Epidemiologic approach to the etiology of Type I Diabetes Mellitus and its complications. N Engl J Med 1987; 317: 1390–1398.

[2] Rothman KJ. Measures of disease frequency. In: Modern Epidemiology. Boston: Little, Brown and Co, 1986; 23–49.

[3] Palmberg P, Smith M, Waltman S et al. The Natural History of retinopathy in insulin-dependent juvenile-onset diabetes. Opthalmology 1981; 88: 613–618.

[4] Klein R, Klein BEK, Moss SE et al. The Wisconsin Epidemiologic Study of Diabetic Retinopathy. II. Prevalence and risk of diabetic retinopathy when age at diagnosis is less than 30 years. Arch Opthalmol 1984; 102: 520–526.

[5] Rand LI, Prud'homme GJ, Ederer F et al. Diabetic Retinopathy Study Group. Factors influencing the development of visual loss in advanced diabetic retinopathy: Diabetic Retinopathy Study (DRS) report no. 10. Invest Opthalmol Vis Sci 1985; 26; 983–991.

[6] Krolewski AS, Warram JH, Rand LI et al. Risk of proliferative diabetic retinopathy in juvenile-onset type I diabetes: a 40-year follow-up study. Diabetes Care 1986; 9: 443–452.

[7] Rand LI, Krolewski AS, Aiello LM et al. Multiple factors in the prediction of risk of proliferative diabetic retinopathy. N Engl J Med 1985; 313: 1433–1438.

[8] Janka HU, Warram JH, Rand LI et al. Risk factors for progression of background retinopathy in long-standing IDDM. Diabetes 1989; 38: 460–464.

[9] Klein R, Klein BEK, Moss SE et al. Glycosylated hemoglobin predicts the incidence and progression of diabetic retinopathy. JAMA 1988; 260: 2864–2871.

[10] Viberti GC, Jarrett RJ, Mahmud U et al. Microalbuminuria as a predictor of clinical nephropathy in insulin-dependent diabetes mellitus. Lancet 1982; 1: 1430–1432.

[11] Mogensen CE, Christiansen CK. Predicting diabetic nephropathy in insulin-dependent patients. N Engl J Med 1984; 311: 89–93.

[12] Mathiesen ER, Oxenboll B, Johansen K et al. Incipient nephropathy in Type I (insulin-dependent) diabetes. Diabetologia 1984; 26: 406–410.

[13] Bangstad HJ, Hanssen KF, Kierulf P et al. Elevated albumin excretion is common among poorly controlled adolescent insulin dependent diabetics. Diabetes Research 1987; 6: 43–46.

[14] Viberti G. Etiology and prognostic significance of albuminuria in diabetes. Diabetes Care 1988; 11: 840–845.

[15] Mogensen CE. Microalbuminuria as a predictor of clinical diabetic nephropathy. Kidney International 1987; 31: 673–689.

[16] Krolewski AS, Warram JH, Christlieb AR et al. The changing natural history of nephropathy in type I diabetes. Am J Med 1985; 78: 785–794.

[17] Andersen AR, Christiansen JS, Andersen JK et al. Diabetic nephropathy in Type I (insulin-dependent) diabetes: an epidemiological study. Diabetologia 1983; 25: 496–501.

[18] Deckert T, Poulsen JE, Larsen M. Prognosis of diabetes with diabetes onset before the age of thirtyone. II. Factors influencing the prognosis. Diabetologia 1978; 14: 371–377.

[19] Feld-Rasmussen B, Mathiesen E, Deckert T. Effect of two years of strict metabolic control on the progression of incipient nephropathy in insulin-dependent diabetes. Lancet 1986;: 2: 1300–1304.

[20] Dahl-Jorgensen K, Hanssen KF, Kierulf P et al. Reduction of urinary albumin excretion after 4 years of continuous subcutaneous insulin infusion in insulin-dependent diabetes mellitus. Acta Endocrinol 1988; 117: 19–25.
[21] Viberti GC, Bilous RW, Mackintosh D et al. Long-term correction of hyperglycemia and progression of renal failure in insulin-dependent diabetes. Br Med J 1983; 286: 598–602.
[22] Blythe WB. Natural history of hypertension in renal parenchymal disease. Am J Kidney Dis 1985; 5: A50–A56.
[23] Wiseman M, Viberti GC, Mackintosh D et al. Glycaemia, arterial blood pressure and micro-albuminuria in type I (insulin-dependent) diabetes mellitus. Diabetologia 1984; 26: 401–405.
[24] Christiansen CK, Mogensen CE. The course of incipient diabetic nephropathy: studies on albumin excretion and blood pressure. Diabetic Med 1985; 2: 97–102.
[25] Oakley, WG, Pyke DA, Tattersall RB et al. Long-term diabetes: a clinical study of 92 patients after 40 years. Q J Med 1974; 43: 145–156.
[26] Borch-Johnson K, Nissen RN, Nerup J. Blood pressure after 40 years of insulin-dependent diabetes. Diabetic Nephrop 1985; 4: 11–12.
[27] Krolewski AS, Canessa M, Warram JH et al. Predisposition to hypertension and susceptibility to renal disease in insulin-dependent diabetes mellitus. N Engl J Med 1988; 318: 140–145.
[28] Mangili R, Bending JJ, Scott G et al. Increased sodium-lithium countertransport activity in red cells of patients with insulin-dependent diabetes and nephropathy. N Engl J Med 1988; 318: 146–150.
[29] Hilton PJ. Cellular sodium transport in essential hypertension. N Engl J Med 1986; 314: 222–229.
[30] Viberti GC, Keen H, Wiseman MJ. Raised arterial hypertension in parents of proteinuric insulin dependent patients. Br Med J 1987; 295: 575–577.
[31] Kofoed-Enevoldsen A, Borch-Johnsen K, Kreiner S et al. Declining incidence of persistent proteinuria in Type I (insulin-dependent) diabetic patients in Denmark. Diabetes 1987; 36: 205–209.
[32] Laffel LMB, Laffel GL, Valsania P. Diabetic nephropathy is an independent risk factor for cardiovascular (CV) death. Diabetes 1987; 36 (suppl 1): 203A (abstract).
[33] Laffel LMB, Krolewski AS, Rand LI et al. The impact of blood pressure on renal function in insulin-dependent diabetes. Kid Int 1987; 31: 207 (abstract).
[34] Parving HH, Hommel E. High blood pressure is a major risk factor in progression of diabetic nephropathy. J Diabetic Complications 1988; 2: 92–95.
[35] Brenner BM. Hemodynamically mediated glomerular injury and the progressive nature of kidney disease. Kidney Int 1983; 23: 647–655.
[36] Bending JJ, Dodds RJ, Keen H et al. Renal responses to restricted protein intake in diabetic nephropathy. Diabetes 1988; 37: 1641–1646.
[37] Krolewski AS, Kosinski EJ, Warram JH et al. Magnitude and determinants of coronary artery disease in juvenile-onset, insulin-dependent diabetes mellitus. Am J Cardiol 1987; 59: 750–755.
[38] Sorlie P. The Framingham Study. Section 32; Cardiovascular disease and death following myocardial infarction and angina pectoris – 20 year follow-up. Washington DC: DHEW Publ. No. (NIH) 77 to 1247, 1977.
[39] Crall FV, Roberts WC. The extramural and intramural coronary arteries in juvenile diabetes mellitus. Analysis of nine necropsy patients aged 19 to 38 years with onset of diabetes before age 15 years. Am J Med 1978; 64: 221–230.
[40] Valsania P, Kowalchuk GJ, Zarich SW et al. Severity of coronary artery disease in young insulin dependent patients with insulin-dependent diabetes. for publication).
[41] McGill HC, Jr. Persistent problems in the pathogenesis of atherosclerosis. Atherosclerosis 1984; 4: 443–451.

[42] Enos WF, Holmes RH, Beyer J. Coronary disease among United States soldiers killed in action in Korea; preliminary report. JAMA 1953; 152: 1090–1093.
[43] McNamara JJ, Molot MA, Stremple JF et al. Coronary artery disease in combat casualties in Vietnam. JAMA 1971; 216: 1185–1187.
[44] Lerner DJ, Kannel WB. Patterns of coronary heart disease morbidity and mortality in the sexes: a 26-year follow-up of the Framingham population. Am Heart J 1986; 111: 383–390.
[45] Robertson WB, Strong JP. Atherosclerosis in persons with hypertension and diabetes mellitus. Lab Invest 1968; 18: 78–91.
[46] Becker RC. Cardiovascular disease in patients with chronic renal failure. Cleve Clin J Med 1988; 55: 521–530.
[47] Jensen T, Borch-Johnsen K, Kofoed-Enevoldsen A et al. Coronary heart disease in young Type I (insulin-dependent) diabetic patients with and without diabetic nephropathy: incidence and risk factors. Diabetologia 1987; 30: 144–148.
[48] Borch-Johnsen K, Kreiner S. Proteinuria: value as predictor of cardiovascular mortality in insulin dependent diabetes mellitus. Br Med J 1987; 294: 1651–1654.
[49] Colwell JA, Lopes-Virella M, Halushka PV. Pathogenesis of atherosclerosis in diabetes mellitus. Diabetes Care 1981; 4: 121–133.
[50] Ruderman NB, Haudenschild C. Diabetes as an atherogenic factor. Prog Cardiovas Dis 1984; 26: 373–412.
[51] Juhan I, Buonocore M, Jouve R et al. Abnormalities of erythrocyte deformability and platelet aggregation in insulin-dependent diabetics corrects by insulin in vivo and in vitro. Lancet 1982; 1: 535–538.
[52] Jones RL, Peterson M. The fluid phase of coagulation and the accelerated atherosclerosis of diabetes mellitus. Diabetes 1981; 30 (suppl 1): 33–38.
[53] Sosenko JM, Breslow JL, Miettinen OS et al. Hyperglycemia and plasma lipid levels. A prospecvtive study of young insulin-dependent diabetic patients. N Engl J Med 1980; 302: 650–654.
[54] Lopes-Virella MF, Sherer K, Lees AM et al. Surface binding, internalization and degradation by cultered human fibroblasts of low density lipoproteins isolated from Type I (insulin-dependent) diabetic patients: changes with metabolic control. Diabetologia 1982; 22: 430–436.
[55] Semenkovich CF, Ostlund RE, Schechtman KB. Plasma lipids in patients with Type I diabetes mellitus. The influence of race, gender, plasma glucose control: Lipids do not correlate with glucose control in black women. Arch Intern Med 1989; 149: 51–56.
[56] Bent-Hansen L, Deckert T. Metabolism of albumin and fibrinogen in Type I (insulin-dependent) diabetes mellitus. Diabetes Res 1988; 7: 159–164.
[57] Lorenzi M, Maliero ZE, Toledo S. Glucose toxicity for human endothelial cells in culture. Delayed replication, disturbed cell cycle, and accelerated death. Diabetes 1985; 34: 621–627.
[58] Ross R. The pathogenesis of atherosclerosis – an update. N Engl J Med 1986; 314: 488–500.

Epidemiology and clinical impact of diabetic late complications in NIDDM

H.U. Janka

In all societies the overwhelming majority of people with diabetes have non-insulin dependent diabetes mellitus (NIDDM) [1]. Since these patients, if not adequately controlled, are nearly equally subject to the devastating complications of diabetes mellitus, the total number of diabetic late complications is higher for NIDDM than for IDDM. In NIDDM, however, there are specific characteristics in rate of occurrence and clinical impact of diabetic retinopathy, nephropathy, neuropathy, and macrovascular disease which will be addressed in this review.

Retinopathy

Proliferative diabetic retinopathy (PDR) and diabetic maculopathy are the major causes of blindness in diabetic patients [2]. PDR is generally considered to be a more important problem in IDDM, and macular edema more important in NIDDM. Accurate comparisons have been difficult because of uncertainties in the clinical assessment of diabetes type, the paucity of studies that have evaluated patients of both types with the same methods, and the even greater rarity of population-based studies [3]. In the Wisconsin Epidemiologic Study it was found that 40% of patients who were > 30 of age at diagnosis and had had the disease for < 5 years had some degree of retinopathy when treated by insulin whereas only 28% of these patients not taking insulin [4] showed this complication. Prevalence of retinopathy rose steeply to 80% in older-onset insulin-treated persons with 15 years of diabetes; in the non-insulin-treated persons prevalence rose to 50%. In the insulin-taking group, prevalence of PDR rose fairly steadily from 2% in persons with < 5 years of diabetes duration to more than 25% in those with > 20 years, whereas in the non-insulin-taking group, prevalence remained about 2–5% regardless of duration. In this epidemiologic study, prevalence of macular edema did not vary substantially by diabetes type, but PDR was significantly more common in younger-onset individuals. Because diabetes with onset after the age of 30 years was more common than the younger-onset type, the majority of individuals with PDR or macular edema were NIDDM patients. As expected, various clinic populations have a somewhat different distributions. Among patients attending the Eye Unit at the Joslin Clinic, the age at diabetes diagnosis was 40 years or more in only 22% of patients with PDR [5]. In a cross-sectional study in the out-patient clinic of the Massachusetts General Hospital, screening of NIDDM patients in the age range 55–75 years showed prevalence of retinopathy to be 25%, most of these with background retinopathy [6]. Duration of diabetes and hemoglobin A_{1c} (HbA_{1c}) concentration were the two major predictors of the presence of retinopathy. A similar prevalence and the relationship to duration of diabetes was recently reported by a British diabetic clinic [7].

There are, however, various pitfalls in using such data to suggest causation. We have assumed that the relationship of exposures and prevalence is a fair estimate of the relationship of exposures and incidence. The relationship of putative risk factors to the incidence of diabetic retinopathy, therefore, has to be proven in a prospective manner. There are three prospective studies which should be cited in this context [8–10]: The UGDP study accumulated much data on the occurrence of complications in NIDDM, but the data were analysed largely on the basis of treatment assignment rather than blood glucose [8]. There were no significant differences in the development of retinopathy among the four treatment groups despite lower mean fasting blood glucose levels in the variable-insulin treatment group. A direct comparison between blood glucose and other tentative risk factors, however, was not performed. In the British study examining outcome in diet-treated NIDDM randomized to either a low-carbohydrate or low-fat diet, the overall incidence of retinopathy increased as metabolic control worsened [9]. The third study examined a genetically distinct NIDDM population, i. e., the Pima Indians [10]. There was almost no retinopathy in subjects with a 2 hour post-OGTT blood glucose < 200 mg/dl. The prevalence of retinopathy tended to increase with higher blood glucose as well as with higher blood pressure values [11]. The Whitehall Study also showed that blood pressure was substantially elevated years in advance of the diagnosis of diabetes in the group which developed retinopathy [12]. These findings provide some evidence for an independent effect of hypertension on diabetic eye disease.

It can be concluded from all these studies that the quality of metabolic control and the level of blood pressure are probably major risk factors for the development of retinopathy in NIDDM. This relationship was also documented in several studies in the recent past in IDDM patients [13, 14, review 15]. The Diabetes Control and Complication Trial (DCCT) is expected to provide definite answers to the question whether stringent blood glucose control can prevent or ameliorate diabetic retinopathy in IDDM [16]. Since a study of this size can hardly be performed in NIDDM, the DCCT results will probably have to be applied to all diabetic patients regardless of diabetes type and treatment.

Diabetic nephropathy

Knowledge about the renal disease that complicates NIDDM is very small in comparison to knowledge of renal disease that complicates IDDM. Although glomerulosclerosis has frequently been observed, hyperfiltration of the kidney and increased glomerular filtration rate seem to be rather rare [17]. Albuminuria in NIDDM is, as in IDDM, predominantly of glomerular origin [18], although it is not strictly correlated with the degree of glomerulopathy [19]. Thus, the pathogenesis of microalbuminuria has not been exactly defined. It is probable that both structural and haemodynamic changes play a role.

There are several recent reports of the prevalence of proteinuria and microalbuminuria in NIDDM patients. In an Italian population-based study, the overall prevalence rates for microalbuminuria (albumin excretion rate 30 – 350 μg/min) were 25.8% and for macroalbuminuria (> 350 μg/min) 3.0% [20]. Within the first 5 years of diabetes the rate of microalbuminuria was already 20.9%. It increased slightly with duration of diabetes up to 10 years and then tended to level off. In a sample of all registered non-insulin-treated NIDDM with a mean duration of diabetes of 5 years in Erfurt/GDR, 6.7% were found to have persistent macroproteinuria and 9.6% signs of pyelonephritis in addition [21]. Other authors reported a prevalence of microalbuminuria of as high as 41 – 59% in NIDDM [22, 23]. The rate of progression of proteinuria to frank clinical diabetic nephropathy in NIDDM is, in contrast to IDDM, rather low [24]. In a Swiss study, 510 NIDDM patients were followed over 8 years [25]. In only one of 122 deceased patients could death be ascribed to end-stage renal disease (ESRD). Approximately 5 – 10% of NIDDM patients develop ESRD [26, 27]. As in diabetic retinopathy, poor metabolic compensation and hypertension contribute to the progression of diabetic nephropathy, also in NIDDM [28, 29]. At present the best predictor for the development of ESRD is persistent proteinuria. Furthermore, a high albumin excretion rate is an even better predictor of macrovascular complications and early mortality in NIDDM (see below).

Although rate of development of ESRD in NIDDM is less than that in IDDM, due to the much greater frequency of the former patients nearly half of all diabetic on renal replacement therapy are NIDDM patients [30, 31]. Apparently, due to aggressive antihypertensive treatment, better blood glucose control, and more appropriate choice of renal replacement therapy the prognosis of these patients has been improved in the last years [31].

Diabetic neuropathy

Diabetic neuropathy is not confined to a single type of diabetes, but can occur in IDDM, NIDDM, and various forms of acquired diabetes [review 32]. Although there is considerable uncertainty as to the prevalence of diabetic neuropathy, it is generally accepted that neuropathy is a very common, and often very troublesome, major complication of diabetes. Diabetic neuropathy is probably just as frequent in NIDDM as in IDDM. The few existing epidemiologic studies, however, are inconsistent in terminology, diagnostic criteria, and study populations [33]. In Pirart's 25-year prospective study of 4400 patients in a diabetic clinic, neuropathy, as defined as a loss of Achilles and/or patellar reflexes combined with diminished vibratory sensation, was present in 12% of patients at diagnosis, particularly in older NIDDM patients. Thereafter, the overall prevalence of neuropathy increased linearly with duration of diabetes to nearly 50% after 25 years [34]. In a group of 503 Mexican patients with NIDDM, 32.2% were found to have symptoms attributable to peripheral neuropathy and 40.8% loss of ankle vibration and/or Achilles tendon reflexes [35]. More refined techniques of clinical neurophysiology show even greater prevalence of neuropathy [32]. Thus, damage to peripheral nerves is the most underestimated of the diabetic complications.

The aetiology of nerve damage is presently explained by two theories: metabolic and vascular. There is considerable evidence that sorbitol and fructose accumulate in nerves and cause a depletion of myo-inositol and the enzyme Na^+/K^+-ATPase. These changes can be corrected by achievement of normoglycemia as well as by application of pharmacologic agents such as aldose reductase inhibitors (ARI). On the other hand, specific microvascular disease with endothelial cell proliferation, occlusion of lumen and thickening of the basal laminia has been detected in the nerves of diabetics. These pathologic changes in peripheral nerves were observed in a series of human biopsy studies. Segmental demyelination is prominent in humans with frequent remyelination, and there is also evidence of axonal degeneration with some regeneration. The changes are undoubtedly patchy and thus suggest focal aspects as well as a diffuse symmetrical abnormality [36]. There is, however, a marked histopathological heterogeneity of the neuropathy in

IDDM and NIDDM [37]. NIDDM patients do not exhibit markedly increased axo-glial dysjunction or axonal atrophy as IDDM do. Furthermore NIDDM patients show significantly more capillary closure of the vasa nervorum.

From a clinical perspective, it is useful to classify diabetic neuropathy into the broad categories of somatic and autonomic neuropathies, each with its own further subdivisions. It is beyond the scope of this article to discuss these entities in detail. Whereas symmetrical distal polyneuropathy is the most common form of diabetic neuropathy in both NIDDM and IDDM, diffuse motor neuropathy is increasingly common in older NIDDM patients. A severe degree of muscle wasting and weakness develops over 3–6 months with apparent good metabolic control. Biopsy studies suggest significant small vessel disease in this condition. Diabetic neuropathy of the lower extremity nerves contributes significantly to the development of paraesthesia, pain, foot ulcerations, medial arterial calcification, osteopenia [38], Charcot's neuroarthropathy, and, consequently, to foot or leg amputation. The amputation rate is particularly high in NIDDM patients. In the population-based prospective study in Pima Indians, amputation rate was 100 times more frequent in the diabetics than in non-diabetics. Medial arterial calcification and impaired vibratory perception-threshold were significant predictors for lower-extremity amputations [39].

Diabetic autonomic neuropathy, also a common complication of diabetes, has been associated with increased mortality. The increased mortality risk has been well publicized, primarily by the work of Ewing et al [40]. Alterations of the autonomic nervous system have been implicated in the pathogenesis of cardiac arrhythmias, myocardial ischemia, and sudden cardiac death. Recent data suggest that diabetic cardiac autonomic neuropathy may result in sympathetic imbalance and QT interval prolongation, predisposing these patients to sudden arrhythmias and death [41]. Until recently, autonomic neuropathy has not been correlated with glycemic control. However, the Diabetes Control and Complication Trial (DCCT) has demonstrated such a relationship [16] implicating that correction of hyperglycemia may be the most promising therapeutic principle in treatment of autonomic as well as somatic neuropathy.

Macrovascular disease

Cardiovascular diseases are the major cause of morbidity and mortality in the diabetic patients, especially in developed countries where atherosclerosis is the most common complication of diabetes. It occurs at a younger age and progresses more rapidly in diabetic than in non-diabetic subjects and frequently culminates in such fatal or disabling complications as myocardial infarction, stroke, or gangrene [42]. The acceleration of atherogenesis occurs in all types of diabetes. In the Whitehall Study, the age-adjusted rate of coronary heart disease mortality was 6.1 in IDDM and 8.3 NIDDM in comparison to 3.9 in non-diabetics [43]. In a recent review of all population-based epidemiologic studies, it was shown that NIDDM subjects exhibit a 3–4 times higher rate of cardiovascular mortality than non-diabetic subjects [26].

The most important macrovascular complication is coronary heart disease. NIDDM patients with this disease have a much poorer prognosis. Survival rate in NIDDM patients after myocardial infarction is markedly reduced [44]. Furthermore, sudden cardiac death and silent myocardial ischemia/infarction are more frequent in diabetic patients [45].

The enhanced risk of macrovascular disease in NIDDM is traditionally ascribed to factors associated with diabetes which aggravate the atherogenic processes. Since it was not possible to explain the excess risk by the generally accepted risk factors such as diastolic hypertension, hypercholesterolemia, and cigarette smoking various other factors have been held responsible. These include certain aspects of blood pressure elevation, lipid abnormalities, hyperinsulinemia/insulin resistence, hyperglycemia and protein glycosylation, abnormal hemostasis and hemorrheology, and impaired kidney function.

Hypertension

A high percentage of NIDDM patients are hypertensive according to the majority of epidemiologic surveys [review 46]. In the Schwabing Study, prevalence of hypertension in diabetics of age 50–60 years was more than 50%, and increased even more with age [47]. Comparable data were reported from Dresden. 53% of NIDDM patients exhibited hypertensive blood pressure values in contrast to 17.3% of age-matched general population [48]. In a study of patients in the offices of general practitioners in Southern Bavaria, hypertension (> 160/95 mmHg) was diagnosed in nearly three quarters of all elderly NIDDM patients [49]. In the Schwabing Study, blood pressure was found to be a strong predictor for cardiovascular complications in NIDDM [50]. A highly significant correlation was found between systolic and diastolic blood pressure readings, although systolic pressure appeared to be a much stronger risk factor. Comparable results were found in the Framingham Study: a marked increase of cardiovascular complications was associated with isolated increase of systolic blood pressure. The authors conclude that isolated systolic hypertension is a powerful contributor to cardiovascular complications, and that the exclusive use of diastolic blood pressure in the elderly for judgement of cardiovascular risk may actually be misleading [51].

Lipid abnormalities

NIDDM is associated with changes in plasma lipids and lipoproteins which can lead to atherogenesis. Several reports have described a closer association of hypertriglyceridemia than of hypercholesterolemia to atherosclerosis in diabetes mellitus [52, 53]. Recent publications described an altered composition of VLDL and LDL particles in NIDDM patients with a higher content of triglycerides in LDL and an increased content of cholesterol esters in VLDL [54]. It was suggested that these alterations may lead to an impairment of lipoprotein-receptor interaction and may, thereby, induce atherogenesis. For NIDDM patients, the recent dietary and therapeutic recommendations of the European Atherosclerosis Society seem appropriate in so far as they are designed to lower not only cholesterol but also triglycerides levels [55].

Hyperinsulinemia/ Insulin resistance

Hyperinsulinemia and insulin resistance have also been proposed as a factor contributing to the increased cardiovascular morbidity. Interaction between plasma insulin levels and lipid metabolism as well as blood pressure values have been well documented [56]. Plasma insulin levels are abnormally high in many NIDDM as well as in the majority of subjects with impaired glucose tolerance. The Schwabing Study found that NIDDM patients with macroangiopathy had elevated plasma C-peptide levels and that the amount of insulin in secondarily insulin-treated NIDDM patients was significantly associated with the development of macrovascular complications [57]. Two large studies in USA have shown that the rate of coronary heart disease was dependent on antidiabetic therapy and that patients on insulin have the most severe forms of atherosclerosis [58, 59]. This implies that severity of diabetes underlies these associations. However, a direct effect of exogenously induced hyperinsulinemia and insulin resistance cannot be excluded.

Hyperglycemia

In patients with insulin resistance, there is very commonly a positive correlation of insulin and blood glucose. However, a series of epidemiologic studies were unable to find a significant relationship between blood glucose at baseline with the cardiovascular end points. The authors of the Framingham Study pointed out that repeated measurements of blood glucose and the introduction of glycosylated hemoglobin in the risk variable set improves prediction of macrovascular complications [60]. In diabetics a large amount of glycosylated protein can be detected in nearly every tissue, e. g., in coronary arteries and aorta [61]. Until recently, it was not clear whether this finding has any clinical impact. The hypothesis of "advanced glycosylated end products", their interaction with macrophages, liberation of lymphokinins, and the subsequent endothelial damage [62] appears to be a very attractive explanation of the link between protein glycosylation and vascular disease, but this relationship has to be proven in further studies. There is, however, no doubt that the increased rate of protein glycosylation can be prevented by improvement of diabetic control.

Hemostatic and hemorrheologic changes

Hemostasiologic and hemorrheologic changes are also dependent on degree of hyperglycemia. Elevated plasma levels of fibrinogen, which are responsible to a large degree for blood viscosity, can be lowered by improvement of metabolic control. Metabolic effects are also suspected to be associated with changes of platelet aggregability [63]. Due to increased turnover of platelets in NIDDM patients with both microangiopathy and macroangiopathy, there are an increased number of platelets with young and particularly reagible forms. Platelets adhere to the vessel wall particularly on sites of turbulent flow, e. g., where arteries branch off and platelets hit the vessel wall perpendicularly [64]. This may explain predilection sites of atherosclerosis, e. g., at the carotid artery bifurcation. Since in all diabetics there is an increased rigidity of the artery wall with changes of the laminar blood flow even without atherosclerosis, mechanical characteristics of the vessel wall and blood flow alone may contribute to the development of macroangiopathy in both NIDDM and IDDM.

Renal disease

For decades there has been a debate as to whether microangiopathy plays an important role in the development of macrovascular disease in diabetic patients. The morphologic changes of the vasa vasorum described so far are, however, not very convincing. On the other hand, the recognition of proteinuria as risk marker for macrovascular disease has led to a strong interest in the microangiopathy of the kidney and, therefore, diabetic nephropathy in

NIDDM. Today, constant microalbuminuria (> 20 μg/min) is one of the best predictors not only for development of end stage renal disease but also for cardiovascular complications in NIDDM [65, 66]. The interaction between kidney disease and atherosclerosis is probably very complex and, at present, cannot be explained by underlying increases of blood pressure and serum lipids. However, since microalbuminuria can be reduced by lowering blood glucose and blood pressure, it is probable that metabolic control is the most important measure for prevention and therapy of macrovascular complications in NIDDM.

References

[1] Keen H. Diagnosis and classification of diabetes mellitus. In: Krall LP ed. World book of diabetes in practice, Vol 2. Amsterdam: Elsevier, 1986; 8–15.

[2] Kohner EM, Sharp PS. Diabetic retinopathy. In: Alberti KGMM, Krall LP, eds. The Diabetes Annual/3. Amsterdam: Elsevier, 1987; 252–288.

[3] Davies MD. Diabetic retinopathy: a clinical overview. Diab/Metab Rev 1988; 4: 291–322.

[4] Klein R, Klein BEK, Moss SE et al. The Wisconsin Epidemiology Study of Diabetic Retinopathy: prevalence and risk of diabetic retinopathy when age at diagnosis is 30 or more years. Arch Ophtalmol 1984; 102: 527–532.

[5] Aiello LM, Rand LI, Briones JC. Diabetic retinopathy in Joslin Clinic patients with adult-onset diabetes. Ophtalmology 1981; 88: 619–623.

[6] Nathan DM, Singer DE, Godine JE et al. Retinopathy in older type II diabetics: association with glucose control. Diabetes 1986; 35: 797–801.

[7] Grey RHB, Malcolm N, O'Reilly D, Morris A. Ophtalmic survey of a diabetic clinic. I. Ocular findings. Brit J Ophtalmol 1986; 70: 797–803.

[8] University Group Diabetes Program. A study of the effects of hypoglycemic agents on vascular complications in patients with adult-onset diabetes. Diabetes 1976; 25: 1129–1148.

[9] Howard-Williams J, Hillson RM, Bron A et al. Retinopathy is associated with higher glycemia in maturity-onset type diabetes. Diabetologia 1984; 27: 198–202.

[10] Pettit DJ, Lisse JR, Knowler WC et al. Development of retinopathy and proteinuria in relation to plasma-glucose concentrations in Pima Indians. Lancet 1980; 1: 1050–1052.

[11] Knowler WC, Bennett PH, Ballintine EJ. Increased incidence of retinopathy in diabetics with elevated blood pressure. N Engl J Med 1980; 302: 645–650.

[12] Jarrett RJ. Duration of non-insulin-dependent diabetes and development of retinopathy: analysis of possible risk factors. Diab Med 1986; 3: 261–263.

[13] Klein R, Klein BEK, Moss S. Glycosylated hemoglobin predicts the incidence and progression of diabetic retinopathy. Diabetes 1988; 37 (suppl 1): 51A.

[14] Janka, HU, Warram JH, Rand LI et al. Risk factors for progression of background retinopathy in long-standing IDDM. Diabetes 1989; 38: 460–464.

[15] Hanssen KF, Dahl-Jorgensen K, Lauritzen T et al. Diabetic control and microvascular complications: the near-normoglycaemic experience. Diabetologia 1986; 29: 677–684.

[16] The DCCT Research Group. Diabetes Control and Complication Trial (DCCT): results of feasibility study. Diabetes Care 1987; 10: 1–19.

[17] Friedman, EA, Sheih SD, Hirsch SR et al. No supranormal glomerulum filtration (GFR) in type II (non-insulin-dependent) diabetes. Amer Soc Nephrol 1981; 14: 102A.

[18] Damsgaard EM, Mogensen CE. Microalbuminuria in elderly hyperglycemic patients and controls. Diabetic Med 1986; 3: 430–435.
[19] Schmitz A, Gundersen HJG, Østerby R. Glomerular morphology by light microscopy in non-insulin-dependent diabetes: lack of glomerular hypertrophy. Diabetes 1988; 37: 38–43.
[20] Garancini P, Gallus G, Calori G et al. Microalbuminuria and its associated risk factors in a representative sample of Italian type II diabetics. J Diab Complic 1988; 2: 12–15.
[21] Zabel-Langhennig R, Fiedler A. Erste Ergebnisse einer Untersuchung zur Häufigkeit der diabetischen Nephropathie bei den nicht-insulinabhängigen Diabetikern einer geschlossenen Population. Workshop „Neue Aspekte des Typ-II-Diabetes". Leipzig: Novo-Berichtsband 1987; 171–176.
[22] Schnack C, Watschinger B, Scheithaner BW et al. Prevalence of microalbuminuria in Type 2 (non-insulin-dependent) diabetes mellitus: effect of duration of disease, glycaemic control, and blood pressure. Diabetologia 1987; 30: 584A.
[23] Standl E, Rebell B, Stiegler H et al. Prevalence and risk profile of incipient diabetic nephropathy in type 2 (non-insulin-dependent) diabetes mellitus. Diabetologia 1987; 30: 584A–585A.
[24] Mogensen CE. Microalbuminuria as a predictor of clinical diabetic nephropathy. Kidney Intern 1987; 31: 673–689.
[25] Fabre J, Balant LP, Dayer PG et al. The kidney in maturity onset diabetes mellitus. A clinical study of 510 patients. Kidney Intern 1982; 21: 730–734.
[26] Panzram G. Mortality and survival in type 2 (non-insulin-dependent) diabetes mellitus. Diabetologia 1987; 30: 123–131.
[27] Editorial. Provision of renal replacement therapy for diabetic patients in the UK. Lancet 1987; II: 21–22.
[28] Allawi J, Rao PV, Gilbert R, Scott G et al. Brit Med J 1988; 296: 462–464.
[29] Hasslacher C, Wolfrum M, Stech G, Wahl P et al. Diabetische Nephropathie bei Typ-II-Diabetes. Einfluß von Stoffwechselkontrolle und Blutdruck auf Entwicklung und Verlauf. Dtsch med Wschr 1987; 112: 1445–1448.
[30] Friedman EA. Diabetes with kidney failure. Lancet 1986; 1: 1285.
[31] Quellhorst E, Mietzsch G, Schünemann B et al. Nierenersatz bei diabetischer Nephropathie. Klin Wschr 1988; 66: 899–905.
[32] Vinik A, Mitchell B. Clinical aspects of diabetic neuropathies. Diab/Metab Rev 1988; 4: 223–253.
[33] Melton III LJ, Dyck PJ. Epidemiology. In: Dyck PJ, Thomas PK, Asbury AK et al, eds. Diabetic Neuropathy. Philadelphia: WB Saunders, 1987; 27–35.
[34] Pirart J. Diabetes mellitus and its degenerative complications: a prospective study of 4,400 patients observed between 1947 and 1973. Diabetes Care 1978; 1: 168–188, 252–263.
[35] Paisey, RB, Arredondo G, Villalobos A. Association of differing dietary, metabolic, and clinical risk facts with microvascular complications of diabetes: a prevalence study of 503 Mexican type II diabetic subjects. Diabetes Care 1984; 7: 428–433.
[36] Ward JD. Diabetic neuropathy. In: Krall LP, ed. World Book of Diabetes in Practice. Amsterdam: Elsevier, 1988; 3: 227–233.
[37] Greene DA, Lattimer SA, Sima AAF. Pathogenesis and prevention of diabetic neuropathy. Diab/Metab Rev 1988; 4: 201–221.
[38] Edmonds ME, Clarke MB, Newton S et al. Increased uptake of bone radiopharmaceutical in diabetic neuropathy. Q J Med 1985; 57: 843–855.
[39] Nelson RG, Gohdes DM, Everhart JE et al. Lower-extremity amputation in NIDDM: 12-yr follow-up study in Pima Indians. Diabetes Care 1988; 11: 8–16.
[40] Ewing DJ, Campbell IW, Clarke BF. The natural history of diabetic autonomic neuropathy. Q J Med 1980; 49: 95–108.
[41] Kahn JK, Sisson JC, Vinik AI. QT interval prolongation and sudden cardiac death in diabetic autonomic neuropathy. J Clin Endocrinol Metab 1987; 64: 751–754.

[42] Kannel WB, McGee DL. Diabetes and cardiovascular disease. The Framingham Study. JAMA 1978; 241: 2035–2038.
[43] Jarrett RJ. Risk factors of macrovascular disease in diabetes mellitus. Horm Metab Res 1985; 15 (suppl): 1–3.
[44] Smith JW, Marcus FE, Serokman R. Prognosis of patients with diabetes mellitus after myocardial infarction. Amer J Cardiol 1984; 54: 718.
[45] Nesto RW, Phillips RT. Asymptomatic myocardial ischemia in diabetic patients. Amer J Med 1986; 80 (suppl 4c): 40–47.
[46] Pyörälä K, Laakso M, Uusitupa M. Diabetes and atherosclerosis: an epidemiologic view. Diabetes/Metabolism Reviews 1987; 3: 463–524.
[47] Janka HU, Standl E, Bloss G et al. Zur Epidemiologie der Hypertonie bei Diabetikern. Dtsch med Wschr 1978; 103: 1549–1555.
[48] Hanefeld M, Schulze J, Fischer S et al. The Diabetes Intervention Study (DIS): a cooperative multi-intervention trial with newly manifested type II diabetics: preliminary results. Monogr Atheroscler 1985; 13: 98–103.
[49] Stiegler H, Rebell B, Standl R et al. Zur Epidemiologie von Risikofaktoren und makrovaskulären Komplikationen bei Typ II-Diabetikern in der Praxis des niedergelassenen Arztes. Akt Endokr Stoffw 1987; 8: 216.
[50] Janka HU, Dirschedl P. Systolic blood pressure as a predictor for cardiovascular disease in diabetes: a 5-year longitudinal study. Hypertension 1985; 7 (suppl II): 90–94.
[51] Kannel WB. Hypertension and other risk factors in coronary heart disease. Am Heart J 1987; 114: 918–925.
[52] Bierman EL. Atherosclerosis and lipoproteins in diabetes mellitus. Diabetes 1979; 28: 580–585.
[53] Janka HU. Herz-Kreislauf-Krankheiten bei Diabetikern: Schwabinger Studie. München: Urban & Schwarzenberg, 1986; 38–43.
[54] Howard BV. Lipoprotein metabolism in diabetes mellitus. J Lipid Res 1987; 28: 613–623.
[55] Study Group, European Atherosclerosis Society. Strategy for the prevention of coronary heart disease: a policy statement of the European Atherosclerosis Society. European Heart J 1987; 8: 77–88.
[56] Stout RW. Hyperinsulinaemia – a possible risk factor for cardiovascular disease in diabetes mellitus. Horm Metab Res 1985; 15 (suppl): 37–41.
[57] Janka HU, Ziegler AG, Standl E et al. Daily insulin dose as a predictor of macrovascular disease in insulin treated non-insulin-dependent diabetics. Diab Metabol 1987; 13: 359–364.
[58] Lemp GF, Vander Zwang R, Hughes JP et al. Association between the severity of diabetes mellitus and coronary arterial atherosclerosis. Am J Cardiol 1987; 60: 1015–1019.
[59] Valsania P, Warram JH, Martin B et al. High risk of coronary artery disease among hypertensive diabetic patients treated with insulin. Diabetologia 1988; 31: 553A.
[60] Wilson PWF. Diabetes and cardiovascular disease: The Framingham Study. International Symposium on cardiovascular complications of diabetes mellitus. Boston, 1988.
[61] Wieland OH. Zur Pathogenese diabetischer Gefäßkomplikationen: Mögliche Beteiligung der nicht-enzymatischen Glucosylierung von Proteinen. Hämostasiologie 1983; 3: 92–96
[62] Brownlee M, Cerami A, Vlassara H. Advanceed glycosylation end products in tissue and the biochemical basis of diabetic complications. New Engl J Med 1988; 318: 1315–1321.
[63] Janka HU. Thrombozytenfunktion bei diabetischer Angiopathie. Stuttgart: Thieme; 1983.
[64] Müller-Mohnsen H, Scholtes L. Auslösung der Thrombogenese durch strömungsmechanische Materialtransporte gegen die Gefäßwand. Hämostasiologie 1982; 2: 3–43.
[65] Mogensen CE. Microalbuminuria predicts clinical proteinuria and early mortality in maturity-onset diabetes. N Engl J Med 1984; 310: 356–360.
[66] Schmitz A, Vaeth M. Microalbuminuria and mortality in non-insulin dependent diabetes. Diabet Metab 1988; 14: 193.

Microalbuminuria and diabetic renal disease

C.E. Mogensen

Introduction

Overt diabetic nephropathy is usually a straight forward clinical diagnosis. It is seen in many insulin-dependent patients after a diabetes duration of usually more than 10 years, most often associated with background and later proliferative retinopathy. Its characteristics are as follows:

a) persistent proteinuria, meaning a total protein excretion of more than 0.5 gram per 24-hour period, measured on several occasions, b) diabetes duration usually more than 10 years, c) presence of diabetic retinopathy, d) no evidence of other renal diseases of non-diabetic origin, e. g., glomerulonephritis and no urinary tract infection.

When caring for patients in a diabetic clinic one may get the impression that diabetic nephropathy by this definition is not very common. However, careful follow-up studies [1 – 6] defining the cumulative incidence of protein-

Table 1 Cumulative incidences of diabetic nephropathy
20 and 40 year cumulative incidence of nephropathy by center, diabetes type and year(s) of diagnosis of diabetes

Institution	Year of diagnosis of diabetes	20 year follow-up	40 year follow-up
Joslin Clinic Boston, young IDDM	1939	≈30%	≈46%
	1949	≈18%	–
	1959	≈16%	–
Steno Clinic Copenhagen, young IDDM	1933 – 42	≈34%	≈47%
	1943 – 52	≈24%	–
	1953 – 62	≈20%	–
Health Center for PIMA Indians, young NIDDM	?	≈50%	–
Osaka Diabetes Clinic, Japan, young NIDDM	?	≈50%	–

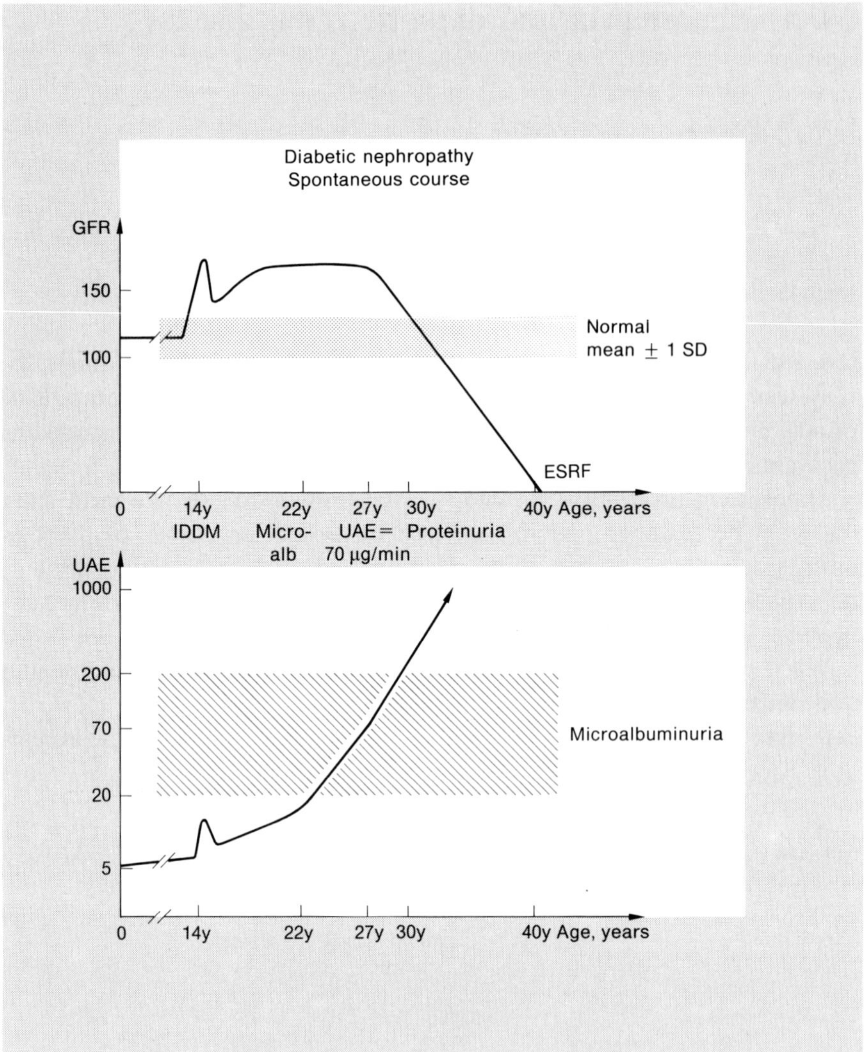

Fig. 1 The figure shows two key parameters, GFR and urinary albumin excretion rate (UAE), in a patient with diabetes diagnosed at the age of 14. At the clinical diagnosis increases in urinary albumin excretion rate and very high GFR are seen. These abnormalities are reversed by good metabolic control. In the course of diabetes GFR is still strongly related to poor or semipoor metabolic control. After about 9 years of diabetes, at 23 years of age, the patient developed microalbuminuria with a rather rapid rise id UAE, associated with poor metabolic control and increasing blood pressure. At a UAE level of around 70 µg/min, GFR started to decline in a linear fashion, continuing into the stage of overt diabetic nephropathy. At 40 years of age the patient developed end-stage renal failure. The hatched area indicates the microalbuminuric level, 20 – 200 µg/min.

uria show that about 35%, or even more, of patients eventually develop nephropathy and subsequent deterioration of renal function. This issue is discussed in more detail in chapter 2 of this book. It is likely that the incidence has declined over the last few years, from about 45 – 50% to about 30 – 35%. In young NIDDM patients in certain populations, diabetic nephropathy is also a serious problem (Table 1). However, in elderly NIDDM patients cardiovascular disease may be a more serious problem and, indeed, many such patients die before development of significant renal disease.

Until recently it has not been possible to predict the development of this serious complication, but new refined laboratory techniques have made it possible to define an early stage of diabetic renal disease. Incipient diabetic nephropathy can be detected by measuring minute amounts of albumin in the urine of diabetic patients. In this way overt diabetic nephropathy with proteinuria can be predicted many years before it actually develops (Fig. 1). Inded, nephropathy can also be prevented in many patients, if more intensified treatment is undertaken.

Definition of microalbuminuria and incipient diabetic nephropathy in IDDM patients

Microalbuminuria is defined as abnormally increased urinary albumin excretion rate (UAE) in the absence of clinical proteinuria as measured, for example, by the Albustix® test or by measurement of total proteinuria, for example, by the sulfosalicylic acid test. In order to standardize measurements, a number of workers in this field have agreed upon the following levels for defining microalbuminuria, incipient diabetic nephropathy, and overt diabetic nephropathy [7 – 8] (Table 2).

Microalbuminuria is considered to be present if the urinary albumin excretion (UAE) rate is between 20 and 200 μg/min corresponding roughly to 30 – 300 mg per 24 hour period. Urine samples should be collected when the patient is at rest and his diabetes is under average clinical control. No measurements should be made on patients in ketosis or poor control until proper control is attained. If excretion is lower than 20 μg/min, he is considered to have normoalbuminuria and if excretion is higher than 200 μg/min he is considered to have macroalbuminuria or clinical proteinuria.

It has been proposed that the term incipient diabetic nephropathy be used when microalbuminuria is persistent or, as is usually the case, increasing [7 – 8]. Microalbuminuria should be present in at least two of three urine samples collected over a period of several months. Other workers prefer the

Table 2 Microalbuminuria and diabetic nephropathy (DN): Stages in diabetic renal involvement and nephropathy in IDDM patients

Stage	Designation	Main characteristics	Main structural changes	GFR (ml/min)	Albumin excretion (UAE)	Blood pressure	Suggested main patho-physiological change
Stage 1 At clinical diagnosis	Hyperfunction and hypertrophy stage*	Large kidneys and glomerular hyperfiltration*	Glomerular hypertrophy; basement membrane thickness	≈150	May be increased	N	Glomerular volume expansion and increased intra-glomerular pressure
Stage 2 In short-term diabetes	"Silent" stage with normal UAE but structural lesion present	Normal UAE	Increasing basal membrane (BM) thickness and mesangial expansion	With or without hyperfiltration**	N (often increased in stress situations)	N	Changes as indicated above but quite variable (dependent on metabolic control); in addition, increased accumulation of BM and BM-like material
In long-term diabetes			No or few studies	With or without hyperfiltration[b]	N (often increased in stress situations)	N or slightly elevated	
Stage 3 Early	Incipient DN (or "at-risk-patient")	Persistently elevated UAE (20 – 200 μg/min)	Severity probably between stages 2 and 4	≈160	20 – 70 μg/min	Often elevated by 5 – 10% compared to healthy subjects and increasing by 3.5% per year. Blood pressure elevated during exercise	Glomerular closure probably starts in this stage. In some patients high intra-glomerular pressure
Late				≈130	70 – 200 μg/min		

Stage 4			Further increase in basement membrane thickening and mesangial expansion.			Blood pressure increase by ≈7% per year	
Early		Clinical proteinuria or UAE >200 μg/min	Increasing rate of glomerular closure.	≈130–70	>200 μg/min	Often definate hypertension	High rate of glomerular closure and advancing mesangial expansion
Intermediate	Overt DN		Hypertrophy of remaining glomeruli	≈70–30		Hypertension almost ubiquitous	
Advanced				≈30–10		Hypertension almost ubiquitous	Hyperfiltration in remaining glomeruli (deleterious?)
Stage 5	Uremia	End-stage renal failure	Generalized glomerular closure	0–10	Decreasing (due to nephron closure)	High, but often controlled by dialysis treatment	Advanced lesions and glomerular closure

* Changes present probably in all stages when control imperfect
** Possible marker of future nephropathy (if GFR >150 ml/min)
GFR = glomerular filtration rate; N = normal; UAE = urinary albumin excretion; DN = diabetic nephropathy

designations: at-risk-for-nephropathy-patients, high-risk-patients or simply microalbuminuria [8].

However, since microalbuminuria may be caused by other factors not related to renal disease, it is reasonable to have a distinction between microalbuminuria and incipient diabetic nephropathy [8]. Since the risk of subsequent nephropathy is rather high, around 80%, the term incipient nephropathy seems justified. Overt diabetic nephropathy is defined as urinary albumin excretion above 200 μg/min or 300 mg/24h, found in at least 2 our of 3 urine samples collected over a period of several months.

Urinary albumin excretion rate has been studied in many normal persons and a rather close agreement on normal ranges has been found by various groups [9–11]. When measuring excretion rate at rest in young persons, a mean value of about 5 μg/min is usually found with a range from 2–13 μg/min. We found that values for 24 h collection are around 7 mg/24 h (range 1.7–30, n = 43), with no sex difference. There is some difference between excretion rate at rest and while being up and about, the excretion rate being about 25–50% higher in the latter situation. Also physical exercise may increase excretion rate considerably, although quite hard exercise is needed to produce a profound increase in healthy persons. It is important to know that excretion rate is usually somewhat lower in normal children [12], around 3–4 μg/min, with a wide range. In healthy adult persons there seems to be no increase with age. However, in elderly patients urinary tract infection, hypertension, and cardiac decompensation may be seen quite often. These diseases are known to increase urinary albumin excretion rate, and should, therefore, be born in mind.

The coefficient of UAE variance is rather large, between 30–40%, both in normals and diabetics. Therefore, multiple collections are advisable, especially in the case of elevated values.

Techniques for measuring urinary albumin in small quantities and urine sampling for screening and for quantitative follow-up

The first widely used technique for measuring urinary albumin excretion rate in small quantities was radioimmuno-assay, which was used quite extensively. In later years new techniques have been developed, such as ELISA, nephelometry, fluoroimmuno and other immuno techniques [13–32]. All these procedures have their specific advantages and all are usually sensitive enough to evaluate urinary albumin excretion rate in diabetic patients. The choice of method will depend upon the general experience in the laboratory as well as the laboratory equipment available, i.e., Elisa, radioimmuno-assays or for immuno-precipitation equipment.

Other procedures have been developed for measuring small amounts of urinary albumin for screening purposes, e.g., a newly introduced tablet method. The basis of this technique is the so-called indication error of proteins, meaning that the presence of proteins, especially albumin, will change the color-change point for various pH-indicators, the so-called protein error [33]. Agglutination inhibition techniques may also be used for qualitative detection of microalbuminuria [34].

There are several proposals for suitable urine samples for screening diabetic patients for early renal involvement [35–41]:

A) *A random urine sample* is not very useful because there may be great variations in urine volume output due to fluid intake, and, therefore, excretion rate may not be very closely correlated to concentrations.

B) *Random early morning urine sample.* The first urine sample voided in the morning is usually rather concentrated and by using this sample there is usually a rather good correlation between excretion rate and concentration of albumin. Such a sample is, therefore, suitable for screening purposes. If concentration is above 20–25 μg/l the risk of an abnormal excretion rate is rather high. Measuring creatinine in such a sample and expressing albumin concentration over creatinine concentration may make such a test somewhat more exact, since this corrects for urine volume [41].

C) *An overnight urine sample* is used by many centers and is probably the method of choice. If a diabetic clinic is planning to perform screening for early renal disease this method is recommended [35, 41].

D) Some centers prefer *24-hour urine collection* but more so by tradition, since 24-hour urine collection used to be used for glucose measurements for the evaluation of diabetic control.

E) *A short-term urine collection* may also be used, e.g., while patients are waiting in the clinic. Measurements can also be done in connection with clearance studies. In this way a complete measurement of renal function is performed, but care should be taken to avoid the first urine samples after water-drinking and high urine output due to the early wash-out effect after starting water drinking [42].

Predictive power of microalbuminuria for overt diabetic nephropathy incidence and prevalence of microalbuminuria in diabetic populations

Longterm follow-up studies have been undertaken by three diabetes centers which evaluate the power of microalbuminuria to predict overt diabetic nephropathy defined as clinical proteinuria [43–45]. The technique used, the urine sample used, and the follow-up time differ among centers and, therefore, it is not surprising that there are some differences in predictive level, as seen in Table 3. However, generally speaking, the results are quite consistant, documenting that an elevated urinary albumin excretion rate, in fact, predicts overt diabetic nephropathy with a rather high degree of accuracy. The results obtained are without any intervention. It may, however, be expected that microalbuminuria may, in many cases, reverse by more intensive screening and treatment.

Overt diabetic nephropathy is always preceded by microalbuminuria or incipient diabetic nephropathy. Indeed the transition from microalbuminuria to clinical proteinuria is quite slow, often lasting 5–10 years (Fig. 1). Theoretically, it can, therefore, be assumed that the cumulative incidence of microalbuminuria is the same as the incidence of overt diabetic nephropathy

Table 3 Predictive power of microalbuminuria
Summary of studies of development of overt diabetic nephropathy (DN) based on early microalbuminuria

	London*	Copenhagen**	Aarhus***
Female/male	22/41	42/29	0/43
Follow-up (%)	75	100	98
Mean age at screening (yr)	40 (17–60)	30 (13–50)	25 (18–31)
Mean duration of diabetes at screening (yr)	10 (1–41)	12 (2–36)	12 (7–20)
Follow-up period (yr)	14	6 (mean)	10 (mean)
Proposed discrimination value (μg/min)	30	70	15
Development of DN above discrimination value	7/8	7/7	12/14
Development of DN below discrimination value	2/55	3/64	0/29
Urine sample	overnight	24-hour	short-term at hospital
No. of urine samples	≥1	≥3	≥3
Methods	RIA	radial immune diffusion	RIA

* Viberti et al. [43]
** Mathiesen et al. [45]
*** Mogensen et al. [44]
RIA = radioimmunoassay

Table 4 *Prevalence of microalbuminuria in non-proteinuric IDDM patients, studies from 1987*

Institution	Number of non-protein-uric patients tested	Urine sample	Age years	Age at diagnosis of diabetes years	Diabetes duration years	% with Normo-albuminuria (1–29 mg/24 h)	% with Micro-albuminuria (30–299 mg/24 h)	% with "Borderline elevation" (30–49 mg/24 h)	% with "Incipient diabetic nephropathy" (50–299 mg/24 h)
Steno Copenhagen	652	One/24 h	18–50	<30	>0	76%	24%	8%	16%
Hvidøre Copenhagen	777	At least one/24 h	>18	<41	>5	72%	28%	?	?
Danderyd Stockholm	102	Two over-night sample	mean ≈35 y	mean ≈11 y	>10	84%	16%		
England	1735	One over-night sample	16–60	<40	<35		>30 μg/min 6%*		

* *Selection criteria:*
1) Willingness to participate in trial
2) No BP >160/95
3) <3 episodes of diabetic ketoacidosis/12 months
4) <120 U insulin/24 h
5) No major illness

with a lag time. According to most recent studies, about 20% of diabetic patients will at the present develop clinical proteinuria after 20 years of diabetes, probably 30–35% after 40 years.

The prevalence (not incidence) of microalbuminuria (Table 4) has been studied in several diabetic populations, mainly in insulin-dependent patients and the prevalence is between 16% and 28% in large diabetic populations [46–49]. When patients with hypertension and patients not suitable for intensified treatment are excluded the prevalence is considerably lower, around 6–7%.

In diabetic children older than 15 years quite a dramatic number of patients may show microalbuminuria, around 30% [12]. On the other hand microalbuminuria is quite rare under this age. Microalbuminuria is also quite common in diabetic pregnancy. Increasing albumin excretion during pregnancy indicates a greater risk of development of pregnancy-related complications [50].

The transition from normoalbuminuria to microalbuminuria

The transition from normoalbuminuria to micro-albuminuria is a very important phase in the course of IDDM. Longitudinal studies have now revealed that patients who develop microalbuminuria already show albumin excretion in the upper normal range before the microalbuminuric level is reached (Fig. 1) [51]. It has also been shown that patients developing microalbuminuria have a higher level of glycated hemoglobin. Indeed, the study by Mathiesen and co-workers [51] showed that glycated hemoglobin in these patients is always above 7.5–8%, as evaluated by multiple measurements. If glycated hemoglobin is below 8% the risk of developing microalbuminuria is very small (Fig. 2). On the other hand, there are patients who maintain excretion rate in spite of a rather high level of glycated hemoglobin.

Blood pressure, on the other hand, appears to be normal before the development of microalbuminuria but rises a few years after microalbuminuria is clearly established. The Mathiesen group's data was based on a few measurements of blood pressure in the clinic, and not on 24-hour blood pressure recordings [51]. Importantly, this study suggests that the early phase of microalbuminuria is more closely related to poor metabolic control rather than to blood pressure elevation. However, soon after development of microalbuminuria an elevation in blood pressure, although small, is clearly established. The blood pressure rise early in microalbuminuria is not large, but the increase rate in blood presure, e. g., per year, is probably as important as actual level of pressure [52, 53]. Longitudinal follow-up of blood pressure measurement at regular intervals seems, therefore, very important.

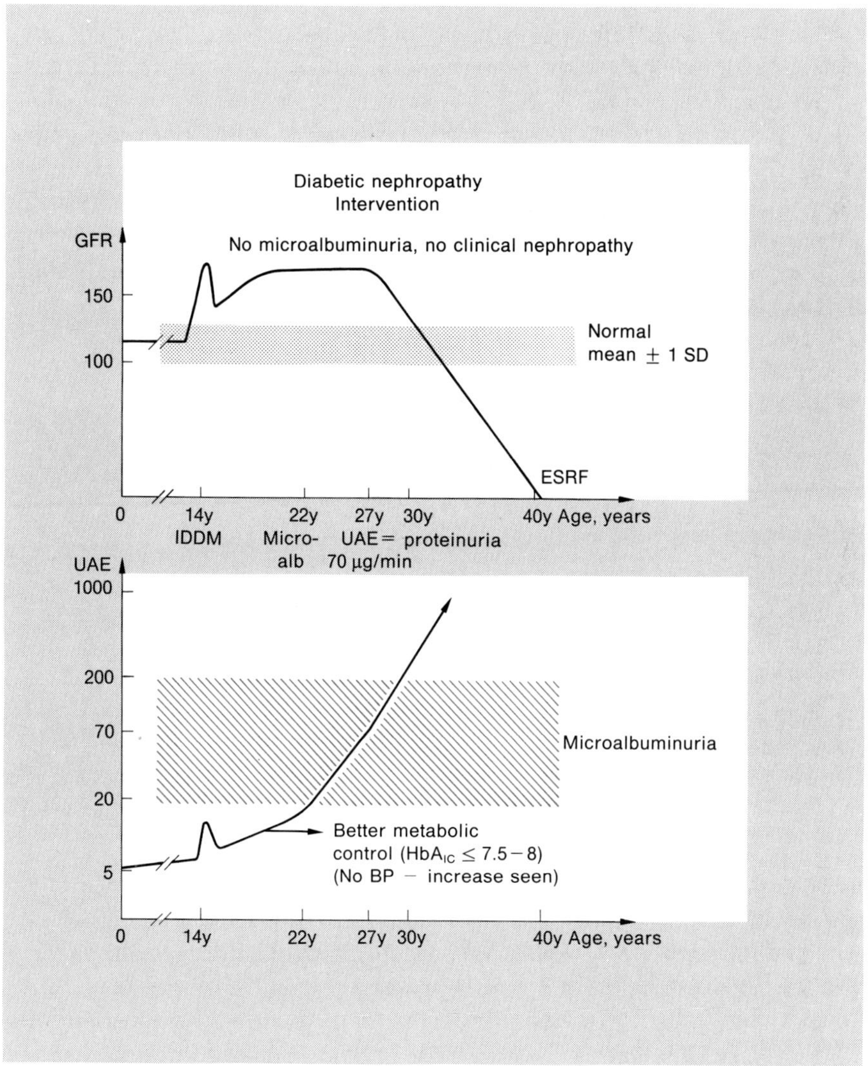

Fig. 2 If patients are maintained at the glycated hemoglobin level of HbA_{1c} less than 7.0–8%, the risk of progression to microalbuminuria is very small. Therefore, it can be anticipated that such patients will only develop microalbuminuria very late if at all.

Progression of microalbuminuria in incipient diabetic nephropathy

The same two main factors have been identified as determinants for the rate of progression of established microalbuminuria, namely quality of glycemic control as measured by HbA_{1c} and blood pressure level, as evaluated by multiple measurements. Unidentified factors probably also exist.

There is no major difference in quality of metabolic control between normo- and microalbuminuric diabetic patients, although the latter tend to have poorer metabolic control (Table 5). However, the progression of microalbuminuria, e. g. the rate of increase per year, is correlated to glycemic control as measured by level of HbA_{1c} [52]. Such a correlation was only identified when intensified metabolic control was introduced in some of the patients in a controlled clinical trial. In this way there was a rather wide range of quality of metabolic control and thus a correlation could more easily be established. If HbA_{1c} values were below a level of 7.5%, progression rate was generally slow, and regression can often be observed [52].

Table 5 Comparison of normoalbuminuric and microalbuminuric IDDM (Cross-sectional study)

	Normo-A (n = 62)	Micro-A (n = 19)
UAE µg/ml	2.4 – 13.8	20.1 – 125.0
HbA_{1c}%	7.9 ± 1.3	8.7 ± 1.5*
GFR ml/min	136 ± 18	146 ± 21*
Syst. BP mmHg	117 ± 8	127 ± 12*
Dia. BP mmHg	75 ± 6	81 ± 7*

* Significantly elevated

The other important factor is level of blood pressure or increase in blood pressure level during the observation period. If mean arterial blood pressure is below 100 mmHg (e. g. approximately corresponding to a systolic value of 130 and a diastolic value of 85), patients remain stable or progression is quite slow. Another related parameter is the rate of increase in blood pressure with time. If a patient shows a consistent rise in blood pressure during 2 years of observation (even with lower values than indicated above) the risk of progression is higher. The relative importance of the two abnormalities, blood pressure and metabolic control, has not yet been defined exactly (Table 6).

Table 6 Elevated blood pressure and poor metabolic control: risk factors for progression in incipient diabetic nephropathy

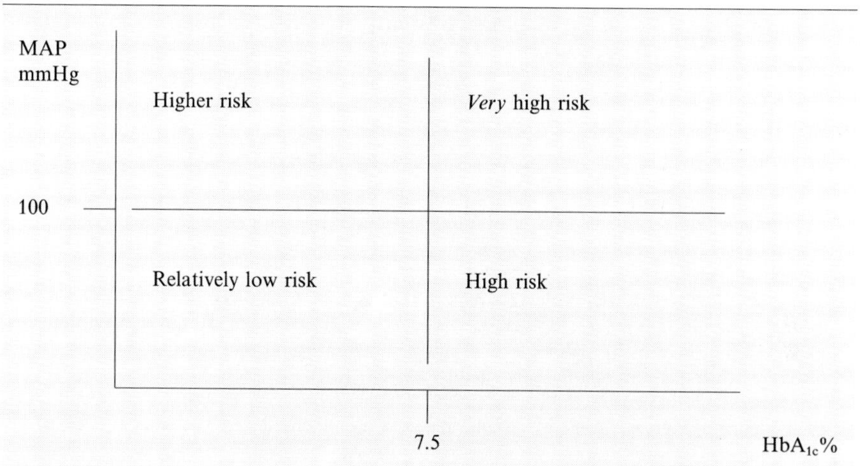

(Additional risk factors:
High protein and salt intake?
Smoking)

Structural and functional correlates of microalbuminuria in the kidney and associated abnormalities

The microalbuminuria range is between 20 and 200 μg/min and cross-sectional and follow-up studies have revealed that GFR is quite often elevated early in the course of microalbuminuria, namely between 20 and 70 μg/min. Thereafter, a fall in GFR is usually seen, at least when GFR is measured by an exact constant infusion technique using inulin or labelled iothalamate as a filtration marker [53] (Fig. 1). This means that the microalbuminuria stage is a very crucial one, namely the stage where renal function starts to deteriorate in diabetic patients.

These observations are in good agreement with structural studies on biopsy material. A study from Japan [54] has revealed that histological changes are found quite extensively in patients with microalbuminuria (Table 7). Whereas patients with normal albumin excretion rate show some lesions, patients with microalbuminuria show both diffuse glomerular lesions and arteriolar changes with a severity between normoalbuminuria and overt nephropathy. Surprisingly, electron microscopic studies have not shown a good correlation between level of microalbuminuria and basement membrane thickening or mesangial expansion. Further studies are being undertaken within this field, including studies of the significance of blood pressure elevation in relation to the level of microalbuminuria [55, 56].

Table 7 Abnormalities associated with microalbuminuria in incipient diabetic nephropathy

1) Glycemic control poorer than in normoalbuminuria, but with considerable overlap
2) Renal structural damage already present (degree of abnormality between normo- and macroalbuminuria)
3) Renal function still well preserved; hyperfiltration early in diabetic nephropathy
4) Increased blood pressure, increasing by about 3 to 4% per year without intervention
5) Development of overt diabetic nephropathy in 80% without intervention
6) More advanced retinopathy, predicted to worsen
7) More advanced neuropathy
8) Evidence of increased general vascular damage, e.g., increased transcapillary escape of albumin
9) Decreased aerobic working capacity
10) Unfavorable lipid profiles

Studies during the last few years have revealed that patients with microalbuminuria generally show much more extended vascular damage in other organs than do patients with normoalbuminuria. For instance, retinopathy is usually more pronounced in these patients [57], and, indeed, proliferative retinopathy can be predicted on the basis of early microalbuminuria [58]. However, there is an inconsistent relationship between microalbuminuria/ proteinuria and retinopathy [59]. A few patients may show rather advanced retinopathy without clinical relevant renal disease, whereas renal disease without retinopathy is very rare. Patients with microalbuminuria may also show early changes in cardiac function [60, 61], as well as more pronounced evidence of neuropathy [62]. These patients show also evidence of more generalized vascular damage, e. g., increased permeability to plasma proteins in general, not only in the kidney, as measured by transcapillary escape rate for albumin [63]. Reduced working capacity [61] and unfavorable lipid profiles are also often seen in diabetics with microalbuminuria [64].

There is usually a huge overlap in level of glycemic control between normoalbuminurics and patients with microalbuminuria, although the tendency is quite clear that somewhat poorer metabolic control is found in microalbuminuria patients. Patients with overt diabetic nephropathy usually show even poorer metabolic control, as measures by HbA_{1c}.

The differential diagnosis of incipient and overt diabetic nephropathy

In young patients the problems regarding differential diagnosis of incipient nephropathy are limited, but in certain cases there may be some difficulties. Patients in severe metabolic derangement and in poor control often show an increase in urinary albumin excretion rate. These changes are quite easily reversible by ordinary clinical control of diabetes. Therefore, urinary albumin excretion rate should not be measured when patients are in too poor control, but rather when the patient is under his or her usual management. Urinary tract infection may cause increases and, therefore, this should be excluded. On the other hand, since urinary tract infection is not common in young well-treated patients with insulin-dependent diabetes, it is usually sufficient to make a test-strip analysis. Severe physical exercise may induce increases in urinary albumin excretion rate and, therefore, urine should be collected at rest. Urinary albumin excretion rate usually normalizes a few hours after physical exercise.

Systemic disease should also be considered. A few patients with insulin-dependent diabetes may develop essential hypertension, that is, increased blood pressure unrelated to renal disease. Such patients show marked increases in blood pressure and, of course, values above 160/95 mm Hg by standard definition, but often a close-to-normal urine albumin excretion rate [65].

Sometimes is may also be difficult to determine whether signs of overt nephropathy are compatible with the course of diabetic renal disease or warrant further diagnostic evaluation [66]. Ultrasonography is often able to define kidney size and shape clearly enough to identify tumors, cysts, and anomalies such as a dilated renal pelvis and ureter. However, when glomerulonephritis is suspected, percutaneous renal biopsy should be performed to clarify diagnosis. Chronic glomerulonephritis, mainly mesangial proliferative and membranous glomerulopathy, and diabetic nephropathy commonly coexist, although the exact prevalence is unknown. Figures of approximately 20%, as published in recent extensive studies, obviously are an overestimate, since it is not general practice to biopsy diabetic patients unless dual pathology is suspected on clinical grounds.

There is agreement that an atypical course of diabetic nephropathy such as (a) clinical proteinuria despite a short history (less than 6 to 10 years) of insulin-dependent diabetes mellitus; (b) nephropathy without the presence of retinopathy; (c) rapid deterioration of renal function; and (d) impairment of renal function without antecedent proteinuria may demand further diagnostic evaluation. In contrast, it is disputable whether an abnormal urinary sediment

Table 8 Effects of intervention modalities

	Metabolic intervention	Antihypertensive intervention			Dietary intervention
Test parameter	Insulin pump-treatment	ACE inhibition (+ diuretics in some case)	β-blockers + diuretics	ACE inhibitors + β-blockers + diuretics (small doses)	Low-protein diet
Hyperfiltration (and elevated filtration fraction)	GFR reduced by about 5% in long-term studies (Aarhus)	Filtration fraction may be reduced by ACE-inhibition (Aarhus)	No studies	No studies	Hyperfiltration reduced (Aarhus)
Borderline elevated UAE	Total normalization in a 4-year follow-up study (Oslo)	No studies	No studies	No studies	No studies
Persistent microalbuminuria: (30 – 300 mg/24 h)	Stabilization (Gentofte)	Microalbuminuria reduced, stable GFR (Paris)	Longterm regression of microalbuminuria, stable GFR (Aarhus)	Regression in a 6-months study, stable GFR (Aarhus)	Microalbuminuria reduced in a small series on a short-term basis (London)
Proteinuria without high BP, possible with reduced GFR	No effect seen in a small series (does not rule out an effect) (London)	Studies ongoing	No studies	No studies	Reduction of fall-rate in GFR and reduced proteinuria according to preliminary studies (London)
Proteinuria, high BP, reduced GFR	No effect seen in a small series (does not rule out an effect) (London)	Rate of decline in GFR lower than in historical controls (Hvidøre)	Longterm treatment with cardioselective β-blockers, diuretics and vasodilators reduces decline in GFR considerably (Aarhus/Hvidøre)	In patients conventionally treated, additional ACE inhibitor may reduce progression (Göteborg)*	Reduction of fall-rate in GFR and reduced proteinuria according to preliminary studies (London)

* The combination not used in all patients

containing microscopic hematuria or red cell casts is an atypical feature of diabetic nephropathy. In recent reports based on a large number of renal biopsies in diabetic patients [67], hematuria was found in about 35% of patients with diabetic nephropathy alone. On the other hand, the necessity of biopsying diabetic patients with permanent or recurrent microscopic hematuria even when no evidence of urinary tract diseases is present was recently emphasized by Hommel and coworkers [68]. In a group of insulin-dependent diabetic patients, biopsies were done solely because of erythrocyturia. These biopsies demonstrated not only diabetic glomerulosclerosis in all of the patients, but also superimposed non-diabetic glomerular disease in 69% of them. Currently, it is unknown to what extent non-diabetic glomerular injury affects the course (or the treatment) of diabetic nephropathy. Patients with non-diabetic renal disease usually benefit from antihypertensive treatment, which, in these patients, also appears to reduce rate of decline of GFR [69].

Prevention and intervention

Results of a number of clinical trials are summarized in Table 8. These trials included intervention trials with optimized metabolic control (especially insulin pumps), trials with various antihypertensive agents (alone or in combination), and, finally, trials with low protein diet.

Trials with optimized insulin treatment

Most studies have been carried out with continuous subcutaneous insulin administration using pumps. Usually a fair reduction in glycated hemoglobin is obtained in comparison to a controlled group. However, it should be emphasized that the level of glycated hemoglobin is by no means totally normalized, the mean intervention value being two to four or even more standard deviations above the normal mean. A considerable overlap between insulin pump treatment and conventional treatment is also often found. However, most studies find a sustained effect even after some years of insulin pump treatment, although it is often difficult to maintain a marked difference in a very longterm study. Also patients are offered important new kinds of intensive treatment, e.g., insulin pen treatment, which to some extent mimics the advantages of insulin pump treatment although the degree of metabolic control is usually not quite as good.

The longest study now presently available is the Oslo study [70]. In this study a small reduction of GFR was also seen, probably as a consequence of better metabolic control in the CSII group. It appeared that in patients with albumin excretion rates in the upper normal range UAE was reduced by longterm treatment compared to conventional treatment. There was a significant difference between pump-treated patients and conventionally treated patients in this respect. Only a few patients on pump treatment showed UAE in the microalbuminuria range. It should be emphasized that patients were not initially strictly randomized with respect to UAE, but still it appears that the two groups of patients were comparable, and the outlook for longterm normalization of UAE by optimized treatment is certainly optimistic. As discussed earlier, patients with high normal values will develop microalbuminuria a few years later, and, thereafter, nephropathy [51].

The Steno Study II [52] deals with patients with persistent microalbuminuria, according to an international consensus [7]. Urine was collected as 24-h specimens and certain microalbuminuria was defined as a level between 30 and 300 μg/24 h period in at least two of three urine specimens. 18 patients were given pump treatment and an 18 patients unaltered conventional treatment. A significant difference with respect to progression was found between the two groups. Excretion of albumin was calculated as fractional clearance, that is a fraction of GFR, and patients on pump treatment were found to be stabilized, whereas to those with conventional treatment were not (Fig. 3). Importantly, 5 patients in the conventionally treated group and none of those on pump treatment developed nephropathy, as defined as clinical proteinuria (> 300 μg/24 hours). It was also observed that rate of progression of microalbuminuria was correlated not only to degree of metabolic control but also to increase in blood pressure level [52]. Indeed patients on conventional treatment show a higher tendency to increase in blood pressure than those on intensified treatment with pumps. The reason for this difference was not apparent, but it may be related to greater sodium retention. This study was not continued for longer than two years, primarily because many patients had to be treated with antihypertensive agents which are likely to decrease UAE more than optimized insulin treatment. The result of the study is optimistic but underlines the confounding effect of blood pressure elevation. New trials must take into consideration not only glycemic control but also level of blood pressure with a pre-planned treatment program. Therefore, the designs of such studies are rather complicated and the studies require either a large number of patients or well-defined patient stratification at entry into the study, especially with respect to blood pressure elevation.

In patients with clinical proteinuria, optimized insulin treatment produced no dramatic effects. Data from a small series of patients at the Guy's Hospital in London showed no statistically significant beneficial effect [71]; it should be born in mind, however, that it is likely that large groups of patients are required to document such an effect. In other studies an association has been found between progression in nephropathy and metabolic control; glycemic control may, therefore, still play an important role in progression of renal disease [72]. It should be noted that optimized treatment is more difficult in these patients, but this author still feels that best possible conventional treatment should be implemented in these patients, possibly by means of the insulin pen.

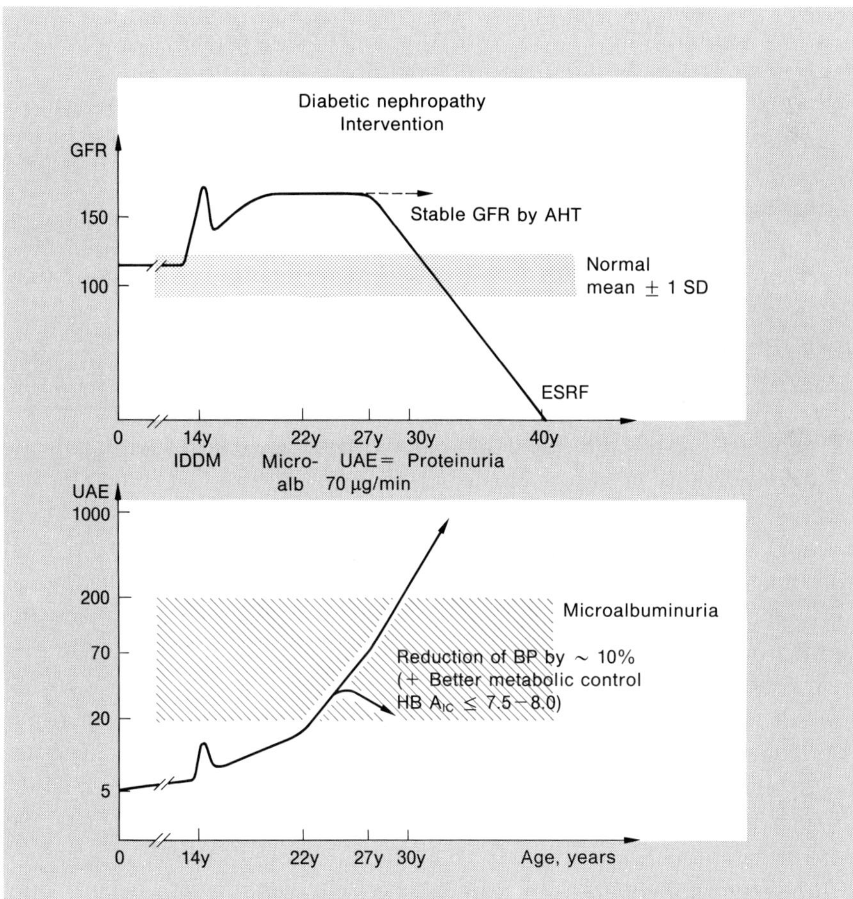

Fig. 3 Antihypertensive treatment using betablockers and diuretics or ACE inhibitors produces a reduction in microalbuminuria in IDDM patients. Combination therapy can also be used. New studies suggest that calcium antagonists can also reverse abnormally increased urinary albumin excretion rate in NIDDM patients. Studies carried out so far suggest that GFR is maintained when microalbuminuria is reduced.

Blood pressure control

It is clear from many studies that patients with microalbuminuria show higher blood pressures than do normoalbuminuric patients; diastolic elevation of blood pressure is especially characteristic. They also show a greater tendency towards increasing blood pressure. Without intervention (under conventional insulin treatment) blood pressure, in fact, increases in such patients 3–4 mm HG per year. The increase in blood pressure is also correlated to an increase in UAE [52, 53].

At the present time a number of studies are being carried out which are designed to firmly establish the effect of antihypertensive treatment. However, one 12 month study testing ACE inhibitors found that this treatment caused regression of microalbuminuria in patients with only borderline blood pressure elevation or normal blood pressure [73]. Patients on placebo showed a further increase in microalbuminuria. A longitudinal study in which patients were followed for an average of 5 years before and 5 years during antihypertensive treatment with beta-blockers and diuretics is also interesting. Before treatment increase rate was, on the average, 18% per year, which is quite typical for such patients; during antihypertensive treatment there was a considerable drop of 19% per year which was sustained over the years (Fig. 3) [74].

Therefore, it is recommended that blood pressure be reduced when patients show considerable increase in blood pressure with time or when blood pressure exceeds 140/90 mm Hg at repeated measurements. This means that blood pressure should be reduced in patients with only borderline hypertension according the WHO criteria. There can be little doubt that reduction of microalbuminuria by antihypertensive treatment will be beneficial to patients. In the two studies [73, 74] mentioned above, GFR was well preserved during treatment, but fell with placebo [74]. Obviously, it is important that there are few side effects of antihypertensive treatement. We have had good experience with young patients with microalbuminuria treated with cardioselective beta-blockers and/or thiazide diuretics and/or ACE-inhibitors as single, dual, or triple treatment, in the latter case in rather small doses. Side effects and possible additional beneficial effects are summarized in Table 9.

It has been demonstrated that in patients with overt diabetic nephropathy conventional treatment with cardioselective beta-blockers and diuretics, in some cases supplemented with vasodilatators, induce a dramatic reduction in the progression of nephropathy, as measured by fall rate in GFR (Fig. 4) [75–76]. Indeed the new 6 year follow-up studies of Parving suggest that the rate of progression is reduced by longterm antihypertensive treatment [76].

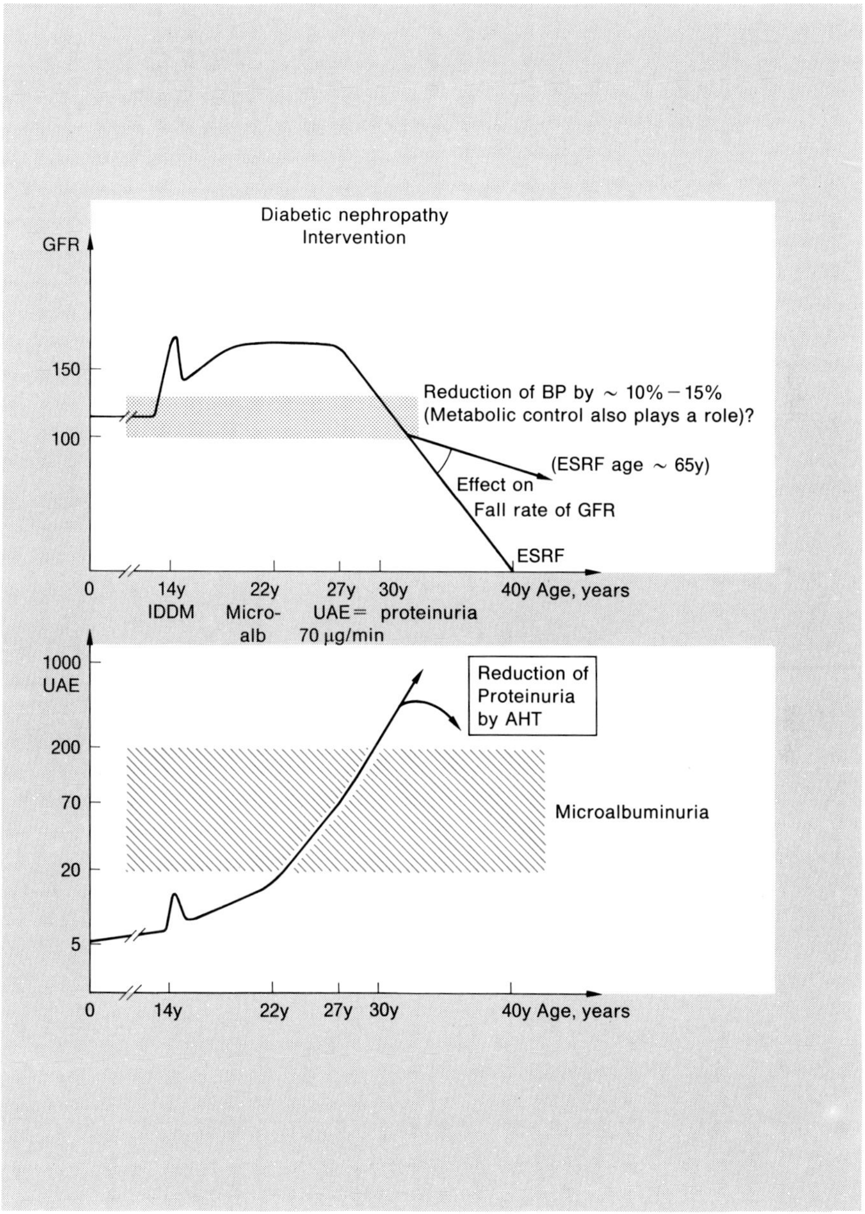

Fig. 4 The rate of decline of GFR in patients with overt diabetic nephropathy can be reduced considerably by antihypertensive treatment, and end-stage renal failure can be postponed. Recent studies have also documented that since the implementation of effective antihypertensive screening and treatment mortality has declined very considerably, as could be anticipated.

Table 9 Diabetes-related side effects and favorable and non-favorable effects related to antihypertensive treatment in diabetics

	Diuretics (Thiazid or loop)	Non-cardio-selective β-blockers	Cardio-selective β-blockers	ACE-inhibitors	Triple treatment: (diuretic β-blockers/ ACE inhibitors	Calcium blockers
Glucose intolerance	Yes (NIDDM related to hypokalemia)	No problem	No problem	No side effects	Limited (with small dosage)	No
Hypoglycemic masking	No	Yes in IDDM	A problem, but limited, seen in few patients	No effects	Limited (with small dosage)	No
Unfavorable lipid profits	Yes	Likely	?	No effects	?	No
Other unfavorable effects	May cause sodium depletion	Less physical exercise capacity	Less physical exercise capacity	Cough and drug-related side effects	Limited (with small dosage)	Foot edema seen in few patients
Favorable effects (apart from BP reduction)	Elimination of edema	Reduction of cardiovascular morbidity/mortality? Normalization of cardiac arrhythmias	Reduction of cardiovascular morbidity/mortality? Normalization of cardiac arrhythmias	Elimination sodium excess and possibly restoration of glomerular pressure gradients	Probably also combination of favorable effects	Effect on certain arrhythmias No potentiation of peripheral ischaemia

New studies also indicate that ACE inhibition is also useful [77, 78]. At the present time it may be concluded that ACE inhibitors, cardioselective beta-blockers combined with diuretics, and triple therapy, are all useful in slowing down the progression of renal disease in diabetic patients with overt nephropathy. Table 10 summarizes combination possibilities in antihypertensive treatment in diabetics. In most studies patients were included irrespective of the blood pressure level. Rate of progression was reduced considerably when mean blood pressure was reduced to a level of around 135/85. Calcium antagonists have also been reported to produce a reduction of deterioration of renal function in non-diabetic renal disease [79]. Microalbuminuria in NIDDM patients can been reduced in a 3 month study [80].

Table 10 How antihypertensive agents may be combined in diabetes

β-blockers	Yes				
ACE-inhibition	Yes	Yes	Yes		
NIFEDIPINE	Yes	Yes	Possibly	Yes (pronounced BP-drop may occur)	
VERAPAMIL	Yes	No	No	Yes (pronounced BP-drop may occur)	No
	Diuretics	β-blockers	β-blockers + diuretics	ACE-inhibition	NIFEDIPINE

Careful clinical metabolic and BP monitoring always required, including control of serum-electrolytes and serum-creatinine or GFR index

Low protein diet

It has been suggested that a low protein diet is able to retard progression of renal insufficiency, irrespective of the original disease process [81]. This concept is certainly also relevant in diabetic patients where hyperfiltration is a very prominent phenomenon, already present at the time of the diagnosis of diabetes. Therefore, a reduction of the protein content of the diet is an important approach retarding progression of renal disease. Although a number of studies have been performed to test this approach, still it is difficult to achieve consensus, and many questions are still unanswered [81].

It is well established that a high protein diet induces high GFR in non-diabetic persons. Recently it has been shown that a reduction of the protein content of the diet from a high to moderate protein intake is able to reduce GFR elevation [82]. Indeed, the traditional dietary treatment in which carbohydrates and later fats were considered inappropriate exposes many diabetics to a rather high protein diet [83].

Short-term studies indicate that microalbuminuria can be reduced by a low protein diet; we still need longterm follow-up studies [84]. In the case of overt diabetic nephropathy, preliminary studies also suggest that the rate of progression can be reduced. A comparison of the rate of decline in GFR of patients on a normal diet and a low protein diet suggests that the low protein regimen indeed reduces rate of progression [85, 86]. Since glycemic control and blood pressure level are unaltered in some of these studies, it is suggested that the low protein content of the diet is responsible for the retarded progression of renal disease. Interestingly, the reduction of phosphate and fat intake, which accompany a reduction in protein intake, may be equally important. Urinary protein excretion usually falls during low protein diet [85, 86].

Microalbuminuria in non-insulin-dependent diabetes

Urinary albumin excretion rate has also been studied quite extensively in patients with non-insulin-dependent diabetes. In these patients, however, there may be a number of factors beside early renal disease that can cause an increase in urinary albumin excretion rate. Thus the classification used in the insulin-dependent patients can not be applied to these patients. For instance, it is suspected that cardiovascular disease, including essential hypertension and cardiac decompensation, can cause an increase in urinary albumin excretion rate which is independent of glomerular disease in diabetes [87].

However, it has been found quite consistently that microalbuminuria is the best marker not only of development of proteinuria, but also of early mortality in these patients (Fig. 5). Three studies have documented that even a slight degree of microalbuminuria can predict a rather considerable increase in mortality even during a rather short observation period. There are two retrospective studies, one from London and one from Aarhus, and one prospective study from Fredericia which document the increased mortality in patients with microalbuminuria [88–91].

Therefore, there can be no doubt that microalbuminuria is a strong prognostic indicator in these patients. On the other hand, it has not been established whether intervention, for instance, intensified control of diabetes by insulin, oral agents, or diet has any influence on outcome. Also it is not known whether antihypertensive treatment is effective, although it has been shown that microalbuminuria can be reduced. So far there have been no studies regarding use of diuretics, digitalis or ACE inhibitors. It has been shown that NIDDM patients with microalbuminuria often have unfavorable lipid profiles and therefore dietary intervention may be important.

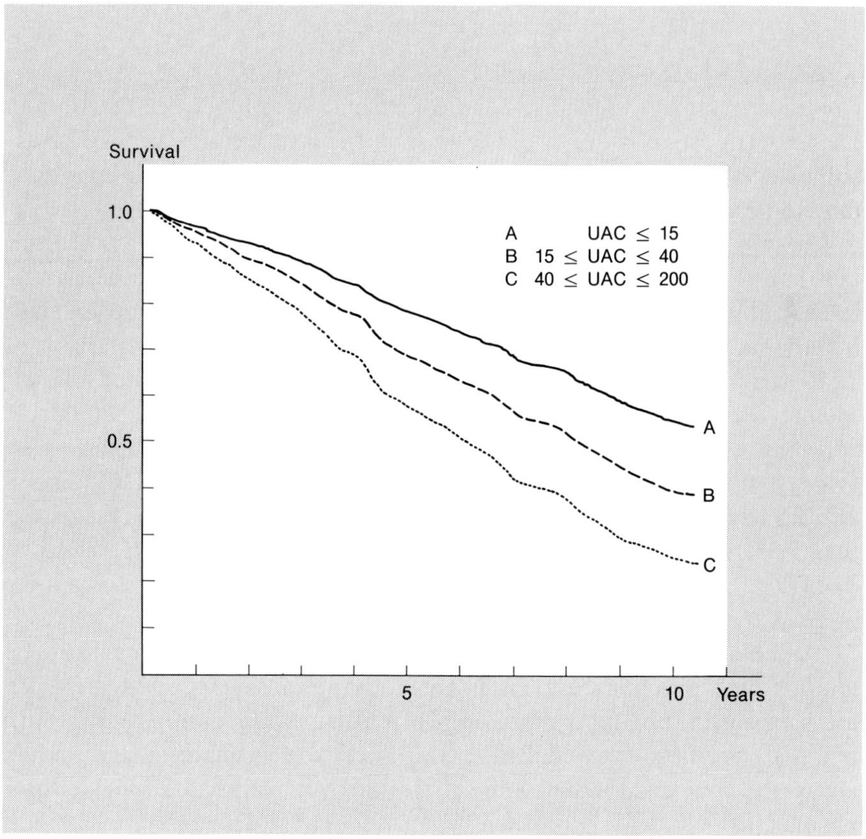

Fig. 5 Mortality in NIDDM patients (n = 503) with various levels of urinary albumin concentration (UAC µg/ml) in morning urine at the initial examination. Patients with high UAE have a much poorer survival rate than those with UAE close to normal.

Proposal for practical guidelines for the management of young IDDM-patients to prevent or postpone diabetic nephropathy

The following guidelines for glycemic, antihypertensive, and dietary control are recommended on the basis of recent studies:

Glycated hemoglobin is a key parameter and the reference interval for HbA_{1c} is clearly important. In agreement with others we have found that the reference interval is 5.4 ± 1.0% ($\times \pm 2SD$) using both BIO-RAD HbA1c mini-columns and a method using high pressure liquid chromatography. Thus using the reliable methods the level 7.5% is roughly equal to 4 standard deviations above the mean of the reference value.

The normoalbuminuric patient (< 20 μg/min or < 30 mg/24 h period)

A. HbA_{1c} < 7.5%–8%

Continue treatment modality. Take care that control does not deteriorate. Diabetes education is important as well as frequent measurement of glycatedhemoglobin. Numerous blood glucose measurements are also important in monitoring patients.

The level 7.5–8% was chosen because hyperfiltration (GFR > 150 ml/min/1.73 m^2), a risk factor for overt nephropathy, is rarely seen below this level. It is also rare that patients with normoalbuminuria develop microalbuminuria, provided that HbA_{1c} is below this level. Patients below HbA_{1c} of 7.5% were generally stable without progression in the Steno Study II, although these patients already had microalbuminuria. HbA1c should, of course, not be so low that many hypoglycemic attacks occur. There is no evidence that HbA1c level needs to be totally normalized in IDDM. This is also in agreement with the finding that patients with a HbA_{1c}-level of less than 7.5% with glucose intolerance do not develop microvascular lesions.

B. HbA_{1c} > 7.5–8%

Try to obtain better control either by conventional insulin treatment or by multiple daily injections, e. g., using one of the new insulin pen systems which are inexpensive, non-hazardous, and easy to handle (in contrast to insulin-pumps). General diabetes education is always extremely important and should always be conducted along with all treatment modalities. Although some patients, namely those "protected" against longterm diabetic complications, may be "over-treated" it is not readily possible to distinguish the "protected" patients from the "non-protected" (Table 2). However, treatment with pen systems is without side-effect, and preferred by many patients as a convenient and flexible way of insulin injection. Insulin pump treatment might be considered but should only be introduced in highly motivated and well disciplined adult diabetics with family or spouse who can help when ketoacidosis develops.

Hypertension or borderline hypertension (BP $\geq$ 140/90 mmHg) should be managed as indicated below. However, blood pressure elevation is not commonly found in patients with normal albumin excretion rate.

Although normoalbuminuric patients generally have a good prognosis over the subsequent decade, they are probably not protected against nephropathy in the long run. Retinopathy and other complications may certainly develop although at a smaller risk rate. Furthermore, it is not always easy to determine whether patients with values from 15 to 30 µg/min at rest have normo- or microalbuminuria, so that follow-up of patients is clearly important.

Patients with persistent or increasing microalbuminuria (20 – 200 µg/min or 30 – 300 mg/24 h by repeated measurements)

Glycemic control should be achieved as in the normoalbuminuric patients, but even more aggressively in view of the results or the Steno Study II. This study showed that microalbuminuria could be arrested by good metabolic control ($HbA_{1c} \leq 7.5-8\%$). If resources are limited, as they are in most centers, effort towards better metabolic control should be allocated to these patients, who have a very high risk of subsequent nephropathy, namely around 80%, without intervention. As indicated above, insulin pump treatment can be introduced but only in very selected diabetics.

Blood pressure elevation is often found in these patients, and may reach a value of $\geq$ 140/90 mmHg with the risk of a further subsequent rise. Blood pressure should be carefully monitored along with albumin excretion rate. In incipient diabetic nephropathy, blood pressure usually increases by around 3 – 4 mmHg per year.

Blood pressure should be reduced to less than 140/90. Elevation of diastolic pressure is especially characteristic of these patients; a slightly elevated systolic blood pressure is probably not important. This means that patients defined by the WHO as borderline hypertensive should be treated. A pressure of 130 – 135/80 – 85 in young persons is probably appropriate. It should also be born in mind that blood pressure should not be so low that renal ischemia and other side effects can occur. Blood pressure and urinary albumin excretion rate should be monitored to document both the short-term and the longterm effect of treatment. Initially, a non-pharmacological approach may be attempted. If pharmacological intervention is required side-effects should be minimized using low doses of cardioselective betablockers and/or diuretics most often with potassium supplementation, and/or ACE-inhibitors as single, dual, or triple therapy. Frequent assessment of other complications is required, especially evaluation of retinopathy.

The proteinuric patients

Adapt the glycemic and antihypertensive treatment program as indicated above although glycemic control may be less rigid. Higher antihypertensive doses and/or triple treatment are often needed to reduce blood pressure to around 135/85 mmHg. Loop diuretics should be used in patients with advanced nephropathy and ACE inhibitors may be useful. Hypoglycemic masking and ortostatic hypotensive discomfort or other side effects may be a problem, especially in patients with advanced neurological or vascular involvement so that treatment in such patients may be difficult. Antihypertensive treatment will slow progression of the nephropathy in most patients. Effects of treatment should be monitored by measuring urinary protein excretion, serum creatinine, and even GFR in addition to blood pressure.

Regarding the diatary approach, longterm results are not yet available. Still we can say that a high protein diet should not be proposed. In patients with somewhat reduced renal function, a low protein-diet (40 – 50 g/day) may be advocated if GFR remains stable and if compliance is not a problem. Such a diet may also be useful in some patients to improve lipid profiles. However, consensus has not yet been reached on the value of such diets.

Brief guidelines for the older NIDDM patient

So far, there have been no clinical trials on the longterm effects of optimized diabetes treatment and of antihypertensive treatment in patients with NIDDM. However, theoretically the guidelines for IDDM patients also apply to these patients. Higher blood pressure values should, of course, be accepted in the case of patients above the age of 45. Allowance for increasing blood pressure levels should be made before start of pharmacological treatment. About 5 mmHg per decade after the age of 45 can be added so that a patient aged over 65 years of age should be treated when diastolic blood pressure exceeds 100 mmHg on repeated measurements. However, it must be stressed that there are no longitudinal follow-up studies showing that antihypertensive treatment affects morbidity and mortality. Antihypertensive treatment will, therefore, remain a matter of debate until studies are available. Guidelines for non-diabetic hypertensives may be used until such time.

References

[1] Knowler WC, Kunzelman CL. Population comparisons of the frequency of diabetic nephropathy. In: Mogensen CE, ed. The Kidney and Hypertension in Diabetes Mellitus. Boston: Martinus Nijhoff Publishing, 1988; 25–32.

[2] Borch-Johnsen K. Incidence of nephropathy in insulin-dependent diabetes as related to mortality. In: Mogensen CE, ed. The Kidney and Hypertension in Diabetes Mellitus. Boston: Martinus Nijhoff Publishing, 1988; 33–40.

[3] Borch-Johnsen K, Kreiner S. Proteinuria: value as predictor of cardiovascular mortality in insulin-dependent diabetes mellitus. Br Med J 1987; 294: 1651–1654.

[4] Borch-Johnsen K, Kreiner S, Deckert T. Diabetic nephropathy – susceptible to care? A cohort-study of 641 patients with type I (insulin-dependent) diabetes. Diabetes Res 1986; 3: 397–400.

[5] Borch-Johnsen K, Nissen H, Henriksen E. et al. The natural history of insulin-dependent diabetes mellitus in Denmark: 1. long-term survival with and without late diabetic complications. Diabetic Med 1987; 47: 363–370.

[6] Krolewski AS, Warram JH, Rand LI et al. Epidemiologic approach to the etiology of type I diabetes mellitus and its complications. N Engl J Med 1987; 317: 1390–1398.

[7] Mogensen CE, Chachati A, Christensen CK et al. Microalbuminuria: an early marker of renal involvement in diabetes. Uremia Invest 1985–86; 9: 85–96.

[8] Mogensen CE. Microalbuminuria as a predictor of clinical diabetic nephropathy. Kidney Int 1987; 31: 673–689.

[9] Hemmingsen L, Skaarup P. The 24-hour excretion of plasma proteins in the urine of apparently healthy subjects. Scand J Clin Lab Invest 1975; 35: 347–353.

[10] Marre M, Claudel JP, Ciret P et al. Routine measurement of urinary albumin excretion by laser-immunonephelometry. Diabete & Metab 1988; 14: 181–182.

[11] Christensen CK. The concept of incipient diabetic nephropathy and the longitudinal course of microalbuminuria: effect of antihypertensive intervention. In: Mogensen CE, ed. The Kidney and Hypertension in Diabetes Mellitus. Boston: Martinus Nijhoff Publishing, 1988; 165–174.

[12] Mathiesen ER, Saurbrey N, Hommel E. et al. Prevalence of microalbuminuria in children with type 1 (insulin-dependent) diabetes mellitus. Diabetologia 1986; 29: 640–643.

[13] Watts GF, Albano JDM, Bennett JE et al. Assessment of new radioimmunoassay kit for determining urinary albumin at low concentrations: comparison with radial immunodiffusion. J Clin Pathol 1986; 39: 1151–1154.

[14] Brodows RG, Nichols D, Shaker G et al. Evaluation of a new radioimmunoassay for urinary albumin. Diabetes Care 1986; 9: 189–193.

[15] Di Mario U, Pietravalle P, Napoli A et al. A sensitive routine assay for urinary albumin based on the competitive binding to anti-albumin antibodies in solid phase. Horm Metab Res 1986; 18: 689–692.

[16] Marre M, Claudel J-P, Ciret P et al. Laser immunonephelometry for routine quantification of urinary albumin excretion. Clin Chem 1987; 33: 209–213.

[17] Harmoinen A, Vuorinen P, Jokela H. Turbidimetric measurement of microalbuminuria. Clin Chim Acta 1987; 166: 85–89.

[18] Kearney EM, Mount JN, Watts GF et al. Simple immunoturbidimetric method for determining urinary albumin at low concentrations using Cobas-Bio centrifugal analyser. J Clin Pathol 1987; 40: 465–468.

[19] Bakker AJ. More on immunoturbidimetry of urinary albumin (Letter to the Editor). Clin Chem 1987; 33: 198–199.

[20] Lloyd DR, Hindle EJ, Marples J et al. Urinary albumin measurement by immunoturbidimetry. Ann Clin Biochem 1987; 24: 209–210.

[21] Silver A, Dawnay A, Landon J et al. Immunoassays for low concentrations of albumin in urine. Clin Chem 1986; 32: 1303–1306.

[22] Gillery P, Rousselle P, Malgras A et al. A sensitive fluoronephelometric assay of slight albuminuria. Clin Chem 1987; 33: 717–718.
[23] Chesham J, Anderton SW, Kingdon CFM. Rapid, competitive enzyme immunoassay for albumin in urine. Clin Chem 1986; 32: 669–671.
[24] Torffvit O, Wieslander J. A simplified enzyme-linked immunosorbent assay for urinary albumin. Scand J Clin Lab Invest 1986; 46: 545–548.
[25] Townsend, JC. A competitive immunoenzymometric assay for albumin in urine. Clin Chem 1986; 32: 1372–1374.
[26] Krämer BK, Jesse U, Ress KM et al. Enzyme-linked immunosorbent assay for urinary albumin at low concentration. Clin Chem 1987; 33: 609–611.
[27] Coppo R, Amore A, Roccatello D et al. A solid phase enzyme immunoassay for the measurement of urinary albumin and the detection of microalbuminuria. J Diab Complications 1987; 1: 58–60.
[28] McBain AM, Brown IRF. An improved enzyme-immunoassay method suitable for screening to detect microalbuminuria. Ann Clin Biochem 1987; 24: 207–208.
[29] Watts GF, Bennett JE, Rowe DJ et al. Assessment of immunochemical methods for determining low concentrations of albumin in urine. Clin Chem 1986; 32: 1544–1548.
[30] Dezier JF, Jouanolle AM, Le Reun M et al. Comparaison de deux méthodes de dosage de la microalbuminurie L'immunonéphélémétrie et la radioimmunologie. Ann Biol Clin 1987; 45: 78–84.
[31] Fioravanti M, Solerte SB, Patti AL et al. Determination of albuminuria in type 1 and type 2 diabetic patients with microproteinuria and overt nephropathy. Comparative evaluation between a radial immunodiffusion procedure and a highly sensitive radioimmunoassay. La Ricerca Clin Lab 1987; 17: 171–179.
[32] Feldt-Rasmussen B, Dinesen B, Deckert M. Enzyme immunoassay: an improved determination of urinary albumin in diabetics with incipient nephropathy. Scand J Clin Lab Invest 1985; 45: 539–544.
[33] Schmitz A. Microalbutest®: A new screening method for detecting microalbuminuria in diabetes mellitus. Uremia Invest 1985–86; 9: 79–84.
[34] Spooner RJ, Weir RJ, Frier BM. Detection of microalbuminuria in diabetic patients using a simple latex agglutination test. Clin Chim Acta 1987; 166: 247–253.
[35] Gatling W, Rowe DJF, Hill RD. Microalbuminuria: an appraisal of assay techniques and urine collection procedures for measuring urinary albumin at low concentrations. In: Mogensen CE, ed. The Kidney and Hypertension in Diabetes Mellitus. Boston: Martinus Nijhoff Publishing, 1988; 41–50.
[36] Nathan DM, Rosenbaum C, Protasowicki VD. Single-void urine samples can be used to estimate quantitative microalbuminuria. Diabetes Care 1987; 10:; 414–418.
[37] Marshall SM, Alberti KGMM. Screening for early diabetic nephropathy. Ann Clin Biochem 1986; 23: 195–197.
[38] Eshøj O, Feldt-Rasmussen B, Larsen ML et al. Comparison of overnight, morning and 24 hour urine collections in the assessment of diabetic microalbuminuria. Diabetic Med 1987; 4: 531–533.
[39] Cowell CT, Rogers S, Silink M. First morning urinary albumin concentration is a good predictor of 25 hour urinary albumin excretion in children with type 1 (insulin-dependent) diabetes. Diabetologia 1986; 29: 97–99.
[40] Howey JEA, Browning MCK, Fraser CG. Selecting the optimum specimen for assessing slight albuminuria, and a strategy for investigation: novel uses of data on biological variation. Clin Chem 1987; 33: 2034–2038.
[41] Hutchison AS, O'Reilly DStJ, MacCuish AC. Albumin excretion rate, albumin concentration, and albumin/creatinine ratio compared for screening diabetics for slight albuminuria. Clin Chem 1988; 34: 2019–2021.
[42] Viberti GC, Mogensen CE, Keen K et al. Urinary excretion of albumin in normal man. The effect of water loading. Scand J Clin Lab Invest 1982; 42: 147–151.

[43] Viberti GC, Jarrett RJ, Mahmud U et al. Microalbuminuria as a predictor of clinical nephropathy in insulin-dependent diabetes mellitus. Lancet 1982; I: 1430–1432.
[44] Mogensen CE, Christensen CK. Predicting diabetic nephropathy in insulin-dependent patients. N Engl J Med 1984; 311: 89–93.
[45] Mathiesen ER, Oxenbøll B, Johansen K et al. Incipient nephropathy in type I (insulin-dependent) diabetes. Diabetologia 1984; 26: 406–410.
[46] Niazy S, Feldt-Rasmussen B, Deckert T. Microalbuminuria in insulin-dependent diabetes: Prevalence and practical consequences. J Diab Complications 1987; 1: 76–80.
[47] Parving H-H, Hommel E, Mathiesen E et al. Prevalence of microcalbuminuria, arterial hypertension, retinopathy, and neuropathy in patients with insulin-dependent diabetes. Br Med J 1986; 296: 156–160.
[48] Berglund J, Lins P-E, Adamson U et al. Microalbuminuria in long-term insulin-dependent diabetes mellitus. Prevalence and clinical characteristics in a normotensive population. Acta Med Scand 1987; 222: 333–338.
[49] Microalbuminuria Collaborative Study Group, UK. Microalbuminuria and glycaemic control. In: Diabetic Complications '87. Multicentre and/or Prospective Study Session on Diabetic Complications. Rome, Ilaty: Consiglio Nazionale delle Richerche, 1987.
[50] Mogensen CE, Klebe JG. Microalbuminuria and diabetic pregnancy. In: Mogensen CE, ed. The Kidney and Hypertension in Diabetes Mellitus. Boston: Martinus Nijhoff Publishing, 1988; 223–230.
[51] Mathiesen ER, Rønn B, Jensen T et al. Microalbuminuria precedes elevation in blood pressure in diabetic nephropathy (abstract). Diabetologia 1988; 31: 519A.
[52] Feldt-Rasmussen B, Mathiesen E, Deckert T. Effect of two years of strict metabolic control on the progression of incipient nephropathy in insulin-dependent diabetes. Lancet 1986; II: 1300–1304.
[53] Christensen CK, Mogensen CE. The course of incipient diabetic nephropathy: Studies of albumin excretion and blood pressure. Diabetic Med 1985: 2: 97–102.
[54] Inomata S, Oosawa Y, Itoh M et al. Analysis of urinary proteins in diabetes mellitus – with reference to the relationship between microalbuminuria and diabetic renal lesions. J Japan Diab Soc 1987; 30: 429–435.
[55] Ellis EN, Mauer SM. Diabetic nephropathy. In: Alberti KGMM, Krall LP, eds. The Diabetes Annual/1. Elsevier Science Publishers B.V., 1985; 309–322.
[56] Bilous RW, Steffes MW, Goetz FC et al. Diastolic hypertension occurs along with, and not before, the development of the mesangial lesions of diabetic nephropathy (abstract). Diabetologia 1988; 31: 471A.
[57] Barnett AH, Dallinger K, Jennings P et al. Microalbuminuria and diabetic retinopathy. Lancet 1985; I: 53–54.
[58] Vigstrup J, Mogensen CE. Proliferative diabetic retinopathy: At risk patients identified by early detection of microalbuminuria. Acta Ophthalmol 1985; 63: 530–534.
[59] Agardh E, Tallroth G, Bauer B et al. Retinopathy and nephropathy in insulin-dependent diabetics: An inconsistent relationship? Diabetic Med 1987; 4: 248–250.
[60] Thuesen L, Christiansen JS, Mogensen CE et al. Cardiac hyperfunction in insulin dependent diabetic patients developing microvascular complications. Diabetes 1988; 37: 851–856.
[61] Jensen T, Richter EA, Feldt-Rasmussen B et al. Impaired aerobic work capacity in insulin-dependent diabetic patients with increased urinary albumin excretion. Br Med J 1988; 296: 1352–1354.
[62] Berglund J, Adamson U, Eliasson K et al. Autonomic neuropathy – the cause of blood pressure disturbances in microalbuminuric diabetics? In: Diabetic Complications '87. International Symposium, October 1987. Rome, Italy: Consiglio Nazionale delle Ricerche, 1987; 12.
[63] Feldt-Rasmussen B. Increased transcapillary escape rate of albumin in type 1 (insulin-dependent) diabetic patients with microalbuminuria. Diabetologia 1986; 29: 282–286.
[64] Jensen T, Stender S, Deckert T. Abnormalities in plasmas concentration of lipoproteins

and fibrinogen in type 1 (insulin-dependent) diabetic patients with increased urinary albumin excretion. Diabetologia 1988; 31: 142–145.

[65] Christensen CK, Krusell LR, Mogensen CE. Increased blood pressure in diabetes: essential hypertension or diabetic nephropathy? Scand J Clin Lab Invest 1987; 47: 363–370.

[66] Mogensen CE, Schmitz O. The diabetic kidney: From hyperfiltration and microalbuminuria to end-stage renal failure. Med Clin North Am 1988; 72: 1465–1492.

[67] Chihara J,. Takebayashi S, Taguchi T et al. Glomerulonephritis in diabetic patients and its effect on the prognosis. Nephron 1986; 43: 45–49.

[68] Hommel E, Carstensen H, Skøtt P et al. Prevalence and causes of microscopic haematuria in type 1 (insulin-dependent) diabetic patients with persistent proteinuria. Diabetologia 1987; 30: 627–630.

[69] Alvestrand A, Gutierrez A, Bucht H et al. Reduction of blood pressure retards the progression of chronic renal failure in man. Nephrol Dial Transplant 1988; 3: 624–631.

[70] Dahl-Jørgensen K, Hanssen KF, Kierulf P et al. Reduction of urinary albumin excretion after 4 years of continuous subcutaneous insulin infusion in insulin-dependent diabetes mellitus. Acta Endocrinol (Copenh) 1988 (In press).

[71] Viberti GC, Bilous RW, Mackintosh D et al. Long term correction of hyperglycaemia and progression of renal failure in insulin dependent diabetes. Br Med J 1983; 286: 598–602.

[72] Nyberg G, Blohmé G, Nordén G. Impact of metabolic control in progression of clinical diabetic nephropathy. Diabetologia 1987; 30: 82–86.

[73] Marre M, Chatellier G, Leblanc H et al. Prevention of diabetic nephropathy with enalapril in normotensive diabetics with microalbuminuria. Br Med J 1988; 297: 1092–1095.

[74] Christensen CK, Mogensen CE. Antihypertensive treatment: long-term reversal of progression of albuminuria in incipient diabetic nephropathy. A longitudinal study of renal function. J Diab Complications 1987; 1: 45–52.

[75] Mogensen CE. Long-term antihypertensive treatment inhibiting progression of diabetic nephropathy. Br Med J 1982; 285: 685–688.

[76] Parving H-H, Andersen AR, Smidt UM et al. Effect of antihypertensive treatment on kidney function in diabetic nephropathy. Br Med J 1987; 294: 1443–1447.

[77] Parving H-H, Hommel E, Smidt UM. Protection of kidney function and decrease in albuminuria by captopril in insulin dependent diabetics with nephropathy. Br Med J 1988; 297: 1086–1091.

[78] Björck S, Nyberg G, Mulec H et al. Beneficial effects of angiotensin converting enzyme inhibition on renal function in patients with diabetic nephropathy. Br Med J 1986; 293: 471–474.

[79] Eliahou HE, Cohen D, Hellberg B et al. Effect of the calcium channel blocker nisoldipine on the progression of chronic renal failure in man. Am J Nephrol 1988; 8: 285–290.

[80] Schmitz A, Pedersen MM, Mogensen CE. Effects of Felodipine on urinary albumin excretion and metabolic control in hypertensive non-insulin-dependent diabetics (Submitted for publication).

[81] El Nahas AM, Coles GA. Dietary treatment of chronic renal failure: ten unanswered questions. Lancet 1986; I: 597–600.

[82] Pedersen O, Schønau Jørgensen F, Pedersen MM et al. The effect of moderate protein restriction on kidney function in normoalbuminuric Type 1 (insulin-dependent) diabetic patients (abstract). Diabetologia 1988; 31: 530A.

[83] Wood FC, Bierman EL. Is diet the cornerstone in management of diabetes? N Engl J Med 1986; 315: 1224–1227.

[84] Cohen D, Dodds R, Viberti GC. Effect of protein restriction in insulin dependent diabetics at risk of nephropathy. Br Med J 1987; 294: 795–798.

[85] Evanoff GV, Thomson GS, Brown J et al. The effect of diatary protein restriction on the progression of diabetic nephropathy. A 12-month follow-up. Arch Intern Med 1987; 147: 492–495.

[86] Bending JJ, Dodds R, Keen H et al. Lowering protein intake and the progression of diabetic

renal failure (abstract). Diabetologia 1986; 29: 516A.
[87] Yudkin JS, Forrest RD, Jackson CA. Microalbuminuria as predictor of vascular disease in non-diabetic subjects. Lancet 1988; II: 530–533.
[88] Mogensen CE. Microalbuminuria predicts clinical proteinuria and early mortality in maturity-onset diabetes. N Engl J Med 1984; 310: 356–360.
[89] Jarrett RJ, Viberti CG, Argyropoulos A et al. Microalbuminuria predicts mortality in non-insulin-dependent diabetes. Diabetic Med 1984; 1: 17–19.
[90] Schmitz A, Væth M. Microalbuminuria: A major risk factor in non-insulin-dependent diabetes. A 10-year follow-up study of 503 patients. Diabetic Med 1988; 5: 126–134.
[91] Damsgaard EM, Frøland A, Mogensen CE. Microalbuminuria is a strong predictor of 6-year mortality of elderly Type 2 (non-insulin-dependent) diabetic patients and non-diabetic subjects. A prospective study (abstract). Diabetologia 1988; 31: 483A.

Diabetic retinopathy

E.M. Kohner

There are several chapters and review articles written each year on diabetic retinopathy. In order to avoid too much repetition this chapter will not aim to cover all aspects of the condition. After describing the clinical features, treatment, and the size of the problem, it will describe the newer ideas about the pathogenic mechanisms. Where possible, recent new knowledge will be emphasized.

The retinal vessels can be easily seen, and fluorescein angiography allows detailed examination. It is, therefore, not unexpected that the natural history of this disease is well established. While examination of the eye is easy, obtaining tissue for examination of pathological processes in the early stages is difficult, and this may be the cause of our woeful lack of knowledge of the underlying mechanisms of diabetic retinopathy. The need for special permission to remove eyes for postmortem examination at least in the UK only adds to this difficulty.

Lesions and their evolution

The earliest clinically recognizable lesions are microaneurysms. They may arise anywhere in the retina, but are usually first seen in the macular area, or lateral to the macula. Even when well established and extensive, most are usually at the posterior pole, and only rarely are they seen in large numbers at the retinal periphery. Microaneurysms are always associated with capillary non-perfusion, but in the early stages these can only be identified by fluorescein angiograms.

Haemorrhages, characteristically blot haemorrhages are the next feature to appear. Flame shaped haemorrhages are seen in the nerve fibre layer near the disk, and were thought to represent associated hypertension. It was Harrold [1] who first noted that he could not differentiate between hypertensive and normotensive diabetics on the basis of haemorrhages. By themselves, a few haemorrhages have no specific prognostic significance. However, in type II non-insulin dependent diabetes (NIDD) the number of haemorrhages in relation to hard exudates are prognostically important. In this condition as well as when there are clusters of large blot haemorrhages they are indicative of ischaemia, and are therefore classified as pre-proliferative lesions.

The next most commonly seen lesions are hard exudates. They are most frequently seen between the superior and inferior temporal vessels, usually starting some distance from the fovea, but gradually approaching it. They start as scattered lesions, but tend to coalesce and form rings and plaques (Fig. 1). Hard exudates invariably indicate leakage. They are not seen on fluorescein angiograms, but the leakage from micro-vascular abnormalities associated with the hard exudates is usually clearly recognizable. Hard exudates are associated with "retinal thickening" on stereo colour photographs and oedema on examination. The advancing oedema preceeding the exudates affects the fovea and is responsible for macular oedema in the exudative type of diabetic maculopathy.

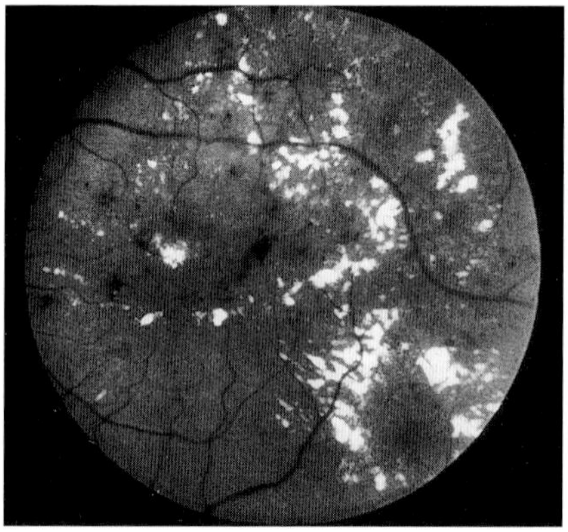

1

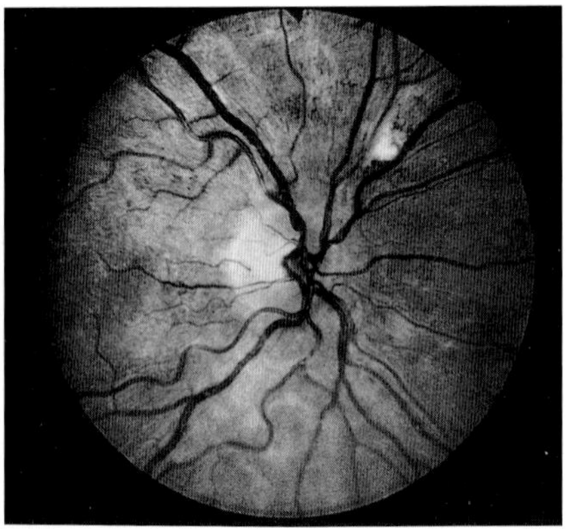

2

Fig. 1 Right macular region of a patient with diabetic maculopathy. Hard exudates form rings and plaques lateral to macula. At centre of hard exudate rings there are haemorrhages and microvascular lesions.

Fig. 2 Right disc region of young patient with preproliferative retinopathy. Note venous dilatation and beading, especially the superior nasal vein, one cotton wool spot and the many IRMA.

Venous abnormalities such as dilatation are common, especially in type I, insulin dependent (IDD) diabetes, but are not of any importance. However, venous beading, loops and reduplication are prognostically important pre-proliferative lesions. They are usually associated with other pre-proliferative lesions such as intra-retinal microvascular abnormalities (IRMA) and cotton wool spots (Fig. 2). IRMA are dilated capillaries, often with microaneurysms, and are seen in retinas in which many capillaries are not perfused. Cotton wool spots indicate interruption of axoplasmic transport [2], which could occur from capillary non-perfusion alone, but is usually associated with occlusion of arterioles and venules [3]. One or two cotton wool spots in an eye are not of prognostic importance, but multiple cotton wool spots, usually in excess of 8 – 10, indicate a more rapidly advancing retinopathy in which proliferative lesions will develop within one year.

The lesions so far described are non-proliferative or background lesions. They only cause visual loss if the fovea is involved in a haemorrhage or, more commonly, in oedema. Macular oedema is, in fact, the commonest cause of visual loss in diabetes, as it is frequently seen in NIDD. Worldwide, NIDD is much more common than IDD and, therefore, macular oedema as a cause of visual loss is important. Macular oedema may cause visual loss in IDD as well, but in this condition, unless associated with renal impairment, it only rarely causes *severe* loss of vision. In some instances macular oedema occurs in the absence of hard exudates, from generalized leakiness of microaneurysms or dilated capillaries. Ischaemia of the macular area also causes visual loss and ischaemic oedema, again seen more commonly in the older patients. Young patients can maintain good vision for considerable time even when there is a huge loss of capillaries in the perifoveal area.

Visual outcome in IDD and in some 20% of NIDD patients is determined by the appearance of proliferative lesions. New vessels arise from the retinal vessels (Fig. 3a), primarily veins, and from the optic disk. They invariably indicate the presence of large areas of non-perfusion in the midperiphery and far periphery of the retina. At first they grow on the surface of the retina and may be difficult to differentiate from IRMA, but invariably they break through the internal limiting membrane, and then use the posterior surface of the vitreous as a scaffold. The retracting vitreous pulling on the vessels is the primary cause of vitreous haemorrhage. New vessels have some fibrous tissue covering from their earliest days. With time, the fibrous tissue increases and, as all fibrous tissue, tends to contract, exert traction on the retina, and, eventually, causes detachment (Fig. 3b). Fibrous tissue can also form a thin sheet over the posterior vitreous face or the internal limiting membrane. It should perhaps be emphasized that new vessels themselves are not a cause of visual loss, but rather the complications the vessels cause, haemorrhage (Fig. 4), and tractional consequences, which cause the visual loss. Since new vessels have no symptoms, and since once complications are present treatment may be difficult, it is important to screen patients for the presence of new vessels, and for pre-proliferative lesions.

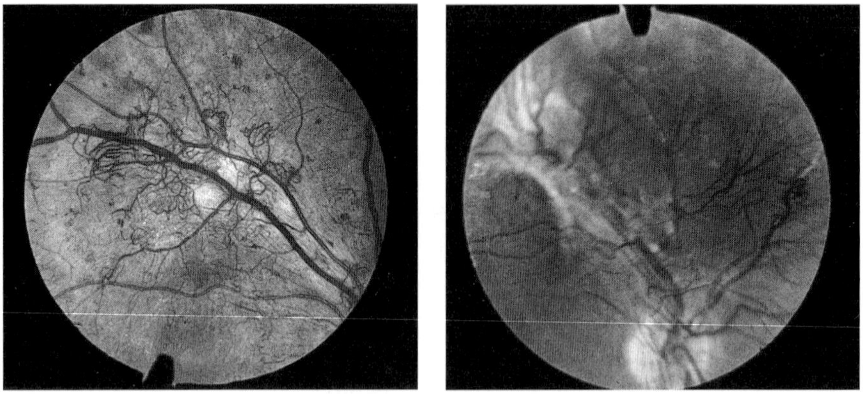

a b

Fig. 3a Right superior temporal region showing new vessels surrounding the vein — visual acuity 6/6.

Fig. 3b Same as Fig. 3a but 2 years later showing fibrous tissue replacing new vessels causing detachment of the macula. Visual acuity counting fingers.

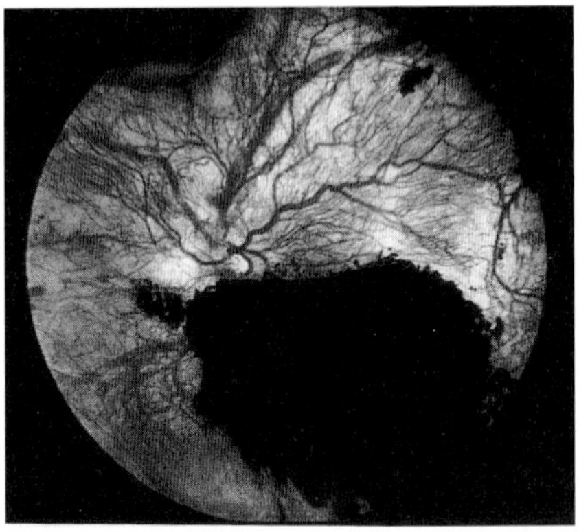

Fig. 4 Preretinal haemorrhage in one eye with extensive disc new vessels causing visual loss as it lies in front of the fovea.

With the availability of photocoagulation as a treatment for sight threatening retinopathies, proliferative retinopathy, and maculopathy, interest has focused on the early lesions, and in particular the quest for the identification of a "pre retinopathic stage". Is there a recognizable stage which indicates that retinopathy is likely to develop in the absence of intervention, similar to the stage of increased microalbuminuria in diabetic nephropathy? Is there a stage when intervention will prevent the development of clinically obvious retinopathy? In 1975 when Cunha-Vaz and coworkers [4] first described vitreous fluorophotometry, hopes were indeed high that such a stage did exist. Cunha-Vaz described a sensitive technique for measuring leakage of fluorescein into the vitreous, in small quantities not picked up by the photographic film. This leakage was present in long-term diabetes even in the absence of retinopathy. Cunha-Vaz and coworkers confirmed their findings in a larger study [5], and the hope for the identification of a pre-retinopathic stage was heightened by the work of the St. Louis group [6] who also reported improvement in leakage with the improved diabetic control achieved by continuous subcutaneous insulin infusion (CSII) [7]. It was, therefore, disappointing when the Hammersmith group reported that there was some leakage in normals and that there was no difference between normals and diabetics without any retinopathy [8]. This work was confirmed by the elegant studies of Lund-Andersen and coworkers [9], and more recently by Roy and coworkers from the National Eye Institute [10]. Thus, in spite of high hopes and a lot of work at present there is no recognizable pre-retinopathic stage in diabetic retinopathy.

Histological changes

Histological changes predate changes seen on clinical examination. The earliest changes probably affect the basement membrane. Thickening of the basement membrane affects all capillary beds. It is probably due to both increased formation and reduced removal of basement membrane material. There are also alterations in the collagen composition of the basement membrane with increased cross linking. The cause of the abnormalities is not known. One current theory is that there is increased glycosylation of proteins which alters the composition and, therefore, the removal of basement membrane. Another is that aldose reductase is somehow involved. Since basement membrane is secreted by endothelial cells, this theory pre-supposes that aldose reductase is present in the endothelial cells, a fact by no means universally accepted. The evidence for the role of aldose reductase is also not very strong. It has been shown that galactosaemic animals do indeed have increased amount of basement membrane, and this increase is prevented by aldose reductase inhibitors, such as sorbinil, provided one is given early in the disease. However, whether sorbinil has a similar effect in diabetic patients has not yet been proven.

Detailed histological evaluation of diabetic retinopathy only became possible after the pioneering work of Cogan and Kuwabara in the 1960 s [11]. These workers developed the technique of retinal digest preparation, which allowed the visualisation of the individual cells in the vessel wall. They were then able to demonstrate that already in early diabetes there is an imbalance between the two types of cells composing the capillary wall, the pericytes and the endothelial cells. In normal capillaries there is a one to one relationship between the two, in diabetes pericytes are lost preferentially and early. This is followed by uncontrolled increase in the number of the endothelial cells, leading to microaneurysm formation and dilatation of some of the capillaries. We do, however, know that before microaneurysms can form capillaries must occlude. The cause of the endothelial cell abnormality has not been clearly established. That endothelial abnormality may occur early is demonstrated by abnormal von Willebrand Factor levels [12], abnormal prostacyclin synthesis [13], and abnormal fibrinolytic activity [14]. These, together with increased platelet aggregation [15], may well lead to capillary occlusion and subsequent cell death. Since the turnover of retinal capillary endothelium is slow, damaged endothelial cells are not easily replaced in the early stages of the disease, though this may change after the loss of the pericytes.

It is also not known at what stage the integrity of the blood-retinal barrier is broken. In vitro fibrin clots adhering to the vessel wall damage the endothelial cells by causing alteration in the cytoskeletal elements responsible for cell to cell contact. In longterm diabetic dogs Wallow and coworkers observed penetration of horseraddish peroxidase into the interendothelial tight junctions of the retinal capillaries [16]. It is, however, likely that in the early breakdown of the blood-retinal barrier leakage is through the endothelial cells and not through the tight junctions. Since a few days of high glucose medium did not cause this increased permeability, other factors are probably also necessary. This is the reason why King and coworkers did not demonstrate increased permeability in their cell culture work [17].

In any case, eventually endothelial cells die and capillaries are lined by empty basement membrane tubes. Indeed, new vessels never develop, unless there are large areas of capillary non-perfusion. The initial step of new vessel formation is dissolution of the basement membrane by endothelial cells entering them. Further cells migrate into this break and replicate at a rapid rate, forming solid tubes of cells which have the ability to canalize. Capillary loops are formed by fusion of the leading edge of the canalized tubes. The newly formed capillaries have both endothelial cells and pericytes in their walls. The role of the pericytes in these newly formed vessels is not known. Fibrous tissue formation follows the development of the new vessels, but little is known about the stimulus for this lesion. Similarly, it is not known what causes the capillary tubes to break through the internal limiting membrane, though it could be the uninhibited growth and replication of the cells.

Epidemiology

Although there is a wide variation of occurence of diabetes in various populations, there is no evidence of any variability in the presence of diabetic retinopathy [18]. The largest and most carefully conducted epidemiological study in a Caucasian population comes from Wisconsin, where the records of the entire diabetic population of southern Wisconsin were examined. All patients whose diabetes was diagnosed before the age of 30 were examined [19], while a stratified randomized sample of those diagnosed after the age of 30 and presumed to be NIDDs was examined [20]. Visual acuity was checked and clinical examination was supplemented by stereo photographs of seven standard fields which were assessed at the Madison Reading Centre. In many points the study confirmed previous less well-documented data, but some new information also arose.

In Type I, IDD retinopathy is uncommon before about 5 – 10 years diabetes duration. Thereafter its frequency rises steeply, so that by 15 years duration over 80% have retinopathy, and by 20 years 97% of this population had at least one microaneurysm. However, it must be emphasized that on photographic assessment the tendency is for the overestimation of the presence of microaneurysms unless very experienced graders were used. (At the Hammersmith Reading Centre, whose graders are less experienced than those at Madison, the disagreements between graders are almost invariably limited to the presence or absence of a single microaneurysm). Thus almost all patients are likely to develop at least minimal lesions of diabetic retinopathy after 20 years diabetes duration. Proliferative retinopathy in this group of patients also increased with duration of diabetes, and reached 60% by 25 years diabetes duration. It tended to fall after about 30 years, probably because many with the most severe microvascular disease had died by that time.

In those whose diabetes was diagnosed after the age of 30, retinopathy was common even in the first 5 years, reaching almost 20%. Among these patients those on insulin had a higher prevalence of retinopathy, reaching 80% among those who had the disease for 20 years, but only about 40% among those treated with diet only or diet and oral hypoglycaemic agents. In this group of patients, proliferative retinopathy never reached more than 20%. The authors did not discuss why patients were on insulin. It is possible that those with the more severe complications were given insulin, in the hope of ameliorating their retinopathy. Certainly this has been fashionable and still is so among many diabetologists and general practitioners. Alternately, it is possible that those with the more severe diabetes are the ones who have a higher risk of developing retinopathy. The United Kingdom Prospective Diabetes Study (UKPDS) [21] has only recorded the presence of retinopathy and its severity at entry into the study, which includes 1111 patients so far. Over 23% had retinopathy at entry. In the great majority of the patients retinopathy was minimal, that is, manifested by the presence of one or two microaneurysms only. Those with retinopathy differed from those without in that they were older, leaner, had higher systolic and diastolic blood pressure, and more impaired age-adjusted vibration sense using biothesiometry. Increasing severity of retinopathy was seen with increasing age and systolic blood pressure. Whether diabetic control affects severity of retinopathy has not yet been clearly established, but the Wisconsin study indicated that a definite independent risk of severity of retinopathy is related to blood glucose control (measured by HbA_1 and blood glucose levels) in both IDD and NIDD patients [19, 29].

Prevalence of retinopathy in populations with high risk of developing diabetes, usually NIDD, is not unlike that found by Klein and coworkers [20]. In studies of diabetes in underdeveloped countries it appears that cataract is a much more common and important cause of blindness than is the retinopathy, even in the IDD patients.

Treatment of diabetic retinopathy

Many treatments have been tried for diabetic retinopathy, but only a few have proven to have a beneficial effect.

The treatment of early diabetic retinopathy

There is, at present, no treatment that can reliably arrest the advancement of early diabetic retinopathy. In animal studies Engerman has shown that excellent diabetic control over a 5 year period prevented the development of retinopathy in dogs [22]. But the degree of control achieved in the dogs was far better than what we can hope to achieve in humans. The question remains whether improved control can prevent development of retinopathy or at least delay it. A large multicenter study which is now being carried out in the US, the Diabetic Control and Complications Trial, should eventually answer the question. But even if answered positively, the fact that centers have to advertize for patients suggests that not many patients are willing to submit to the rigours of really very strict control, frequent clinic visits, and frequent blood tests.

Has control a role in slowing or arresting the progression of the lesions once retinopathy is established? With the introduction of CSII, home monitoring of blood glucose, and availability of HbA_1 estimations, it has become possible to find answers for this question. Three randomized controlled clinical trials were set up, in which CSII was compared with conventional treatment [23, 24, 25]. In all three trials the CSII patients achieved significantly better control than those on conventional treatment. It was, therefore, both upsetting and unexpected, when all three trials indicated that during the first 6 to 12 months the retinopathy deteriorated more in those on CSII than in the control group. The retinopathy in all these patients was mild, and it was, therefore, expected to be reversible. The lesions that developed or worsened in the CSII patients were cotton wool spots, haemorrhages, and microaneurysms (Fig. 5a, b). In some even IRMA developed. However, in spite of the appearance of these pre-proliferative lesions, new vessels did not develop more frequently in the CSII group. When the studies were continued for a further period of time the situation changed. While in the conventionally treated patients retinopathy continued to deteriorate at a steady rate, in the CSII patients the deterioration was reversed, so that at the end of 2 years or

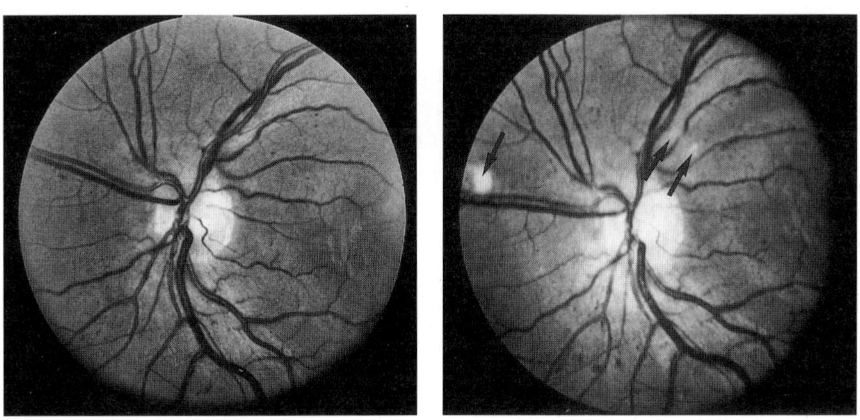

a b

Fig. 5a Left disc area of patient with mild diabetic retinopathy before starting CSII.

Fig. 5b Same as Fig. 5a but 8 months after starting CSII. Note increased haemorrhages in inferior nasal area and 3 cotton wool spots (arrows).

longer the retinopathy in these strictly controlled patients became milder [26, 27]. On fluorescein angiograms especially, the retinopathy looked quiescent in the CSII patients. It is, therefore, possible that studies of much longer duration would show that retinopathy does benefit from good control.

Of the many drugs tried in the amelioration of retinopathy, not one has been shown to have a really striking effect. In a randomized controlled clinical trial of 475 patients, aspirin alone, aspirin together with dipyramidole, and placebo were compared in mild retinopathy in both insulin-treated and non-insulin-treated patients [28]. To evaluate treatment effect, the number of microaneurysms in the macular field of fluorescein angiograms were counted. The results showed that aspirin alone significantly reduced the formation of microaneurysms by about 50% in comparison with the control group. Adding dipyridamole further reduced the number of microaneurysms, but the difference was not significant. The dose of aspirin in this study was 1gm/day, a higher dose than thought to be beneficial in inhibiting platelet aggregation. The Early Treatment of Diabetic Retinopathy Study (ETDRS), a large randomized study, used aspirin in much smaller doses [29]. This study used the relatively insensitive method (when compared with microaneurysm count on fluorescein angiograms) of color photographic grading and retinopathy levels as described by Klein et al [30]. Details of their results are not yet available, but one sentence of the report states that aspirin had no effect [29].

Treatment of sight-threatening retinopathy

For the sight-threatening forms of retinopathy, proliferative retinopathy and diabetic maculopathy, photocoagulation is now the treatment of choice, and this treatment has stood the test of time. The Diabetic Retinopathy Study Group [31] and the British Multicentre Group [32] have both shown that in proliferative retinopathy treatment was significantly better than no treatment. This was particularly so when patients had "high risk characteristics", i.e., new vessels on the disk or within one disk diameter of the disk of more than minimal severity, with or without haemorrhage, or new vessels arising in the retinal periphery associated with vitreous haemorrhage. As a result most centers now treat such patients with the minimum of delay. There is less agreement as to whether new peripheral vessels without haemorrhage should be treated. Many American centers tend to just keep such patients under observation until a complication arises. In the UK the practice is to treat all new vessels as soon as possible, especially when they are forward. Once vitreous haemorrhage is present, treatment can be difficult and is often not very successful. There is also not very good agreement how the patients should be treated. Pan-retinal photocoagulation is the accepted method of treatment for new disk vessels, but the intensity of treatment and the number of burns applied at any one session is not agreed upon (Fig. 6a, b). Generally it is agreed that older patients should be given fewer burns in each session, as these patients are more likely to develop macular oedema as a complication when treatment is too heavy. It is also agreed that treatment should be continued as long as there are active new vessels present. This may mean as many as 5000 or 6000 burns in some patients, although much smaller number usually suffices if the lesions are treated early. In peripheral new vessels it used to be common to treat only the quadrant with the new vessels. Surveying the results of the Hammersmith Hospital, Turner and coworkers [33] found that most patients had wide-spread ischaemia and developed new vessels in other quadrants soon after the initial ones were treated. Pan-retinal photocoagulation is, therefore, advisable even in patients with peripheral new vessels only. In patients who develop new vessels after treatment has been completed need for re-treatment is not common, and visual acuity is maintained over the years.

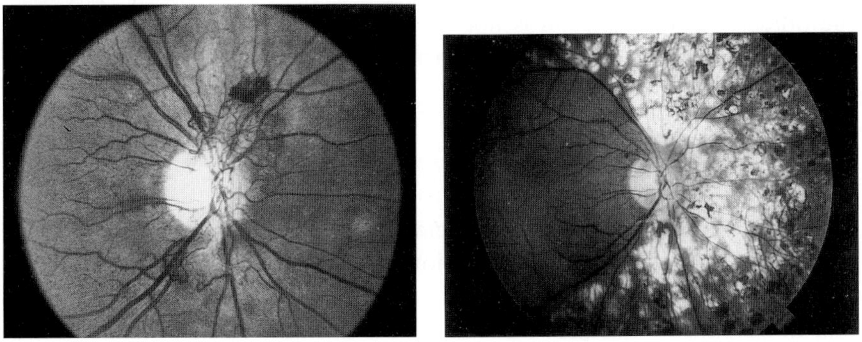

a b

Fig. 6a New vessels arising from the right optic disc before treatment.

Fig. 6b Following panretinal photocoagulation new vessels have gone.

There is less agreement on the treatment of diabetic maculopathy. Focal treatment for hard exudate rings in the perifoveal or even foveal area, treatment of leaky spots on fluorescein angiograms and areas of non-perfusion have been found to be effective by the ETDRS [29]. The problem with diabetic maculopathy is that the ischaemic and oedematous group, the ones starting with impaired vision, do not respond so well. Furthermore, the 10 year follow-up indicates that many patients who had good vision to start with do not maintain this for long periods of follow-up. Thus in the Hammersmith Center out of 113 eyes only 62 were still available for assessment after 10 years. While at entry only 2 eyes with exudative maculopathy had poor vision (6/60 or less), after 5 years 10 out of 37 eyes had poor vision and after 10 years 6 out of 26 eyes had poor vision. At the same time, of the 51 eyes with exudative lesions followed for 10 years, 31 (60%) had good vision (6/12 or better) at entry. 13 of these (50%) of these still had good vision after 10 years. The results were worse in the ischaemic and edematous group. In this group, 17 (30%) eyes had poor vision at entry. Of the 36 followed for 10 years, 44% ended up with 6/60 or worse vision. Only 32 (55%) had good vision at entry; only 6 (16%) of these still had good vision after 10 years. Those who were not followed up mostly died, but some were still alive with severe disabilities.

The problem is that while we can recognize a pre-maculopathy stage in exudative maculopathy when visual acuity is normal and the lesions have developed in the macular field but have not yet reached the edge of the fovea, we can not really recognize such a stage in ischaemic and oedematous patients. In the exudative group early recognition and treatment can stop lesions; in the others early recognition is not possible so that the condition is almost always advanced when we see the patients and treatment is, therefore, always late.

Treatment of advanced diabetic eye disease

Vitrectomy is a relatively new treatment and is used in patients who have severe loss of vision due to the tractional complication of proliferative retinopathy. The techniques of this operation are still being developed and more and more patients not previously treatable can now be helped. In the US, patients are treated relatively early, and even patients with only limited visual loss are offered vitrectomy. In Europe, surgeons are more conservative and only patients with severe visual losses are treated. Although a discussion of the techniques and details of this operation is outside the scope of this chapter, it must be emphasized that this treatment can restore useful vision in patients who are already blind.

Pathogenic mechanisms in the evolution of diabetic retinopathy

The three questions about diabetic retinopathy which have to be answered by any valid theory on the pathogenesis are: 1) why do capillaries close? 2) Why do they become more leaky, and 3) Why do new vessels form?

Capillary closure and leakage

While abnormalities of platelet aggregation are common in diabetes and even more common in those with advanced retinopathy [12], it is now thought, but not yet proven, that the primary defect is in the endothelial lining of the capillaries so that the platelet abnormalities are only secondary to these changes. Damage to the capillary wall is probably caused by the hyperglycemia itself. The most fashionable current theory is that activation of the polyol pathway in the pericytes is probably the most important initiating step. Whether this pathway is also of importance in the endothelial cells is not known. Prolonged hyperglycemia will result in accumulation of sorbitol, and this in itself can damage the pericytes. It is also possible that it is not the elevated sorbitol itself, but some associated phenomenon such as reduced myo-inositol levels or Na/K-ATPase activity which causes the damage. These substances are important for normal neuronal function and their reduced levels are demonstrated by abnormal retinograms which can be corrected by treatment with aldose reductase inhibitors [34]. Early damage to pericytes has been demonstrated by Kador [35] in galactosemic dogs. The loss of the pericytes is followed by focal multiplication of endothelial cells which form microaneurysms. Indeed Kador found that if pericyte loss is inhibited in these dogs by aldose reductase inhibitor, microaneurysm formation does not occur. Recent work by Orlidge and D'Amore suggests that pericytes exert a controlling influence on endothelial cells [36]. In elegant co-culture studies of pericytes with adrenal endothelial cells these workers demonstrated that when there was a direct contact between the two types of cells, pericytes inhibited endothelial cell proliferation. When the cells were separated but exchange of diffusible material was possible, the inhibition did not occur. Other cells did not have this inhibitory effect on endothelial cells; in particular, both pigment epithelial cells and fibroblasts stimulated endothelial cell growth. In further experiments these authors also suggested that the inhibition was due to a stimulation of the activitiy of the endothelial cells' own transforming growth factor β [37]. Even before pericytes are irreversibly damaged, direct contact between them and the endothelial cells may be lost through basement membrane thickening. Basement membrane thickening could result from the polyol pathway activation. As mentioned before, thickening of basement membrane in galactosemic rats can be reduced by aldose reductase inhibitors. Furthermore, using vitreous fluorophotometry in diabetic patients, Cunha-Vaz found breakdown of the blood-retinal barrier to be improved in those patients who were taking aldose reductase inhibitors [38].

While these studies indicate possible causes for the early breakdown of the blood-retinal barrier and the loss of pericytes, it still does not fully explain why endothelial cells are damaged. The most likely cause is the toxic effect of glucose. While endothelial cells have glucose receptors, most of the glucose enters the cells through a facilitated transport of D-glucose. This transport system is affected by Ca^{++} but is unaffected by both Na^{+} and K^{+}. The functioning of this transport system is increased in diabetes, and thus gives rise to high intracellular glucose levels [39]. Lorenzi and coworkers noted that endothelial cells in culture showed reduced replication and increased cell death when glucose levels similar to those seen in diabetes were added to the culture medium [40]. Later work also showed damage to the DNA after 9–14 days exposure to high glucose medium [41]. These workers used umbilical vein endothelium; whether the findings are valid for retinal endothelial cells has yet to be proven.

New vessel formation

In 1948 Michaelson postulated that ischaemic retina produced a vasculogenic factor [42]. Since that time, and especially in the last few years, several angiogenic factors produced by the retina have been isolated, including retina-derived angiogenic factor and retina-derived growth factor [43]. These have been shown to be homologous to acidic and basic fibroblast growth factor (a and b FGF) [44]. Both of these factors stimulate endothelial proliferation in vitro, but bFGF is the more potent [45]. It appears from the coded sequence of the gene of bFGF that there is normally little or no secretion of bFGF by cultured cells [46]. However, bFGF could be a cell-associated angiogenic factor which is only released or activated under circumstances such as ischaemia or cell death. bFGF has been shown to be associated with the extracellular matrix, more specifically, with the heparan sulphate proteoglycan component [47]. bFGF is, of course, not the only growth factor affecting new vessel growth. Insulin-like growth factor-1 (IGF-1), a polypeptide produced by the liver and under the control of growth hormone, is thought to be of importance. One study showed that in the very active proliferative retinopathy of young patients, IGF levels were raised [48], but this study did not correct for age. In a prospective study of pre-proliferative retinopathy patients, Hyer and coworkers [49] showed that in this condition IGF-1 levels were in the normal range. In those patients who developed active new vessels, IGF-1 levels rose transiently (but still stayed in the normal range). Effective treatment of the new vessels resulted in the return of the IGF-1 levels to the pre-proliferative lower level. This suggests at least an association if not a proven causal relationship between proliferative retinopathy and IGF-1 levels. Petty and coworkers identified a plasma factor [50] present in serum from patients with proliferative retinopathy only, which stimulated growth of umbilical vein endothelium. Serum from the same patients did not stimulate bovine retinal endothelial cells [51] suggesting a possible species difference. It is also possible that cells in different parts of the body react differently to the same stimuli.

Stimulation and inhibition of endothelial cells is normally well balanced. A number of substances, vitreous, pigment epithelium, and other growth factors may act as stimulators or as inhibitors, depending on the interaction of these substances. In diabetes the balance between inhibitors and stimulators is upset in favor of the stimulators, resulting in new vessel growth. Although the exact facts are not yet known, we are closer to solving this exciting jigsaw puzzle.

References

[1] Harrold BP. Retinal haemorrhages in diabetes. Brit J Ophthalmol 1971; 55: 225–230.

[2] McLeod D, Marshall J, Kohner EM et al. Pathogenesis of retinal cotton wool spots. Clin Sci and Mol Med 1976; 57: 7–8.

[3] Kohner EM, Dollery CT, Bulpitt C. Cotton wool spots in Diabetic Retinopathy. Diabetes 1969; 16: 691–703.

[4] Cunha-Vaz JG, De Abreau F, Camper AJ et al. Early breakdown of the blood retinal barrier in diabetes. Brit J Ophthalmol 1975; 59: 649–656.

[5] Cunha-Vaz JG, Gray JR, Zeimer RC. Characterisation of early stages of diabetic retinopathy by vitreous fluorophotometry. Diabetes 1985; 34: 53–57.

[6] Krupin T, Waltman SR, Oestrich C et al. Vitreous fluorophotometry in juvenile onset diabetes mellitus. Arch Ophthalmol 1978; 96: 812–814.

[7] White NH, Waltman SR, Krupin T et al. Reversal of abnormalities in ocular fluorophotometry in insulin dependent diabetes after 5–9 months improved metabolic control. Diabetes 1982; 31: 80–85.

[8] Chahal PS, Chowienczyk PJ, Kohner EM. Measurement of blood-retinal barrier permeability: a reproducibility study in normal eyes. Invest Ophthalmol Vis Sci 1985; 26: 977–982.

[9] Krogsaa B, Lund-Anderson H, Mehlsen J et al. The blood-retinal barrier permeability to fluorescein in normal subjects and in juvenile diabetics without retinopathy. Acta Ophthalmol 1986; 64: 173–179.

[10] Roy MS, Bonner RF, Bungay PM. Posterior vitreous fluorophotometry in normal subjects. Arch Ophthalmol 1986; 104: 1004–1007.

[11] Cogan DG, Toussaint D, Kuwabara T. Retinal vascular patterns IV: Diabetic retinopathy. Arch Ophthalmol 1961; 66: 100–112.

[12] Porta M, McCraw A, Kohner EM. Inverse relationship between istocetin cofactor levels and platelet aggregation in insulin dependent diabetics. Thrombosis Research 1982; 25: 507–512.

[13] Harrison HE, Reece AH, Johnson M. Decreased vascular prostacyclin in experimental diabetes. Life Sciences 1978; 23: 351–356.

[14] Almer LO, Pandolfi M, Nilsson IM. Diabetic retinopathy and the fibrinolytic system. Diabetes 1975; 24: 529–534.

[15] Colwell JA. Platelets and diabetic retinopathy. In: Little HL, Jack RL, Patz A et al, eds. Diabetic retinopathy. New York: Thieme Stratton Inc, 1983; 119.

[16] Wallow IHL, Engerman RL. Permeability and Patency of retinal blood vessels in experimental diabetes. Invest Ophthal and Vis Sci 1977; 16: 447–454.

[17] King GL, Berman AB, Bonner-Weir S et al. Regulation of vascular permeability in cell culture. Diabetes 1987; 36: 1460–1467.

[18] Zimmet P, King H, Taylor R et al. The high prevalence of diabetes mellitus impaired glucose tolerance and diabetic retinopathy in Nauru – the 1982 Survey. Diabetes Research 1984; 1: 13–19.

[19] Klein R, Klein BEK, Moss SE et al. The Wisconsin Epidemiology Study of Diabetic Retinopathy. II Prevalence and risk of diabetic retinopathy when age at diagnosis is less than 30 years. Arch Ophthalmol 1984; 102: 520–526.

[20] Klein R, Klein BEK, Moss SE et al. The Wisconsin Epidemiology Study III Prevalence of risk of diabetic retinopathy when age at diagnosis is 30 or more years. Arch Ophthalmol 1984; 102: 527–532.

[21] Kohner EM, Aldington SJ, Nugent Z. United Kingdom Prospective Diabetes Study. Retinopathy at entry in the UK Prospective Diabetes Study. Diabetes 1987; 36 (suppl): 42a

[22] Engerman R, Bloodworth JMB Jr, Nelson S. Relationship of microvascular disease in diabetes to metabolic control. Diabetes 1977; 26: 760–769.

[23] Lauritzen T, Frost-Larsen K, Larsen HW et al. Effect of one year of near normal blood glucose levels on retinopathy in insulin dependent diabetics. Lancet 1983; 1: 200–204.

[24] The Kroc Collaborative Study Group. Blood glucose control and the evaluation of diabetic retinopathy and albuminuria. New Eng J Med 1984; 311: 365–372.

[25] Dahl-Jorgensen K, Brinckmann-Hansen U., Hanssen KF et al. Rapid tightening of blood glucose control leads to transient deterioration of retinopathy in insulin dependent diabetes mellitus. Brit Med J 1985; 290: 811–815.

[26] Dahl-Jorgensen K, Brinckmann-Hansen U, Hanssen KF et al. Effect of near normoglycaemia for 2 years on progression of early diabetic retinopathy, nephropathy and neuropathy: The Oslo study. Brit Med J 1986; 293: 1195–1199.

[27] The Kroc Collaborative Study Group. Diabetic Retinopathy after two years of intensified insulin treatment. JAMA 1988; 260: 37–41.

[28] The DAMAD Study Group. The effect of Aspirin alone and Aspirin-Dipyridamole in early diabetic retinopathy. Diabetes 1989; 38: 491–498.

[29] Early Treatment Diabetic Retinopathy Study Research Group. Photocoagulation for diabetic macular oedema. Arch Ophthalmol 1985; 103: 1796–1806.

[30] Klein BE, Davis MD, Segal P et al. Diabetic Retinopathy: assessment of severity and progression. Ophthalmology 1984; 91: 10–17.

[31] Diabetic Retinopathy Study Research Group. Preliminary report on effects of photocoagulation therapy. Amer J Ophthalmol 1976; 81: 383–397.

[32] British Multicentre Study Group. Photocoagulation for proliferative diabetic retinopathy: a randomised controlled clinical trial using the Xenon Arc. Diabetologia 1984; 26: 109–115.

[33] Turner GS, Ingelsby DV, Shariff B et al. Natural history of peripheral neovascularisation in diabetic retinopathy. Brit J Ophthalmol 1985; 69: 420–424.

[34] MacGregor LC, Matschinsky FM. Treatment with aldose reductase inhibitor or myoinositol arrests deterioration of the electroretinogram of diabetic rats. J Clin Invest 1985; 24: 1250–1258.
[35] Kador PF, Abagi Y, Terubayashi A et al. Prevention of pericyte ghost formation in retinal capillaries of galactose-fed dogs by Aldose Reductase Inhibitors. Invest Ophthalmol Vis Sci 1988; 29 (suppl): 180.
[36] Orlidge A, D'Amore PA. Inhibition of capillary endothelial cell growth by pericytes and smooth muscle cells. J Cell Biol 1987; 105: 1455–1462.
[37] Orlidge A, D'Amore P. Endothelial cell-pericyte coculture produce activated TGF-β which inhibits endothelial growth. Invest Ophthalmol Vis Sci 1988; 29 (suppl): 109.
[38] Cunha-Vaz J, Mota C, Leite E. Effect of Sulindac on the permeability of the blood retinal barrier in early diabetic retinopathy. Arch Ophthalmol 1985; 103: P1307–1311.
[39] Ennis SR, Johnson JE, Pautler EL. In situ kinetics of glucose transport across the blood retinal barrier in normal rats and rats with streptozotocin-induced diabetes. Invest Ophthalmol and Vis Sci 1982; 23: 447–456.
[40] Lorenzi M, Cagliero E, Toledo S. Glucose toxicity for human endothelial cells in culture. Diabetes 1985; 34: 621–627.
[41] Lorenzi M, Montisano DF, Toledo S et al. High glucose induces DNA damage in cultured human endothelial cells. J Clin Invest 1986; 77: 322–325.
[42] Michaelson IC. The mode of development of the retinal vessels and some observations on its significance in certain retinal diseases. Trans Ophthalmol Soc UK 1948; 137: 68–74.
[43] D'Amore P, Klagsburn M. Endothelial cell mitogens derived from retina and hypothalamus: Biochemical and biological similarities. J Cell Biol 1984; 99: 1545–1549.
[44] Baird A, Esch, Gospodarowicz D et al. Retina and eye derived endothelial cell growth factors: partial molecular characterisation and identity with acidic and basic fibroblast growth factor. Biochemistry 1985; 24: 7855–7860.
[45] Gospodarowicz D, Massoglia S, Cheng J et al. Effect of retina derived basic and acidic fibroblast growth factor and lipoproteins on the proliferation of retina derived capillary endothelial cells. Exp Eye Res 1986; 43: 459–476.
[46] Klagsburn M, Sasse J, Sullivan R et al. Human tumour cells synthesise an endothelial cell growth factor that structurally related to basic fibroblast growth factor. Proc Nat Acad Sci USA 1986; 53: 2448–2452.
[47] Baird A, Ling N. Fibroblast growth factors are present in the extracellular matrix produced by endothelial cell In vitro: Implications for a role of Heparinase-like enzymes in the Neovascular response. Biochem Biophys Res Comms 1987; 142: 428–435.
[48] Zapf J, Froesch ER, Humble RE. The insulin-like growth factor (IGF) of human serum: chemical and biological characterisation and aspects of their possible physiological role. Current Top Cell Regul 1981; 19: 257–309.
[49] Hyer SL, Sharp PS, Brooks RA et al. A two year follow up of serum IGF-I in diabetics with retinopathy. Metabolism (In press).
[50] Petty RG, Pearson JD, Morgan DML et al. Stimulation of endothelial cell growth by serum from diabetic patients with retinopathy. Lancet 1988; 30: 208–211.
[51] Kinshuck D, Brooks RA, Kohner EM. Diabetic serum does not affect retinal endothelial cell growth in culture. Current Eye Research (In press).

Neuropathy

D.A. Greene, A.A.F. Sima, M.A. Pfeifer

Introduction

First recognized as a clinical entity more than 200 years ago [1], diabetic neuropathy is now the most common form of peripheral neuropathy in the Western world [2]. Limb-amputation and erectile impotence in diabetic patients are largely attributable to this disorder, which constitutes an unsolved medical problem of enormous proportions. Although originally thought to cause rather than result from the metabolic perturbations of diabetes mellitus by such esteemed scientists as Claude Bernard [3], diabetic neuropathy is now thought to be conditioned by insulin deficiency and/or hyperglycemia, although the specific pathogenetic mechanism(s) that underlie this conditioning effect are not fully understood [4]. Diabetic neuropathy encompasses several distinct syndromes that differ with respect to anatomical distribution of neurological deficit and clinical course. The underlying pathogenetic mechanisms are unknown and remain the object of intense research efforts. Subclinical neuropathy refers to the presence of evidence of impaired nerve function (e. g. slowed nerve conduction velocity, elevated cutaneous sensory thresholds, autonomic dysfunction) in the absence of clinical signs or symptoms consistent with any of the recognized clinical syndromes of diabetic neuropathy. Current therapy for neuropathy is directed firstly at prevention through reduction of putative risk factors such as hyperglycemia, secondly at early diagnosis and prophylaxis to prevent secondary complications such as foot ulceration, and thirdly at palliation of symptoms when they occur. Definitive forms of therapy, targeted against specific underlying pathogenetic mechanisms such as sorbitol pathway activation, nonenzymatic glycation of proteins or microvascular abnormalities, are currently investigative.

Pathogenesis, pathophysiology and pathology

Relationship of clinical and subclinical neuropathy to duration and severity of hyperglycemia

The long-term complications of diabetes including neuropathy are now generally thought to result from the interaction of multiple metabolic, genetic and environmental factors. However, several observations implicate chronic hyperglycemia and/or insulin deficiency as important factors in the causation of diabetic neuropathy [4]. Perhaps Pirart's monumental 25-year prospective study of 4400 unselected patients in a diabetic clinic, plus other less ambitious clinical surveys, provide the most compelling clinical evidence [5]. Clinical neuropathy was present in 12% of patients when diabetes was diagnosed, most commonly in older patients where antecedent undiagnosed hyperglycemia is difficult to exclude (Fig. 1). (Otherwise, clinically detectable diabetic neuropathy is rarely reported within the first five years of diabetes [6].) The cumulative prevalence of neuropathy increased with duration of diabetes independent of age at time of diagnosis of diabetes [7] implying that the development of neuropathy is similar in IDDM and NIDDM (Fig. 2). The similar pattern of neuropathy in IDDM and NIDDM and its occurrence in secondary forms of diabetes (pancreatectomy, non-alcoholic pancreatitis and hemachromatosis) [8], implies that neuropathy is independent of the underlying pathogenetic mechanism of diabetes but instead represents a concomitant or consequence of the diabetic state. The cumulative prevalence of diabetic neuropathy (corrected for duration of diabetes) was higher in patients with chronically poorly controlled diabetes (Fig. 3) [7]; thus the occurrence of diabetic neuropathy correlates with both the duration and severity of insulin deficiency and hyperglycemia [7, 9–11]. Yet, the onset of clinical neuropathy in individual patients is an unpredictable event, neither necessarily reflecting concurrent metabolic control [12] nor following inexorably from prolonged and severe hyperglycemia [7], probably due in part to the indolent and occult nature of the underlying subclinical nerve damage, and/or the presence of other independent pathogenetic variables such as genetic, nutritional, toxic (e. g. alcohol) [13] and mechanical (entrapment and compression) [5, 10].

The link between metabolism and early sub-clinical neuropathy is more well established. For example, the modest slowing of nerve conduction in newly diagnosed IDDM fluctuates with metabolic control, suggesting an initial reversible metabolic contribution to conduction slowing, which is also noted in diabetic animals [14, 15]. The initial improvement in conduction

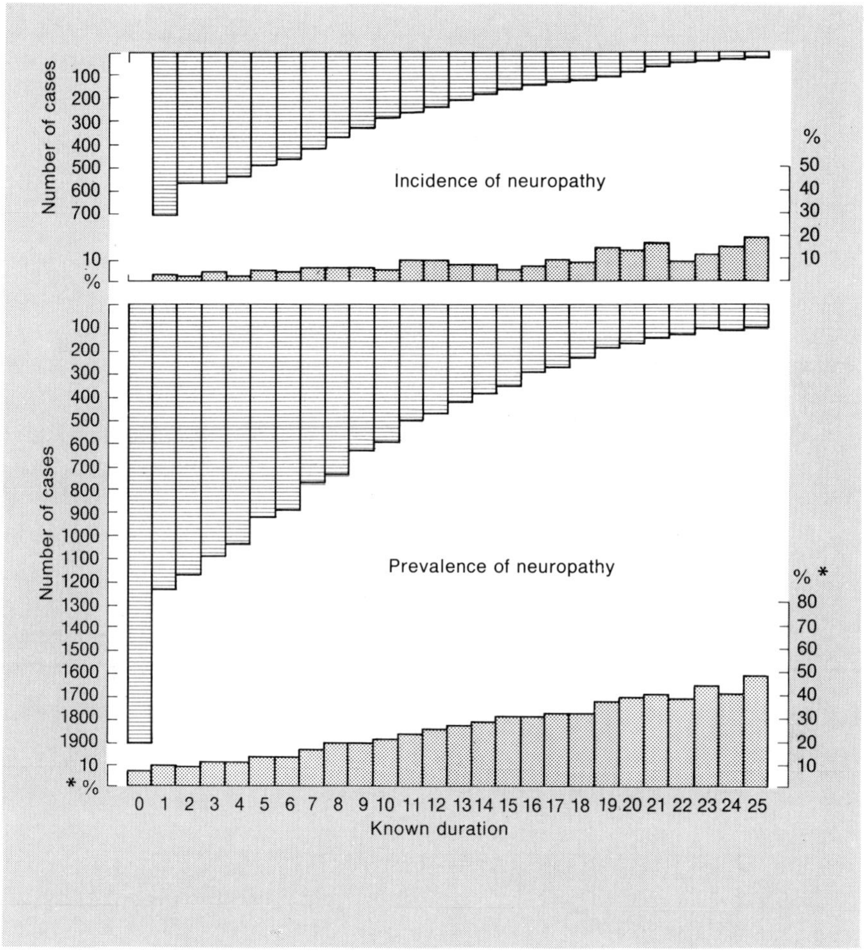

Fig. 1 Increase of annual incidence and prevalence of neuropathy as a function of the known duration of diabetes. The suspended columns show the decrease in the number of subjects over time. This histogram represents the data drawn from the inception cohort (i.e. patients seen from onset of their diabetes) [7].

velocity in response to metabolic intervention parallels improved vibratory perception threshold implying physiological significance [16]. Nerve conduction velocity is inversely correlated with HbA_{1c} [17] and improves slightly but proportionately with HbA_{1c} level in response to conventional metabolic therapy in chronic stable NIDDM [18]. Similarly, intensive treatment statistically significantly improves peripheral nerve conduction in IDDM, but again only slightly [19–22] (however, as discussed below, this may reflect the

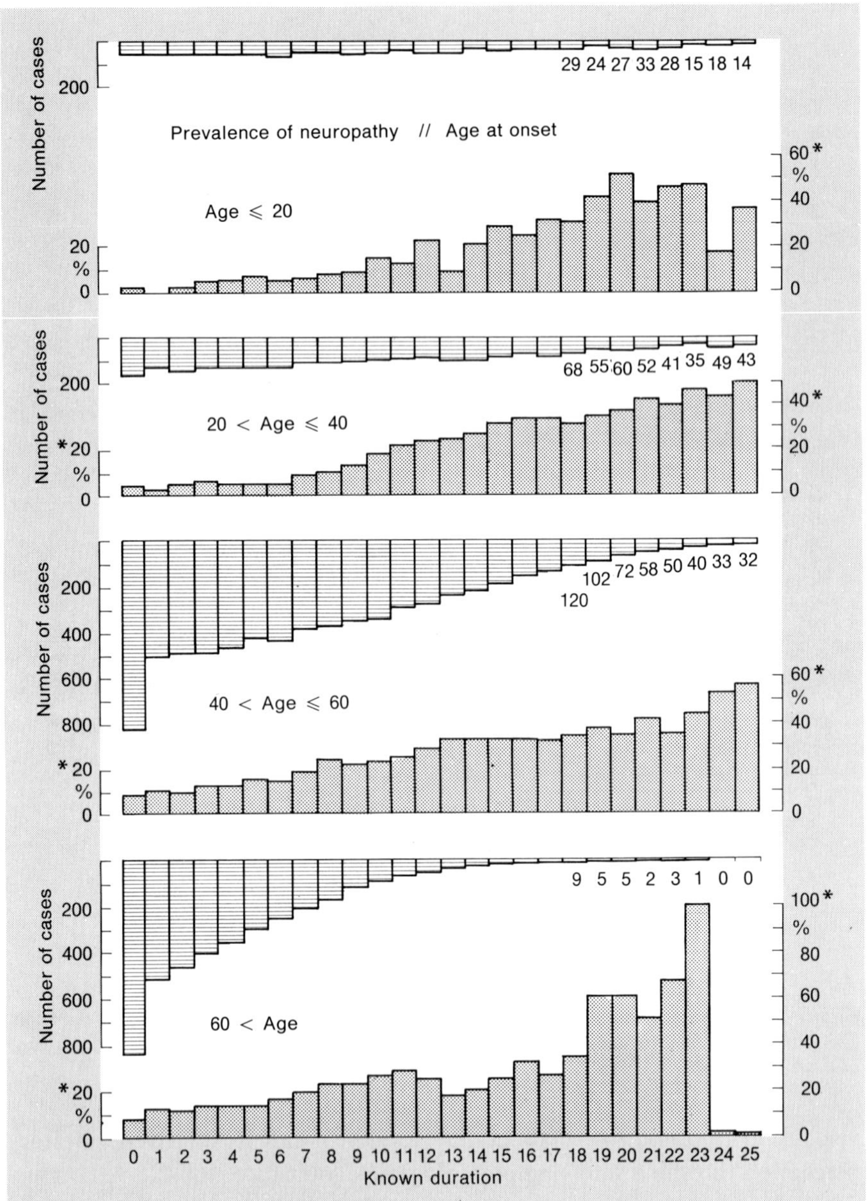

*Fig. 2 Increasing prevalence of neuropathy as a function of the known duration of diabetes in four age groups at the onset of diabetes. If the two below-40 categories are grouped together and compared with the two over-40 grouped together, the differences in prevalence relate to the first nine years, the "young" group being affected later than the "old" group. Statistical significance is given by the starred symbols: *p<0.05, **p<0.01, ***p<0.001 [7].*

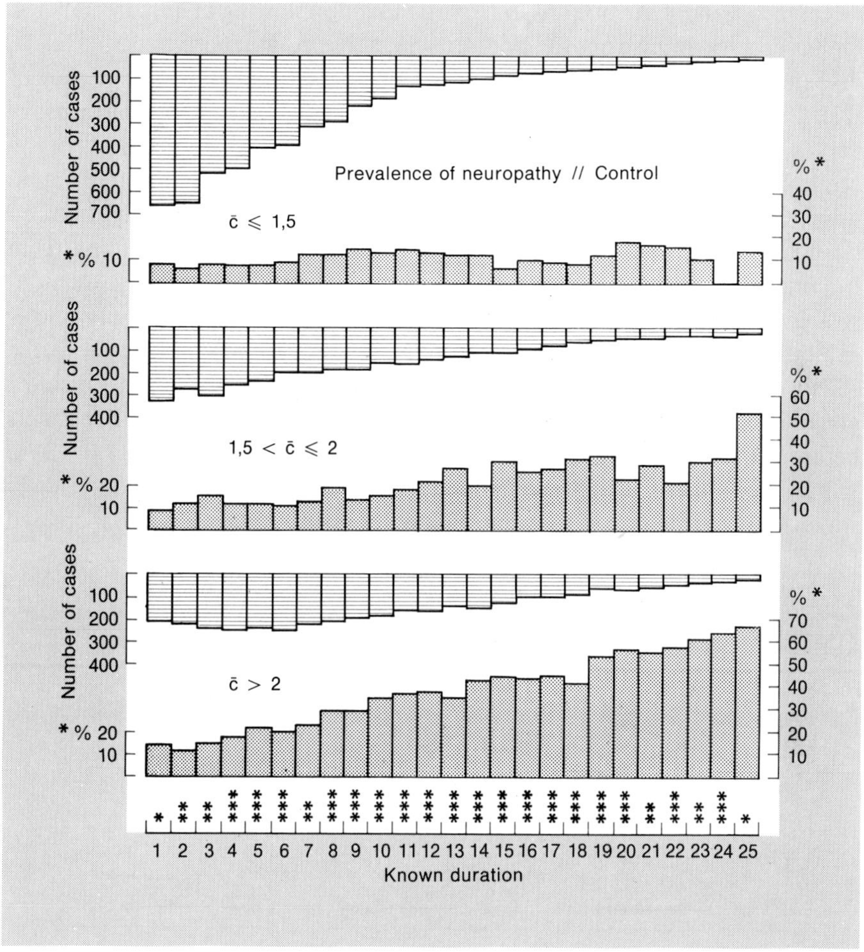

Fig. 3 Increasing prevalence of neuropathy as a function of the known duration of diabetes compared in three groups with various degrees of cumulative glycemic control from good (top) to poor (bottom) (statistical significance, see figure 2). Although the rate of neuropathy remains fairly constant in the "good" control group, it rises with a steep curve for the "poor" control group. Symbols of degree of cumulative glycemic control: C<1.5 = rather good; 1.5<C<2 = fair; C>2 = poor [7].

presence of poorly reversible structural lesions that set an upper limit to nerve conduction in established diabetes). Although these observations suggest a direct metabolic component to conduction slowing even in established diabetes, the time course of the response, extending over several weeks to months, does not completely exclude a significant contribution from structural repair. Acute effects of blood glucose normalization on nerve conduction suggest direct metabolic contributions to nerve conduction slowing in human diabetes. Gallai et al examined motor and sensory nerve conduction velocities in 16 diabetic patients, half with neuropathy, during 3 days of Biostator treatment [23]. Conduction velocity was improved in peroneal, tibial and median sensory nerves but only in patients with neuropathy. Service et al studied 8 hyperglycemic IDDMs before and after 72 hours of Biostator regulation and found improvement in ulnar sensory conduction velocity (+ 3.2 ± 1.4 m/s) but no change in 24 other electrophysiological parameters measured, leading them to conclude that no consistent improvement in nerve function was demonstrable [24]. Troni et al. [25] studied H-reflex conduction velocity, a parameter exhibiting less day-to-day variation than standard nerve conduction, in the soleus muscle in 10 young short-duration IDDMs during 2 days of Biostator glucoregulation. H-reflex conduction velocity was reduced in all patients before Biostator regulation, and increased in all 10 patients from 1.0 – 3 – 0 m/s by 48 hours of Biostator treatment (Fig. 4). H-reflex conduction velocity was acutely normalized in only one patient. H-reflex conduction also increased

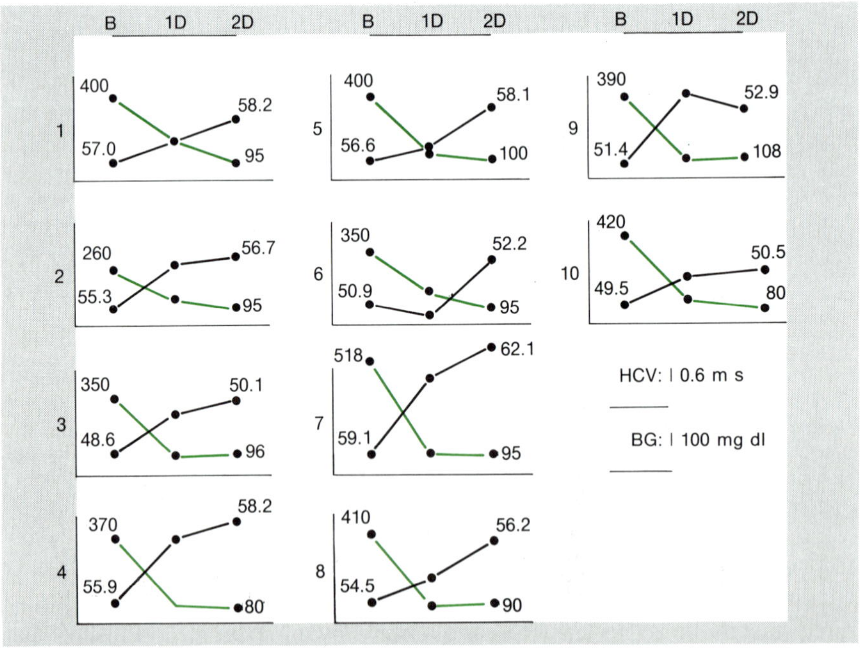

Fig. 4 Changes in mean conduction velocity over the H reflex pathway (n-HCV) and blood glucose during artificial endocrine pancreas treatment in individual patients. B, baseline; D, determination; BG, blood glucose [25].

progressively over 6 months of intensive insulin therapy in 12 other IDDM subjects, with the greatest improvement occurring within the first week; the increase correlated closely with improvement in HbA_{1c}. These observations would strongly suggest that a component of nerve conduction slowing in diabetic patients is rapidly reversible with metabolic therapy, and therefore probably reflects a direct biochemical or biophysical contribution related to metabolic factors rather than structural abnormalities. Although conduction slowing is usually more pronounced in diabetic patients with clinically overt neuropathy, the predictive value of conduction impairment for either the subsequent development or clinical course of diabetic neuropathy has not been established [26]. Therefore, these promising observations that metabolic intervention improves nerve conduction in diabetic patients do not necesarily imply that such treatment will prevent or ameliorate the subsequent development of diabetic neuropathy.

The presumed conditioning role of insulin deficiency and/or hyperglycemia in the pathogenesis of diabetic neuropathy has prompted a broad search for possible underlying mechanism(s) by which these metabolic derangements might selectively destroy elements of the peripheral nervous system. Any generally pathogenetic scheme invoking hyperglycemia and/or insulin deficiency must address the generally positive but variable relationship between metabolic control and the development and progression of clinical neuropathy, the wide clinical spectrum of the disease, the nature of the biochemical defects in peripheral nerve associated with diabetes, and the multiple cell types that appear to be involved in diabetic neuropathy. There are several well-explored metabolic abnormalities in diabetic nerve that result from hyperglycemia [27] and are therefore potential initiating [28] or contributing factors [29] in the pathogenesis of diabetic neuropathy. These abnormalities may occur in several of the cellular constituents of peripheral nerve and its supporting tissues, and may thereby partially account for some of the variability of clinical neuropathy in various subgroups and individual patients with diabets. Metabolic alternations in diabetic nerve that might potentially contribute to the pathogenesis of diabetic neuropathy have been identified primarily through the study of diabetic animals or of nerve tissue or cells in vitro. These studies have led to the generation of four current "metabolic hypotheses" for the pathogenesis of diabetic neuropathy: the sorbitol-accumulation-*myo*-inositol-depletion hypothesis, the hypoxia/ischemia hypothesis, the nonenzymatic glycation hypothesis, and the insulin-neurotrophism hypothesis. It is quite likely that several or all of these mechanisms may be involved in the pathogenesis of diabetic neuropathy at some stage in its development and natural history.

Sorbitol accumulation/myo-inositol depletion hypothesis

The acute and rapidly-reversible slowing of nerve conduction in rapidly-conducting myelinated nerve fibers in acutely diabetic laboratory animals has been attributed to a set of interrelated metabolic abnormalities in diabetic peripheral nerve, resulting from hyperglycemia and involving sorbitol, *myo*-inositol and (Na,K)-ATPase regulation [27]. This conclusion is based on the parallel responses of nerve *myo*-inositol content, (Na,K)-ATPase activity and motor nerve conduction velocity to specific metabolic interventions such as insulin deficiency and insulin replacement, aldose reductase inhibition and dietary *myo*-inositol supplementation in the acutely streptozocin- and spontaneously-diabetic rat (Table 1) [27, 30–32]. Increased metabolism of glucose

Table 1 Parallel responses of rat nerve myo-inositol (MI) content, sodium-potassium ATPase activity, and motor nerve conduction velocity (MNCV) to hyperglycemia and metabolic intervention (from [27])

	Plasma glucose (mg/dl)	Plasma MI (μM)	Nerve MI (mmol/kg)	MNCV (m/s)	Nerve sodium-potassium ATPase (mmol/kg/h)
Nondiabetic	178 ± 7	35 ± 2	3.0 ± 0.2	62 ± 1	97 ± 5
Diabetic	566 ± 30	35 ± 3	2.2 ± 0.1	51 ± 1	55 ± 3
Diabetic + insulin	75 ± 18	30 ± 2	3.0 ± 0.2	63 ± 1	120 ± 7*
Diabetic + MI	600 ± 32	245 ± 27	3.9 ± 0.2	61 ± 1	88 ± 4
Diabetic + sorbinil	623 ± 25	30 ± 3	3.1 ± 0.1	–	96 ± 5

Diabetes leads to, and insulin therapy prevents, a reduction in nerve MI content, MNCV, and sodium-potassium ATPase activity. These changes are also prevented by treatment with aldose reductase inhibitors (e.g., sorbinil), which inhibit the increase in polyol pathway activation in diabetic nerve and, hence, in accumulation of nerve sorbitol and fructose. Dietary MI supplementation is however sufficient to normalize nerve MI, MNCV, and sodium-potassium ATPase in face of persistent hyperglycemia and elevated nerve glucose, sorbitol, and fructose. Hence, changes in diabetic nerve MI metabolism appear central to pathogenesis of the defects in MNCV and nerve sodium-potassium ATPase.

* Data compiled from the streptozocin-diabetic rat and older insulin-replaced spontaneously diabetic BB-Wistar rats whose controls have higher nerve sodium-potassium ATPase activity (117 + 10)

to sorbitol by the enzyme aldose reductase is thought to produce a loss of free *myo*-inositol from some component of peripheral nerve, which in turn is thought to limit the synthesis of inositol-containing membrane phosphoinositides, whose importance in membrane function including (Na,K)-ATPase regulation is becoming increasingly appreciated [27]. (In vitro studies have ascribed diminished utilization of ATP equivalents by an impaired (Na,K)-ATPase in *myo*-inositol-depleted diabetic nerve as the basis for its decreased respiratory activity [33 – 36].) In the acutely diabetic animal, these metabolic abnormalities are closely interrelated: aldose reductase inhibitors prevent not only the accumulation of sorbitol but also the decline in *myo*-inositol, (Na,K)-ATPase activity and nerve conduction velocity, while administration of *myo*-inositol, which does not prevent sorbitol accumulation but does prevent *myo*-inositol depletion, also prevents the reductions in (Na,K)-ATPase activity and nerve conduction in acutely diabetic animals [27]. Reduced availability of diacylglycerol, a phosphoinositide metabolite that activates protein kinase C, an important membrane-bound protein kinase, may be involved in the (Na,K)-ATPase defect in diabetic peripheral nerve, thus providing a biochemical link between *myo*-inositol metabolism and (Na,K)-ATPase regulation [35]. With more prolonged diabetes, and the development of secondary or tertiary structural abnormalities [37], the close parallelism between sorbitol accumulation, *myo*-inositol depletion and the fall in (Na,K)-ATPase activity and conduction velocity do not persist in all instances [38, 39], either due to the development of marked changes in the architecture of the nerve of the superimposition or additional pathogenetic elements or compensatory mechanisms. However, the acute biochemical alterations combined with carefully conducted nodal voltage clamp studies on large myelinated axons support the contention that the rapidly reversible slowing of nerve conduction in acutely diabetic animals is mediated by a specific sequence of biochemical events linking nerve *myo*-inositol content to the function of the (Na,K)-ATPase which, in the axon, develops the sodium gradient necessary for nerve depolarization [32, 37, 40]. This defect results in a 4-fold increase in intra-axonal sodium, sodium-inactivation of voltage-dependent sodium channels, and a selective conduction block in the largest fibers, thereby slowing composite conduction [32]. These early metabolic and functional defects are associated with subtle structural changes involving the node of Ranvier that resemble those of early human diabetic neuropathy [37]. Paranodal swelling occurs within 3 weeks of the onset of diabetes in the spontaneously diabetic BB-Wistar rat, is association with the 4-fold elevation of intraaxonal sodium concentration revealed by voltage clamp studies, and is rapidly reversed by insulin replacement [37], aldose reductase inhibitors or *myo*-inositol supplementation [41]. Prolonged paranodal swelling leads to loss of the junctional complexes that normally anchor terminal myelin loops to the axolemma (Fig. 5) [37], in association with an irreversible decrease in nodal sodium permeability consistent with loss of nodal sodium channels, perhaps by their lateral migration away from the node and into the internodal axolemma [37];

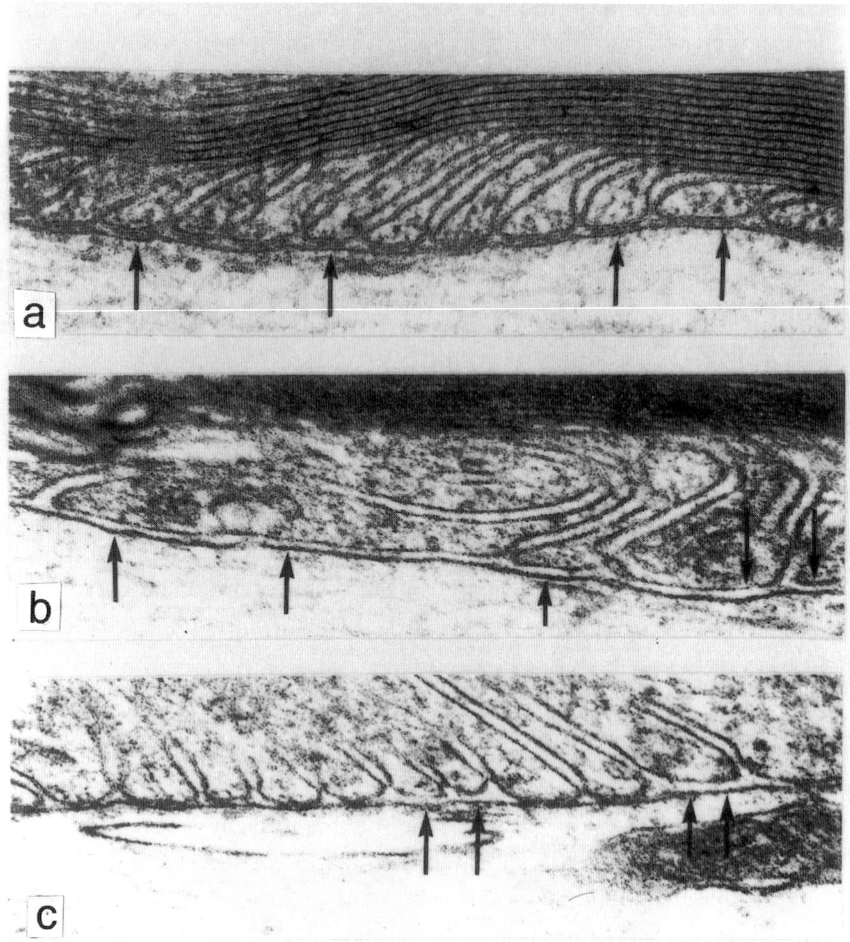

Fig. 5 Effect of spontaneous diabetes and insulin replacement on axo-glial junctional complexes in paranodal terminal myelin loops of large myelinated axons from the sural nerve. Electromicrographs compare terminal myelin loops from a nondiabetic control (a), an insulin-deficient diabetic (b), and an insulin-replaced diabetic (c). Regular junctional complexes between the axolemma and the terminal myelin loops are readily apparent in (a) (arrows), virtually absent in (b), and present in reduced number in (c) [37].

this loss accounts for the component of nerve conduction slowing *not* rapidly reversed by insulin replacement in diabetic rats [37]. Axo-glial dysjunction and paranodal swelling have recently been described in sural nerve biopsies from patients with diabetic neuropathy [42] suggesting that this metabolic, functional and structural sequence observed in the diabetic rat is reproduced in human diabetic neuropathy. In summary, hyperglycemia is known to alter nerve metabolism in several ways. Increased polyol (sorbitol) pathway activity reduces nerve *myo*-inositol content, alters nerve phosphoinositide metabolism and impairs (Na,K)-ATPase activity, further reducing sodium-gradient dependent *myo*-inositol uptake and thereby initiating a self-reinforcing cycle (Fig. 6, right). The impairment of the electrogenic (Na,K)-ATPase secondarily and acutely reduces nerve conduction velocity [32, 37, 40], while probably also inhibiting other sodium-gradient dependent processes such as amino acid uptake [43] and intracellular water homeostasis, leading to paranodal swelling, axo-glial dysjunction, paranodal demyelination and perhaps fiber loss (Fig. 6, left). Other membrane defects may also occur as a consequence of altered

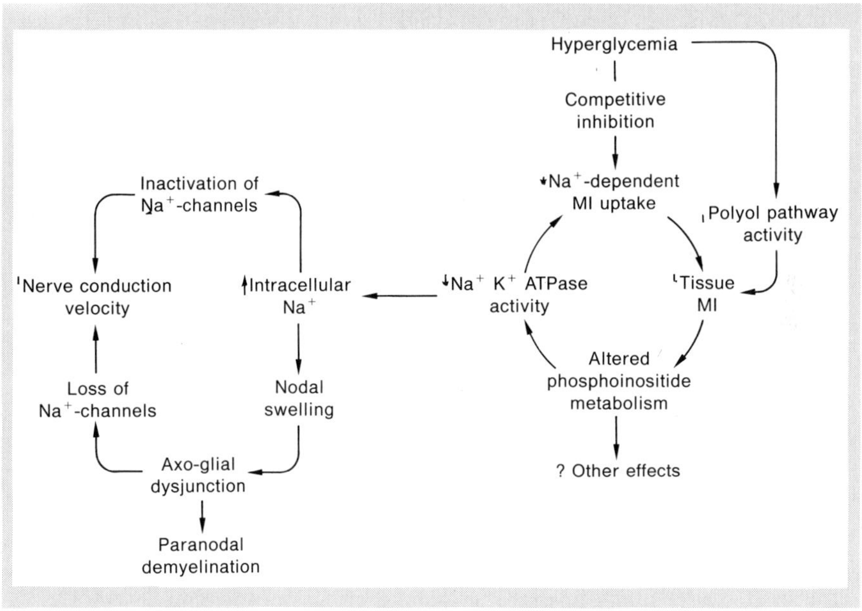

Fig. 6 Postulated relationship between hyperglycemia, polyol pathway, myo-inositol (MI) Na^+/K^+-ATPase, and nerve conduction in diabetes. Hyperglycemia reduces nerve MI by competitively inhibiting its uptake and by an indirect and yet unexplained mechanism related to the increased conversion of glucose to sorbitol by the enzyme aldose reductase. The reduction in nerve MI leads to a decrease in Na^+/K^+-ATPase activity, possibly through an alteration in phosphoinositide metabolism. Since MI uptake in nerve is sodium dependent, a self-reinforcing metabolic cycle involving MI is likely. Acute reduction in nerve conduction velocity in diabetes is ascribed in part to impaired Na^+/K^+-ATPase activity. A further consequence of impaired Na^+/K^+-ATPase activity is a reduction in sodium-dependent amino acid uptake; interference with other sodium-linked processes is probable but as yet unproved. Defects resulting from reduced nerve MI levels other than those mediated by changes in Na^+/K^+-ATPase await further investigation.

inositol phospholipid metabolism, independent of the (Na,K)-ATPase, possibly mediated either by the intracellular calcium-mobilizing action of inositol-1,4,5-triphosphate [44] or the protein kinase C activating capacity of diacylglycerol [45]. While these alterations have been reasonable well characterized in acutely diabetic animals, the extent to which these linked metabolic defects play a role in chronic experimental or human diabetic neuropathy remains to be explored.

Hypoxia/ischemia hypothesis

Vascular as well as metabolic factors have been invoked to explain the structural lesions of human diabetic neuropathy. Both clinical and histopathological features of the rare focal syndromes of diabetic neuropathy (mononeuropathy and mononeuropathy multiplex, cranial neuropathy, lumbosacral plexopathy, radiculopathy) sugggest an acute ischemic element [46]. For instance, admittedly fragmentary but somewhat compelling evidence suggests that focal femoral and cranial neuropathies reflect ischemic injury to diabetic nerve as a result of vascular pathology in susceptible "water-shed" perfusion regions [46]. Endoneurial vascular abnormalities such as basement membrane thickening and reduplication, endothelial cell swelling and proliferation, and platelet aggregation resulting in vessel occlusion have been noted in sural nerve biopsies [47, 48] and at autopsy [2, 49 – 52] in diabetic distal symmetric polyneuropathy. Moreover, the spatially heterogeneous degeneration and loss of distal portions of large and small myelinated nerve fibers that characterized the distal symmetric form of diabetic neuropathy in both man and animals [2, 50, 53 – 60] is accompanied by endoneurial vascular abnormalities [2, 49, 50] and proximal focal lesions resembling those attributed to non-diabetic vascular insufficiency [2, 47, 50] (Fig. 7). A quantitative increase in these vascular abnormalities in association with focal loss of myelinated fibers in older diabetic subjects has been interpreted to suggest hypoxic or ischemic damage to nerve fibers in diabetic distal symmetric polyneuropathy [2, 47, 48]. The possible involvement of microvascular abnormalities in the pathogenesis of diabetic neuropathy is further supported by animal studies indicating faulty regulation of the microcirculation and oxygen delivery in diabetic peripheral nerve by Low and coworkers [61].

Sciatic nerve of chronically diabetic streptozotocin-treated rats exhibit an apparent 30% reduction in blood flow, a near-doubling of vascular resistence, and a significant reduction in the range of measured oxygen tension, all attributed to either rheological and/or microvascular alterations within the vaso nervorum [62]. A concurrent reduction in creatine phosphate energy

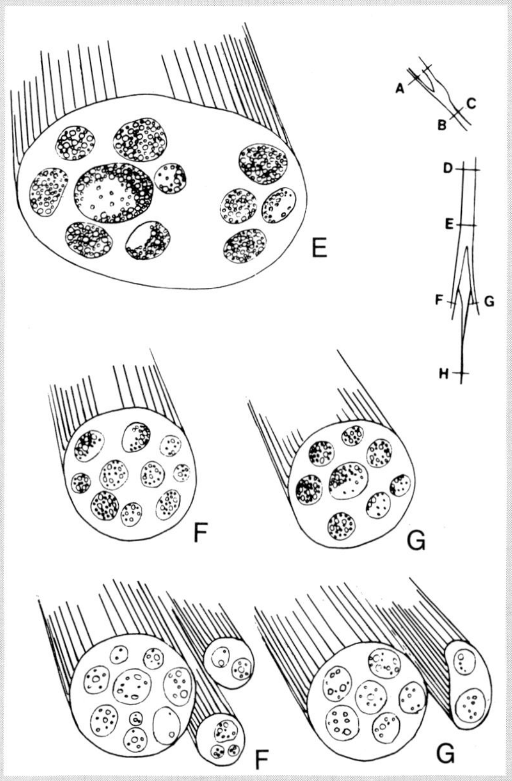

Fig. 7 A line drawing of the spatial distribution of myelinated fiber loss in diabetic polyneuropathy. Multifocal fiber loss begins in the sciatic nerve. At more distal levels (proximal tibial (F) and peroneal (G) nerves), there is greater fiber loss than at the distal sciatic nerve (E), and new multifocal regions of damage are seen. At more distal levels of tibial and peroneal nerves, even greater fiber loss is seen, but it is not possible to identify new multifocal regions of fiber damage. These changes are in keeping with multifocal ischemic injury along the length of nerves [50].

stores and an increase in tissue lactate is consistent with endoneurial hypoxia, and a partially compensatory switch to non-oxidative glycolytic metabolism [63]. However, in vitro studies by Greene and Winegrad using defined nerve preparations from acutely diabetic rabbits had previously demonstrated that reduced creatine phosphate levels and increased lactate concentrations in diabetic nerve persisted during in vitro incubation in 95% oxygen [64].

Furthermore, these studies found that the reduction in creatine phosphate concentration was not due to a change in the "energy charge" of the creatine phosphate energy storage system (i.e. the ratio of creatine phosphate to creatine), but rather represented a net loss of total creatine from the tissue [64]. In addition, the increased lactate production was acutely corrected by insulin in vitro, suggesting that this represented a metabolic effect of insulin deficiency rather than hypoxia [64]. The interpretation of accompanying indirect in situ observations by Low [61] said to indicate that diabetic nerve energy consumption was increased rather than decreased (as suggested by in vitro studies of Greene and Winegrad [64] in support of their conclusion that (Na,K)-ATPase activity is diminished) are subject to alternative interpretations [65]. Low has also demonstrated that exposure of normal rats to chronic hypoxia slows conduction velocity in the specialized caudal nerve [66, 67] and that exposure of normal or chronically diabetic rats to hyperbaric oxygen produces produces numerous metabolic and functional changes in the peripheral nervous system, some of which may be interpreted as a selective partial reversal of some of the elements produced by the diabetic state

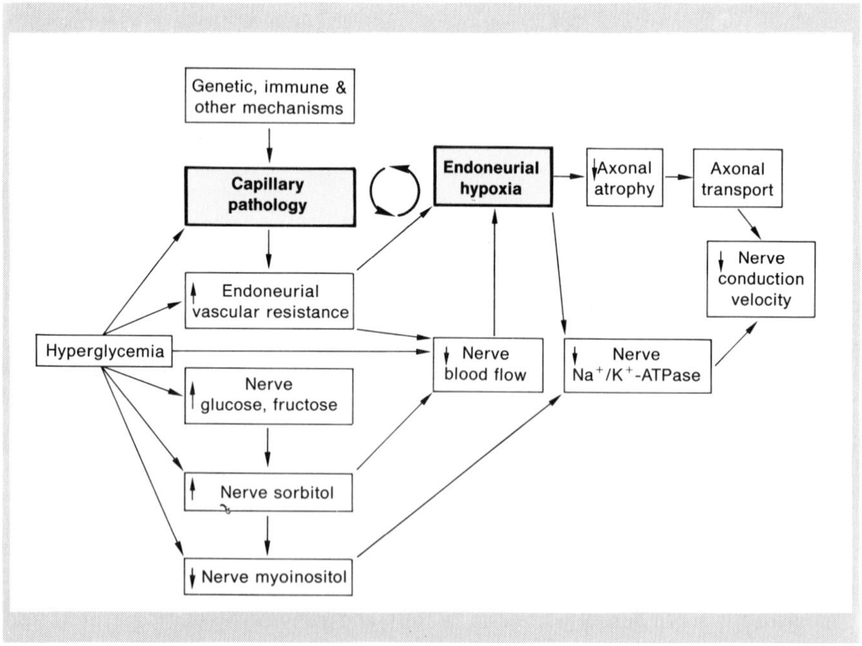

Fig. 8 Suggested pathogenesis of diabetic neuropathy [61].

[68 – 70]. Newrick and colleagues [71] extended these observations to human diabetic neuropathy, wherein they directly measured pO^2 and the tissue-to-venous oxygen gradient in sural nerves in 11 neuropathic diabetics, and 3 non-diabetic individuals and 1 newly-diagnosed non-neuropathic diabetic. The pO_2 was diminished in the neuropathic diabetics, and the oxygen gradient between the sural nerve and blood obtained from the dorsal foot vein was reversed in the neuropathic diabetics (i. e. lower than venous blood) [71]. The subjects were not age-matched, and some of the gradient reversal may represent increased peripheral arterial-venous shunting in the lower extremities of patients with advanced diabetic neuropathy. These exciting and provocative observations suggest that endoneurial hypoxia probably occurs in chronic advanced human diabetic neuropathy, but whether this is a cause or effect of the neuropathy remains unknown (for instance, nerve fibrosis was so severe in 1 of the neuropathic patients that the oxygen electrode could not gain access to the nerve). The ischemia/hypoxia hypothesis, and its possible relationship to other pathogenetic mechanisms is summarized in Figure 8.

Non-enzymatic glycation hypothesis

An additional metabolic abnormality in diabetic nerve is nonenzymatic protein glycosylation, which occurs in a variety of tissue proteins as a result of increased ambient glucose concentration and in some instances protein function is secondarily altered. Peripheral nerve protein glycosylation is increased by acute experimental diabetes [72]. Although glycosylated nerve protein(s) have not been identified, and their function remains unknown, their possible role in the functional and/or structural alterations in diabetic peripheral nerve has not yet been critically examined. Of significant interest is the discovery that brain tubulin may be nonenzymatically glycosylated in vitro and in vivo, with dramatic alteration in its self-assembly and solubility characteristics [73]. Glycosylation of peripheral nerve tubulin might well have important consequences on both fast and slow axonal transport, and on the physical characteristics of the axon cylinder.

Insulin/neurotrophism/axonal-transport hypothesis

A variety of neurotrophic factors are necessary for normal growth and development, maintenance, and regeneration and repair of the nervous system. An impaired maturation of peripheral nerves has been suggested by Thomas and Sharma [74, 75] as an explanation of decreased myelinated fiber size and hence decreased nerve conduction velocity. These investigators have argued that the decreased body weight in streptozotocin diabetic rats would imply an impaired maturation and growth of peripheral nerves. This explanation is unlikely, since metabolic interventions in acute streptozotocin diabetes in rats with either vigorous insulin treatment, *myo*-inositol supplementation or treatment with aldose-reductase inhibitors correct the nerve conduction, whereas *myo*-inositol and aldose reductase inhibitors do not correct the weight deficit. Jacobsen [76] compared streptozotocin diabetic rats with calorie-restricted weight-matched controls but found no comparable decrease in myelinated fiber size, excluding body weight and/or size as a factor in diminished myelinated fiber size of the streptozotocin diabetic rat [76]. Yet, in advanced diabetes in rodents the dominant structural change consists of axonal atrophy and degeneration. Axonal atrophy in streptozotocin-diabetic rats, BB-rats and in the db/db mouse [54, 55, 76–79] appears to progress to a point at which the proximal axon can no longer sustain its distal portion, resulting in Wallerian degeneration [54, 80], but retains its regenerative potential [54]. The mechanism(s) underlying the characteristic axonal atrophy in experimental diabetes is not well understood, and most likely involves several factors such as decreased protein synthesis in the cell soma [81, 82], decreased axonal transport of structural proteins [83–85], as well as a continuous sequestration of axoplasm by the Schwann cell [54, 86, 87], some or all of which could reflect decreased neuronotrophism or neuronotropism. In this regard, altered axonal transport has been invoked in the pathogenesis of diabetic peripheral neuropathy [83–85]. The antegrade fast component (17mm/hr) of axonal transport is responsible for the transport of smooth endoplasmic reticulum, glycoproteins and various enzymes. Antegrade fast axonal transport is probably uneffected by diabetes mellitus [88]. The slow transport of endogenous enzymes such as choline acetyltransferase and acetylcholinesterase is decreased in experimental diabetes [89–91]. Cytoskeletal neurofilaments are transported by the slow component-a (1 mm/day), whereas microfilaments, such as actin, and enolase and calmodulin are transported by the slow component-b of antegrade transport. Slow antegrade transport is slowed 10%–20% in both sensory and motor fibers of the streptozotocin diabetic rat [83, 84]. Structural proteins such as neurofilaments and microtubules are retained in the proximal segments of the axon, which is increased in size, whereas fewer structural proteins reach the distal axon which is reduced in size, and may hence account for the typical axonal atrophy of experimental diabetes [85]. Abnormalities in the transport of structural proteins have been reported in streptozotocin diabetic rats [84, 85], alloxan diabetic rats [89], the spontaneously diabetic BB-rat and db/db mouse [92] and may contribute to non-alignment of neurofilaments in diabetic nerve [54]. Retrograde fast axonal transport (10 mm/hr) is thought to transport material from the distal axon back to the perikaryon for "recycling" and to transport trophic factors and hormones from the periphery to the cell body. Retrograde transport of exogenous nerve growth factor to the dorsal root and superior mesenteric ganglia was decreased in streptozotocin-diabetic rats [93, 94]. Moreover, a variety of neuronotrophic peptides, including nerve growth factor [95, 96], enhance phosphoinositide turnover in neural tissue [97]. Thus, nerve growth factor accessability and action might be diminished in the peripheral nervous system in diabetes due to defective transport [93, 94] and post-receptor signal tranduction [95. 96]. The neurite-promoting effects of insulin and insulin-like growth factors, both increasingly recognized as neuronotrophic agonists, can be duplicated by protein kinase C agonists, suggesting that they too are mediated by the phosphoinositide cascade [98]. Thus, insulin deficiency might impair neuronotrophism by diminishing the availability of and sensitivity to multiple neuronotrophic agonists in the peripheral nervous system, whose action are required not only for a regenerative response to injury, but also for maintenance of the integrity of peripheral nerve axons and Schwann cells. Observations consistent with diminished neurotrophism have been reported in experimental diabetes, including delayed regeneration after nerve transection [99]. One expression of this diminished neuronotrophic tone might well be impaired synthesis and centrifugal transport of axon-specific proteins by slow axonal transport. Additional factors, such as alterations in the endoneurial microenvironment, ischemia etc. might also blunt the ability of the peripheral nervous system to mount a regenerative response to injury in diabetes. Support for a metabolically-mediated impairment of neuronotrophism in human diabetic neuropathy was recently reported from studies of human sural nerve biopsies from patients with diabetic neuropathy following one year of treatment with an aldose reductase inhibitor [100]. A brisk regenerative response yielding a significant increase in fiber number combined with repair of damaged fibers and diminished axonal atrophy resulted from metabolic therapy directed against a specific consequence of hyperglycemia. The denervation produced by fiber loss in diabetic neuropathy should promote the release of neurotrophic factors leading to neurite formation [98], possibly via increased levels of alpha- or beta-tubulin mRNA [98]. Defective phosphoinositide-mediated signalling at the plasma or nuclear membrane might interfere with this sequence either within the dennervated peripheral tissue, at some intermediary site, or at the level of the responding neural tissue in the spinal cord or peripheral nerve. The possibility that glucose-induced *myo*-inositol depletion and diminished insulin and/or insulin-like growth factor synthesis, release or action in diabetes might interact synergistically at the level of agonist-mediated phosphoinositide turnover and generation of second messengers in the peripheral nervous system is worthy of detailed exploration. This hypothetical scheme is illustrated in Figure 9.

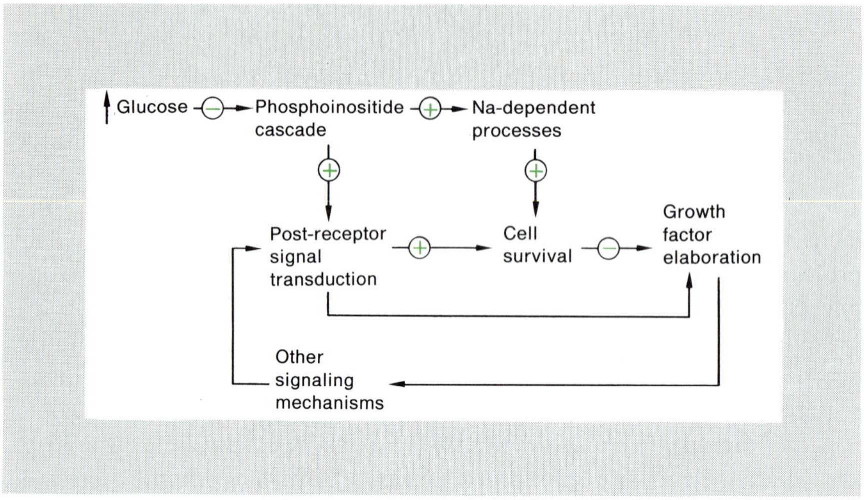

Fig. 9 Self-explanatory.

Histopathology of diabetic neuropathy

Diabetic neuropathy is comprised of several different clinical syndromes (see below) that differ not only in their clinical characteristics, but also in their underlying pathology.

Distal symmetric polyneuropathy

Distal symmetric sensorimotor polyneuropathy is both the most common and also the most pathologically well-studied variant of diabetic neuropathy. While demonstrating that most elements of peripheral nerve are ultimately involved in the disease process, studies of human diabetic distal symmetric polyneuropathy provide no unique pathognomic histopathological lesion, and no conclusive evidence as to the cellular location of the inciting pathogenetic events. The most characteristic pathological finding in diabetic distal symmetric peripheral polyneuropathy is a quantitative reduction in the number of myelinated fibers per unit cross-sectional area of nerve combined with an increased frequency of abnormal nerve fibers whose characteristics suggest a primary but not necessarily specific form of axonal injury [101]. Although this fiber loss exhibits some spatial heterogeneity and accompanies various local structural abnormalities of endoneurial microvessels and connective tissue, the pathogenetic significance of these accompanying lesions in the loss and damage of nerve fibers is unclear, and may differ as a function of type of diabetes and stage of neuropathy. Axons, Schwann cells, perineurial cells and endoneurial vascular elements have all been invoked as the site of the primary processes leading to the development of the peripheral nerve lesions responsible for diabetic neuropathy [2, 39, 47–52, 56, 57, 102–114]. The proximal-to-distal gradient in morphometric abnormalities [2, 50], and the topographic and temporal distribution of neurological signs and symptoms in diabetic distal symmetric polyneuropathy suggest a primary axonopathy preferentially involving longer myelinated axons [52, 102, 111–114]. Lascelles, [107, 108] and others [109, 110], and autopsy studies [39] have emphasized segmental demyelination and remyelination in diabetic distal symmetric polyneuropathy, postulating a primary abnormality of Schwann cells. As discussed above, endoneurial vascular abnormalities such as basement membrane thickening and reduplication, endothelial cell swelling and proliferation, and platelet aggregation resulting in vessel occlusion have been noted in sural nerve biopsies [47, 48] and at autopsy [2, 49–52] in diabetic distal symmetric polyneuropathy. A quantitative increase in these vascular abnormalities in association with focal loss of myelinated fibers in older diabetic subjects has been interpreted to suggest hypoxic or ischemic damage to nerve fibers in diabetic distal symmetric polyneuropathy [2, 47, 48]. Thus, while demonstrating that most tissue elements of peripheral nerve are involved in the disease process at some point, prior studies of human diabetic distal symmetric polyneuropathy provide no consensus as to the location of the initial inciting events leading to the development of diabetic neuropathy.

A recent study of sural nerve biopsies from patients with distal symmetric polyneuropathy was undertaken to evaluate the relative importance of pathological lesions such as axo-glial dysjunction attributable in diabetic animal models to metabolic factors versus those associated with vascular changes in the human material [116]. In order to evaluate effects of age and type of diabetes on sural nerve morphometry, sural nerve biopsies obtained from younger IDDM and older NIDDM patients with neuropathy were compared to strictly age-matched controls and subjected to correction for age-differences by analysis of covariance. The number of myelinated nerve fibers were comparably diminished in IDDM and NIDDM patients compared to their respective age-matched controls (although nerve fiber diminished with age in the non-diabetic controls as well) [116]. The frequency of specific lesions of nerve fibers such as paranodal swelling, demyelination and remyelination; myelin wrinkling; segmental demyelination; and fiber regeneration and remyelination were increased in biopsies from both IDDM and NIDDM patients compared to age-matched or age-corrected controls [116]. IDDM patients exhibited the entire array of morphometric changes described in the rat [117] including paranodal swelling, axo-glial dysjunction [37, 53, 118], and subtle axonal atrophy [55]. NIDDM patients exhibited no increase in axo-glial dysjunction or consistent evidence of axonal atrophy despite comparable degrees of nerve fiber loss, paranodal swelling and paranodal demyelination; this structural discordance persisted after adjustment for age on the basis of age-related changes in the non-diabetic controls [116]. Conversely, Wallerian degeneration and spatial heterogeneity in the pattern of fiber loss compatible with ischemic nerve damage were increased only in NIDDM patients, the latter as a function of duration of diabetes [116]. The increased spatial heterogeneity in sural nerve fiber density in diabetic neuropathy correlates with and has been ascribed to more proximal distinct focal intra- and inter-fascicular regions of fiber loss in autopsy studies (Fig. 7) [2, 50]. This morphological discordance in distal symmetric polyneuropathy complicating IDDM and NIDDM suggests a number of possible differences in the underlying pathogenesis. Firstly, distal symmetrical polyneuropathy in IDDM and NIDDM are unlikely to reflect entirely different pathogenetic processes because of the many shared clinical, biochemical, electrophysiological and morphological characteristics. The population of very large myelinated nerve fibers most susceptible to diabetes-induced axo-glial dysjunction in the BB rat model [37] may have been depleted from the older NIDDM patients by the age-related selective large-fiber loss detected in the non-diabetic control population [116]. Axo-glial dysjunction and subtle fiber atrophy in IDDM, and Wallerian degeneration in NIDDM, may reflect alternative pathways leading from the early metabolic damage to ultimate loss of nerve fibers. Axo-glial dysjunction might be evanescent in NIDDM, progressing rapidly to more advanced stages of fiber pathology such as Wallerian degeneration without being detected with any great frequency in biopsy specimens. Because nerve fiber loss is more focal in NIDDM, and is associated with increased Wallerian degeneration, it is tempting to speculate that superimposed vascular factors in NIDDM patients channel nerve fiber loss through Wallerian degeneration as a sequel or alternative to axo-glial dysjunction. Alternatively, the increased frequency of prolonged undetected antecedent hyperglycemia and the higher prevalence of symptomatic neuropathy at diagnosis in NIDDM patients [7] suggests the possibility that patients with NIDDM may have a longer duration but more indolent neuropathy possibly reflecting a less serious metabolic derangement; this view would be consistent with the significantly lower sural nerve sorbitol levels in NIDDM vs. IDDM despite comparable nerve glucose and HbA_{1c} levels [119]. Finally, because the patients with NIDDM were significantly older than those with IDDM, an interaction of age with diabetes might also contribute to apparent differences in the neuropathy accompanying IDDM and NIDDM. Future prevention and/or treatment studies using specific metabolic intervention, plus additional detailed structural studies in diabetic and non-diabetic subjects will help differentiate among these various pathogenetic possibilities.

Focal diabetic neuropathies

On the basis of admittedly extremely fragmentary but somewhat compelling neuropathological studies, occlusive disease of medium-sized intraneural blood vessels has been invoked in the pathogenesis of focal neuropathy in diabetes at least in selected patients [46]. Because of their rarity, their self-limited course, and the inaccessability for biopsy, the focal diabetic neuropathies have been explored histologically in only a few isolated reports. Serial sections of the third nerve in two diabetic patients dying after developing isolated third nerve palsys revealed focal "acute" demyelinating lesions in the intracavernous watershed area between the intra- and extra-cranial vascular beds in association with local thickening and occlusion of arterioles [120, 121]. A single autopsy study of a diabetic patient dying shortly after developing acute unilateral weakness and sensory loss in the upper and lower leg revealed multiple microinfarcts of bridging fascicles of the ipsilateral obturator, femoral, sciatic and posterior tibial nerves associated with thickening, fibrosis and occlusion of the associated vasa nervorum [122]. These isolated reports associate the focal neuropathies with acute infarctions within the peripheral nervous system.

Autonomic neuopathy

Diabetic autonomic neuropathy has been even less well studied in part because biopsy material is not readily available. The few available autopsy studies demonstrate axonal degeneration and fiber loss in the paravertebral sympathetic chain [123]; the vagus, esophageal and splanchnic nerves [124–126]; and in the intrinsic nerves of the bladder [127]. Swelling and vacuolization of autonomic ganglionic neurons has also been described [128, 129].

Summary

In summary, insulin deficiency and hyperglycemia induce a series of reasonably well characterized acute metabolic and functional defects in the peripheral nervous system including alterations in polyol and *myo*-inositol metabolism, (Na,K)-ATPase activity, microvascular function, axonal transport and electrical function. The relationship between these early and generally reversible metabolic and functional abnormalities to the advanced and poorly reversible histological lesions that underlie the clinical syndromes of diabetic neuropathy are not fully understood. Since it would appear that insulin deficiency and its attendant hyperglycemia are clearly conditioning elements in the pathogenesis of clinical neuropathy, it is reasonable to speculate that these metabolic and functional defects, in conjunction with other poorly defined independent genetic and/or environmental variables, probably are major factors in the pathogenesis of this chronic complication of diabetes.

Early detection and classification

Diabetic neuropathy has been divided into subclinical and clinical stages [130]. The diagnosis of subclinical diabetic neuropathy (Table 1, Class I) requires the demonstration in a diabetic patient of objective measurement of peripheral neural impairment not attributable to a nondiabetic etiology in the absence of detectable clinical signs or symptoms of neuropathy [130]. The diagnosis of clinical diabetic neuropathy (Table 2, Class II) requires the demonstration in a diabetic patient of symptoms or signs plus objective measurement of peripheral neural impairment not attributable to a nondi-

Table 2 Research classification of diabetic polyneuropathy (from [130])

	Clinical assessments		Abnormal physiological tests
	Symptom score	Neurological examination score	
Class I			
A	0	0	0 or AFT or QST
B	0	0	EDX or AFT and QST
C	0	0	EDX and either AFT or QST or both
Class II			
A	+	0	0 or AFT or QST
B	0 or +	+	EDX or AFT and QST
C	0 or +	+	EDX and either AFT
	+	0 or +	or QST or both

+, Abnormal result; 0, normal result
AFT, autonomic function testing; EDX, electrodiagnosis; QST, quantitative sensory testing

Table 3 Common important differential diagnoses of diabetic neuropathy (from [130a])

- Distal symmetrical polyneuropathy
  - Metabolic disorders
    - Diabetes mellitus
    - Uremia
    - Folic acid/cyanocobalamin deficiency
    - Hypothyroidism
    - Acute intermittent porphyria
  - Toxins
    - Alcohol
    - Heavy metals (lead, mercury, arsenic)
    - Industrial hydrocarbons
    - Drugs
  - Infiltrative/inflammatory disorders (nerve biopsy often helpful)
    - Amyloidosis
    - Leprosy
    - Sarcoidosis
    - Periarteritis nodosa
    - Refsum's disease
  - Other diseases
    - Connective tissue diseases, e.g., SLE
    - Dys- and paraproteinemias
    - Leukemias/Lymphomas
    - Paraneoplastic syndrome
- Pains and paresthesias without neurological deficit
  - Depression
  - Hysteria
  - Early small fiber sensory neuropathy
- Autonomic neuropathy without somatic component
  - Shy-Drager syndrome (progressive autonomic failure)
  - Diabetic neuropathy with mild somatic involvement
  - Riley-Day syndrome
  - Idiopathic orthostatic hypotension
- Diffuse motor neuropathy without sensory deficit
  - Guillain-Barré syndrome
  - Primary myopathies
  - Myasthenia gravis
  - Heavy metal toxicity
- Femoral neuropathy
  - Degenerative spinal disc disease
  - Paget's disease of the spine
  - Intrinsic spinal cord mass lesion
  - Equina cauda lesions
  - Coagulopathies
- Cranial neuropathy
  - Carotid aneurysm
  - Intracranial mass
  - Elevated intracranial pressure
- Mononeuropathy multiplex
  - Vasculitides
  - Amyloidosis
  - Hypothyroidism
  - Acromegaly
  - Coagulopathies

abetic etiology [130]. Since there are no distinguishing features unique to diabetic neuropathy, all other likely causes of peripheral neuropathy or disorders that mimic peripheral neuropathy must be excluded by careful history and physical examination and appropriate diagnostic tests (Table 3). Neuropathy must accompany currently accepted diagnostic criteria for diabetes. Since neuropathic symptoms are often vague and nonspecific, confirmatory clinical signs or objective measurements of peripheral nerve dysfunction (somatic or autonomic) must be present.

A subclinical stage of diabetic neuropathy not discernable by careful history and physical examination alone can be identified by a variety of invasive and non-invasive neuropathological and neurophysiological tests including nerve biopsy, nerve conduction studies, quantitative cutaneous sensory tests or autonomic function tests (Table 4).

Table 4A Electrodiagnostic tests (modified from [130])

Motor nerve-conduction studies
Unilateral studies of either ulnar or median nerve including F waves in the upper limb
Unilateral studies of peroneal nerve including F wave in the lower limb
Measurement of muscle-action potential amplitude and latency at each site of stimulation and calculation of segmental conduction velocity
Sensory nerve-conduction studies
Unilateral studies of either ulnar or median nerve in the upper limb
Unilateral studies of either medial plantar or sural nerve in the lower limb
Measurement of nerve-action potential amplitude and latency at each site of stimulation and calculation of segmental conduction velocity
Studies of additional nerves may be necessary to characterize abnormalities based on the distribution of clinical symptoms or signs

Table 4B Autonomic function tests (modified from [130])

Tests of heart-rate control (mainly parasympathetic). Heart-rate response to:
Valsalva maneuver
Deep breathing
Standing
Tests of blood pressure control (mainly sympathetic). Blood pressure response to:
Standing or tilting
Sustained handgrip
Tests of sudomotor control, i.e.:
Temperature-induced sweating
Chemically-induced sweating (e.g., acetylcholine or pilocarpine)

Clinical detection of clinical neuropathy

Clinical neuropathy consists of the superimposition of symptoms and/or clinically detectable neurological deficits that take the form of one or more of the individual clinical syndromes of diabetic neuropathy, each with a characteristic presentation and clinical course (Table 5) [101]. Distal symmetric polyneuropathy, the most commonly recognized form of diabetic neuropathy [131], features sensory deficits and symptoms that overshadow motor involvement [5]. Sensory deficits originate in the most distal portions of the extremities, progress proximally in a "stocking-glove" distribution [5], and in the most advanced cases form vertical bands on the chest as distal portions of truncal nerves become involved [132]. The signs, symptoms and neurological deficits of distal symmetric polyneuropathy vary depending on the classes of nerve fibers that are involved [5] with loss of large sensory and motor fibers diminishing light touch and proprioception and producing muscle weakness, while loss of small fibers diminishes pain and temperature perception and

Table 5 Clinical classification of diabetic neuropathy

A. *Diffuse neuropathy*
  1. Distal symmetric sensorimotor polyneuropathy
    a) Primarily small fiber neuropathy
    b) Primarily large fiber neuropathy
    c) Mixed
  2. Autonomic neuropathy
    a) Abnormal pupillary function
    b) Sudomotor dysfunction
    c) Genitourinary autonomic neuropathy
      (1) bladder dysfunction
      (2) sexual dysfunction
    d) Gastrointestinal autonomic neuropathy
      (1) gastric atony
      (2) gall bladder atony
      (3) diabetic diarrhea
      (4) hypoglycemic unawareness (adrenal medullary neuropathy)
    e) Cardiovascular autonomic neuropathy
    f) Hypoglycemic unawareness
B. *Focal neuropathy*
  1. Mononeuropathy
  2. Mononeuropathy multiplex
  3. Plexopathy
  4. Radiculopathy
  5. Cranial neuropathy

produces paresthesias, dysesthesias and/or neuropathic pain [5]. Diminished or absent deep tendon reflexes, especially the Achilles tendon reflex, may often be an early indication of otherwise asymptomatic neuropathy [5] while undetected but more advanced asymptomatic neuropathy may first present with late complications such as ulceration or neuroarthropathy ("Charcot's joints") of the foot [133]. Diabetic autonomic neuropathy often but not always accompanies distal symmetric polyneuropathy and can impair virtually any sympathetic or parasympathetic autonomic function [133]. Diabetic cardiovascular autonomic neuropathy first compromizes cardiac parasympathetic function diminishing the normal bradycardic responses to sleep and deep inspiration; with progression, sympathetic cardiac and peripheral vascular denervation occurs interfering with normal cardiovascular response to exercise and hypersensitizing the heart to circulating catecholamines predisposing to tachyarrhythmias and sudden death [133]. Gastrointestinal autonomic neuropathy produces the nonspecific gastrointestinal symptoms that afflict the majority of diabetic patients [133]. Esophageal dysmotility and reflux, decreased vagally-mediated gastric acid secretion, and delayed gastric emptying produce anorexia, nausea, vomiting, early satiety and postprandial bloating and fullness [133]. Diabetic enteropathy encompasses the clinical syndromes of diabetic constipation, diabetic diarrhea and fecal incontinence, which all reflect widespread abnormalities in the intrinsic and extrinsic intestinal autonomic nervous system [133]. Retrograde ejaculation, neuropathic erectile impotence and diabetic cystopathy all result from loss of coordination of the autonomic innervation of the genito-urinary tract [133]. Neuropathic impotence is generally but not always accompanied by other manifestations of diabetic neuropathy. The diminished epinepherine response to hypoglycemia in chronic diabetes is generally believed to be the result of autonomic neuropathy of the adrenal medulla, which can blunt the usual adrenergic warning signs of impending hypoglycemia [133]. Diabetic autonomic sudomotor dysfunction produces an asymptomatic distal anhydrosis in a stocking-glove distribution similar to that of distal symmetric polyneuropathy. This diminishes thermoregulatory reserve, predisposes to heatstroke and hyperthermia, and produces a compensatory central hyperhydrosis that is often bothersome to the patient [133].

In contrast to the diffuse distal symmetric polyneuropathy and autonomic neuropathy, focal diabetic neuropathies correspond to the distribution of single or multiple peripheral nerves ("mononeuropathy" and "mononeuropathy multiplex"), cranial nerves, regions of the brachial or lumbosacral plexuses ("plexopathy") or the nerve roots ("radiculopathy") [46]. They are relatively uncommon, of sudden onset, and generally but not always self-limited in diabetic patients, and tend to occur in older age groups [46]. The third cranial nerve is often affected, presenting with unilateral pain, diplopia and ptosis with pupillary sparing in a syndrome termed "diabetic ophthalmoplegia" [46]. Diabetic ophthalmoplegia may occur in the absence of other manifestations of diabetic neuropathy, and may be bilateral and/or recurrent. Radiculopathy presents as bandlike thoracic or abdominal pain, that is often misdiagnosed as an acute intrathoracic or intraabdominal emergency [46]. "Femoral neuropathy" in diabetic patients often involves motor and sensory deficits at the level of the sacral plexus as well as the femoral nerve, with the relative excess of motor versus sensory involvement differentiating diabetic "femoral neuropathy" from that seen in other conditions [46]. Other mononeuropathies mimic the compression neuropathies seen in non-diabetic individuals such as carpal tunnel syndrome [131]. Thus, while distal symmetric polyneuropathy and autonomic neuropathy are common, diffuse, and generally progressive disorders, the focal neuropathies are rare, sudden in onset, often self-limited, and occur primarily in older patients with diabetes.

Nerve biopsy

As mentioned above, sural nerve biopsy, conventionally employed clinically in diagnostically challenging cases of peripheral neuropathy, has been adapted to quantitate and characterize the type and extent of biochemical abnormality [39, 119, 134, 135] and peripheral nerve damage in patients with diabetic polyneuropathy [39, 101, 103, 110, 116] and, in only one instance [57], in patients without significant clinical neuropathy. Because of the extensive structural alterations in sural nerve biopsies from patients with clinically overt neuropathy, biochemical comparisons between intact normal biopsies and diseased diabetic biopsies must be interpreted cautiously, and such studies have not been reported in patients with undamaged nerves. In 2 separate reports [39, 134], Dyck and coworkers found no statistically significant alterations in sorbitol or *myo*-inositol content in sural nerve biopsies from heterogeneous groups of diabetic and mostly neuropathic patients, although sorbitol levels did fall in six subjects treated with an aldose reductase inhibitor as part of a clinical trial with rigorous inclusion criteria [134]. In contrast, studies of sural nerve biopsies from neuropathic diabetic patients recruited under a standardized protocol with rigid inclusion criterial revealed high sorbitol levels that fell with aldose reductase inhibitor therapy [135], and *myo*-inositol levels that were significantly lower than cadaver controls [116]. An "index of pathology" based on quantitative morphometric analysis of fiber populations, and on semi-quantitative analysis of categories of abnormal teased fibers appears to effectively differentiate non-diabetic subjects from subjects with diabetic neuropathy [101] (Fig. 10). Preliminary studies suggest that diabetic subjects without clinical neuropathy may fall intermediate between and overlap these 2 groups. While even detailed quantitative analysis of invasively-obtained sural nerve biopsy material cannot at present completely distinguish diabetic patients with and without neuropathy with absolute diagnostic specificity, sensitivity and reliability, this procedure probably approaches a "gold standard" for the objective and quantitative establishment of the presence of neuropathy in a diabetic subject. Because of their invasiveness, nerve biopsies should be restricted in scientific investigation to "thoughtful well-designed studies aimed at increasing the understanding of basic etiopathogenesis (of diabetic neuropathy) or the mechanism of action of therapeutic agents" [130]. As mentioned below, a recent study employing quantitative morphometric analysis of serial nerve biopsies in patients with diabetic neuropathy treated with an aldose reductase inhibitor revealed what appeared to be a clear-cut treatment response [135].

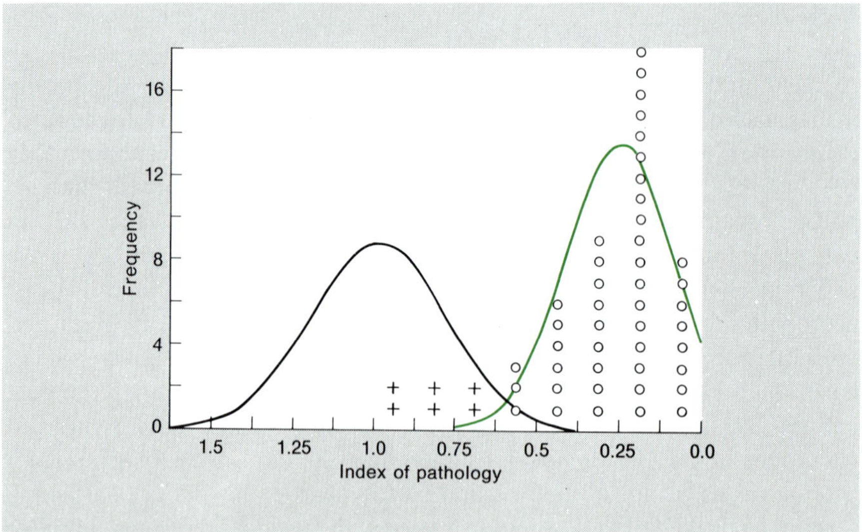

Fig. 10 The indexes of pathology (IP) of diabetics with (open circles) and without (crosses) neuropathy have been plotted as a histogram. The normal distribution curves from healthy subjects (left) and from diabetics with neuropathy (right) are also shown. There is complete separation of diabetic patients with and without neuropathy. One anticipates without having actual data, that with more patients with borderline diabetic neuropathy more overlap of values would occur. For a given patient whose values are at the crossover point of the tails of the two distributions, it is difficult to say whether they are normal or abnormal. This becomes a much greater problem in some clinical measures of neuropathy; therefore it is important to know the sensitivity and specificity of tests used [101].

Nerve conduction tests

Nerve conduction studies and electromyography are generally applied in cases of overt diabetic neuropathy to characterize the type and/or severity of fiber involvment, to differentiate axonal from demyelinative damage, and to localize focal neurological lesions. Electrodiagnostic evaluation is particularly useful clinically to differentiate various disorders within the spectrum of diabetic neuropathy such as mononeuropathy, mononeuropathy multiplex, plexopathy and polyradiculopathy, especially when a diffuse polyneuropathy is also present [130]. In diffuse polyneuropathy, testing of a few nerves adequately reflects the status of the somatic peripheral nervous system [130]. Because nerve conduction measurements and specialized electromyography provides easily quantifiable and objective data concerning the peripheral nervous system, they have been widely applied to the study of both clinical and subclinical neuropathy [130]. Slowing of nerve conduction is readily detectable in groups of patients with diabetes who are free of clinical signs and symptoms of diabetic neuropathy. As summarized above, the modest slowing of nerve conduction in newly diagnosed IDDM that fluctuates with metabalic control is generally ascribed to reversible metabolic abnormalities [14, 15] although its physiological (and potential clinical) significance is underlined by accompanying changes in vibratory perception threshold [16]. In neurologically intact asymptomatic patients with NIDDM, nerve conduction velocity correlates inversely with HbA_{1c} [17] and improves following metabolic intervention proportionately with HbA_{1c} level in response to conventional metabolic therapy in chronic stable NIDDM [18]. Similarly, intensive treatment improves peripheral nerve conduction in IDDM, but again only slightly [19–22]. Following diagnosis of diabetes, nerve conduction velocity slows progressively but modestly in groups of IDDM and NIDDM subjects as a function of duration of disease [102, 136]. However, in diabetic subjects with absent or very mild clinical neuropathy, nerve conduction parameters are influenced by a variety of variables other than the presence or absence of subtle clinical neurological findings, and the severity and duration of diabetes [137, 138]. These include age [137, 138], height [137, 138], and gender [137] as well as pubertal status at time of diagnosis of diabetes [137]. Conventional electromyographic studies using needle electrodes may reveal partial dennervation of intrinsic foot muscles as an early sign of diabetic neuropathy or in patients who are free of symptoms or clinical neurological deficits [130]. A variety of non-standard electrophysiological procedures have been advocated as being more sensitive and/or reliable in detecting impaired electrical conduction in patients with diabetes, such as the

H-reflex latency [139], conduction distribution velocity analysis [140], or resistence to ischemic conduction block [141] but their superior reliability in distinguishing metabolic from structural nerve damage, or in predicting the development of clinically overt neuropathy has not been established.

In patients with overt diabetic neuropathy, nerve conduction abnormalities generally are quantitatively more marked but are not quantitatively different from non-neuropathic diabetic subjects. The more marked [137] slowing of sensory conduction velocity in patients with overt neuropathy correlates largely with loss of large myelinated fibers [103] with only a small residual component attributable to other factors (e.g. "metabolic" factors of demyelination). Therefore, acute improvement of nerve conduction velocity following metabolic intervention in patients with overt neuropathy or even established diabetes is necessarily limited to that component of conduction slowing not attributed to poorly-reversible nerve fiber loss. However, in the absence of prospective studies correlating nerve conduction impairment in asymptomatic individuals with the subsequent development of clinical neuropathy, it is impossible to determine if early functional changes represent detection of early neuropathy, or rather are simply a reflection of the degree of metabolic abnormality at the time that conduction studies were performed. Conversely, since maximum conduction velocity primarily reflects the functional integrity of only the largest and most rapidly conducting nerve fibers, it is only modestly decreased with the selective loss of large fibers since smaller fibers conduct only slightly slower, but it is markedly reduced with widespread demyelination [142]. Therefore, nerve conduction may be impaired in the absence of structurally advanced subclinical neuropathy due to metabolic factors, and yet may be insensitive to axonal loss which is thought to be the pathological hallmark of progressively worsening subclinical neuropathy. A battery of electrophysiological tests including a novel measure of H-reflex conduction velocity in the distal leg, as well as tibial motor and sural sensory conduction velocity and amplitude was able to distinguish normal controls from diabetic subjects, and diabetic subjects with no or mild neuropathy from those having more advanced clinical neuropathy [143]; however, since this cross-sectional analysis was performed in a referral-based population whose general representativeness is undefined, confirmation in a broader population-based study group were be highly desirable before this approach could be widely applied. In general, detailed prospective electrophysiological studies are desperately needed to clarify the clinical relevance and predictiveness of the impaired nerve conduction in subjects with newly-diagnosed or short-duration diabetes as to the subsequent development of clinical disease. Such studies are currently underway in the United States as part of the Diabetes Control and Complications Trial (DCCT) which will follow nerve conduction parameters and the development of clinical neuropathy in 1400 subjects with IDDM over 5–10 years [137].

Quantitative cutaneous sensory thresholds

While assessment of sensory modalities is central to the clinical examination of patients with the predominantly sensory diabetic peripheral polyneuropathy, such clinical measures are inadequate for comparison, quantitation, staging or prospective follow-up of cases due to the intrinsic variation and subjectiveness of the physical examination [144]. Quantitative sensory testing, particularly of vibratory perception threshold, has been used for evaluation of diabetic peripheral neuropathy for generations [144–148]. Vibratory sensation is impaired in newly diagnosed diabetic subjects and improves in conjunction with nerve conduction velocity in response to metabolic intervention [16]. Semi-quantitative corneal light-touch and peripheral vibratory sensory thresholds correlated with the briskness of the Achilles tendon reflex in a cross-sectional analysis of unselected diabetic and non-diabetic subjects [149]. A semi-quantitative cross-sectional survey of "juvenile diabetics" most of whom had no demonstrable neurological deficits on clinical examination and many of whom had diabetes for less than 2 years, revealed multiple sensory deficits (light touch, 2-point discrimination, visual flicker-fusion, auditory fusion and electric taste) even in the group with duration less than 2 years [150]. These intriguing observations, and the apparent ease and convenience of cutaneous threshold measurement has generated a cascade of devices and techniques to quantitate various sensory modalities in subjects with diabetes and diabetic neuropathy that range from rather simple hand-held or portable mass-produced devices [151–153] suitable for field-screening or multi-center trials, to expensive and specialized computer-driven laboratory equipment [144, 154]. While limited follow-up studies suggest that vibratory sensation deteriorates with time in the absence of near-normalization of blood glucose in subjects with IDDM [19], and extensive cross-sectional studies reveal that sensory impairment correlates with other objective and clinical measures of diabetic neuropathy [144], prospective studies indicating whether or not cutaneous threshold parameters predict the development of clinically evident diabetic neuropathy are not available. Yet if quantitatively, sensitively, reproducibly and reliably measured sub-clinical sensory deficits worsen with time, and are continuous with the clinical deficits measured by the neurologist's cotton wisp, pin and tuning fork, then these measures should logically predict the subsequent development of clinical disease. This, however, remains to be proven, and as of the moment, sensory testing cannot be presented as an established screening method to detect early but clinically important neuropathy.

Autonomic function testing

Clinical features of autonomic neuropathy generally occur late in the course of diabetes [155]. Clinical autonomic neuropathy is therefore considered to be a very late complication of diabetes, but patients without autonomic symptoms exhibit impaired autonomic function in a variety of end-organs relatively early in the course of diabetes [155]. The appearance of autonomic symptoms is therefore considered a late stage in a chronic underlying process involving progressively worsening autonomic function. Widespread sub-clinical evidence of autonomic nerve dysfunction is usually easily demonstrable in patients presenting with autonomic symptoms confined to a single organ system. Therefore, a variety of screening techniques have been employed to detect sub-clinical autonomic dysfunction in diabetic patients without autonomic symptoms or with symptoms confined to a single end-organ. The majority of autonomic function tests assess cardiovascular autonomic function, because of its obvious importance and its comparatively straightforward quantification. These methods involve measurement of heart rate response to deep-breathing (sinus arrythmia) [156, 157] Valsalva [158], sustained hand-grip [158] and standing [159]. A sophisticated computerized techinque to quantitate sinus arrythmia ("RR-variation") that focusses on parasympathetic influence and eliminates confounding variables (age, hypovolemia, drugs, hypoglycemia, etc.) clearly distinguishes normal individuals from asymptomatic subjects with even short-duration diabetes (Fig. 11), correlates with other parameters of autonomic and somatic nerve function as well as duration and severity of hyperglycemia, and appears to possibly predict the subsequent development of clinical diabetic neuropathy [157] (this latter supposition needs to be confirmed in larger and longer duration studies such as the DCCT). Less extensively studied and therefore less well characterized as autonomic function tests are a quantitative sudomotor axon reflex test ("QSART") that measures sympathetic post-ganglionic function and which correlates with sinus arrythmia and other parameters of autonomic and somatic function [160], pupillometry [161, 162], the epinepherine and pancreatic polypeptide responses to hypoglycemia [163, 164] and others [164]. Except for the RR-variation test, there are no published studies exploring the extent to which autonomic function tests predict the subsequent development or progression of diabetic neuropathy [157].

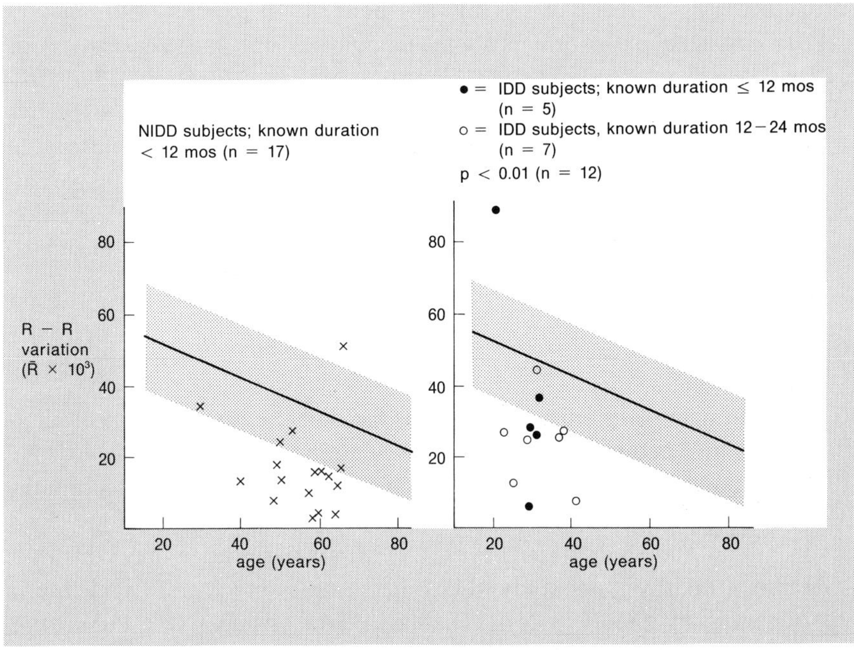

Fig. 11 RR variation in a patient with a recent (less than 24 months) diagnosis of diabetes mellitus. RR variation after beta-adrenergic blockade was determined by the vector analysis technique. The bold lines represent the regression lines and the shaded areas the 70% confidence band for normal subjects. After age adjustment, the group of non insulin-dependent diabetic patients (left panel) and insulin-dependent diabetics (right panel) had significantly smaller RR variation [155].

Summary

Diabetic neuropathy can be classified as being clinical or sub-clinical, based on the presence or absence of signs and/or symptoms consistent with the known clinical syndromes of diabetic neuropathy (Table 2). Diabetic neuropathy, whether clinical or sub-clinical, is a diagnosis of exclusion (Table 3). Clinical neuropathy is further sub-divided on the basis of the anatomic distribution and type of neurological deficit and/or symptoms (Table 5). Subclinical neuropathy is diagnosed and quantified on the basis of abnormalities detected by one or more of several standardized quantitative neurological tests, including electrodiagnostic studies, quantitative cutaneous sensory thresholds, and autonomic function tests (Table 4) [130]. The fact that clinical symptoms, clinical neurological deficits, nerve pathology, and the extent of abnormality of quantitative electrodiagnostic, sensory and autonomic tests correlate closely but not perfectly in patients with diabetes and diabetic neuropathy provides some flexibility in the particular battery of tests employed in any particular clinical study or evaluation [130, 157]. However, with the exception of RR-variation [157], longitudinal prospective studies indicating the predictiveness of any of these tests for the subsequent development of clinically overt diabetic neuropathy are not available, although the relationship between autonomic function tests, nerve conduction tests and the subsequent development of clinical neuropathy is being evaluated in the DCCT.

Risk factors

Reliable estimates of predisposing factors for diabetic neuropathy as well as its impact and frequency within the population are virtually non-existent [131]. The handful of existing epidemiological studies of diabetic neuropathy are heavily criticized for inconsistent and poorly defined terminology, diagnostic criteria and study populations [12]. Minor paresthesia may constitute diabetic neuropathy in one study while others employ much more rigid criteria [8]. A survey by the 1978 NIH Diabetes Data Group (NIH Publication 78–1468) of reported prevalence estimates for clinical or subclinical neuropathy ranged from 10–100% (Table 6). These deficiencies in available data

Table 6 Reported prevalence of symptoms and signs of neuropathy in diabetes (from [131])

Source	Measurement	No. Patients	% Neuropathy
Cleveland 1953	Subjective complaints	261	62
Salford, England 1953	General findings	100	57
Brussels 1965	Objective signs	1,175	21
Stockholm 1950	Objective signs	150	49
Rochester, MN 1961	Electromyography, objective signs	103	42
Philadelphia 1958	Impotence	198	55
New York 1952	Skin vessel dilatation	16	44
London 1960	Abnormal Valsalva maneuver	337	20
Toronto 1961	Objective signs	100	52
Cincinnati 1951	General signs	77	35
Chicago 1966	Objective signs, motor conduction velocity	107	10
Aarhus, Denmark 1968	Motor conduction velocity	14	100
London 1971	Motor conduction velocity	39	100
Edinburgh 1977	Motor conduction velocity, autonomic vascular tests	10	100

U.S. Dept. of HEW: Diabetes data. DHEW Publ. No. (NIH) 78-1468, 1978 stem in large part from a general lack of consensus among experts in the field as to the definition and methods of detection of diabetic neuropathy [131]. Subclinical and clinical diabetic neuropathy are often not clearly distinguished. The diagnostic sensitivity, specificity and reliability of relatively simple objective measures such as the absence of the Achilles tendon reflexes in a person with diabetes is still controversial [131]. Cross-sectional office-based or clinic-based surveys often suffer from significant referral bias, and very few population-based prevalence studies or inception-cohort-based incidence studies exist [131]. Palumbo and coworkers [11] followed the appearance of clinical neuropathy for up to 20 years in a cohort of 995 subjects comprising the entire population of Rochester, Minnesota diagnosed with "maturity onset" diabetes but without accompanying neuropathy between the years 1945 and 1969. The accumulated incidence rate for distal symmetric polyneuropathy in this population-based cohort was 4% after 5 years and 15% after 20 years, with a median time from diagnosis of diabetes to development of neuropathy of 9 years [11, 131]. Comparable data were collected by Pirart [7], who studied the change in prevalence of clinical neuropathy in a referral-based cohort of patients over a 25 year period. The prevalence was 8% in patients with newly-diagnosed diabetes, and over 40% in patients after 20 years of diabetes [7]. This more than 2-fold difference could reflect referral bias in the Pirart study or less complete ascertainment in the Palumbo study, or differences in definition and detection of neuropathy [131]. The basis for these descrepancies in the estimated frequency of diabetic neuropathy, and those evident in Table 6, are regarded as "essentially uninterpretable" [131], severely compromising our ability to grasp additional predisposing risk factors operative within the population on an epidemiological basis.

Despite the lack of good population-based studies, clinical studies suggest that the duration and severity of hyperglycemia are 2 important risk factors for the development of diabetic neuropathy. Clinical neuropathy is rarely detected before the fifth year of diabetes except in NIDDM where preexisting asymptomatic hyperglycemia is difficult to exclude, and it ultimately effects up to 50% of patients with long-duration diabetes [7]. Diabetic neuropathy complicates the secondary forms of diabetes such as that resulting from pancreatectomy, non-alcoholic pancreatitis and hemachromatosis [8], a finding that supports a common pathogenetic mechanism for diabetic neuropathy involving hyperglycemia and/or insulin deficiency at least as permissive risk factors. Yet many patients with very poorly controlled diabetes of long duration do not develop clinically apparent diabetic neuropathy [9], and when it appears, it may take widely differing forms in individual patients. This suggests the presence of independent modifying factors, and the possibility that different pathogenetic variables may be acting in different forms of diabetic neuropathy. As discussed above, histopathological differences in sural nerve biopsies from younger subjects with IDDM and older subjects with NIDDM plus the presence of age-related changes in nerve histopathology in non-diabetic controls would imply that age itself, probably mediated in part by age-related alterations in the endoneurial vasculature, should be an important risk factor in the development of diabetic neuropathy. This supposition is indeed confirmed by the cross-sectional analysis of subjects with IDDM entering the DCCT trial [137] wherein not only age, but also male gender were independent risk factors for the development of clinical diabetic neuropathy. Patients affected with neuropathy had diabetes of longer duration, had lower stimulated C-peptide responses and were also taller and more likely to consume greater than 1 alcoholic beverage per week (these effects were independent of gender). Furthermore, gender, duration of diabetes and HbA_{1c} were also associated with greater impairment of nerve conduction tests, and HbA_{1c} was also an independent risk factor for impaired RR-variation [137]. Previous studies had also suggested that alcoholic intake [165] and height [166, 167] were risk factors for the development of clinical neuropathy, impaired nerve conduction and increased sensory perception threshold in diabetes. Carefully conducted clinical studies to evaluate the interaction of diabetic neuropathy with nutritional factors, cigarette smoking, exercise or other diabetic complications are not available.

Prevention and treatment

A conceptual hierarchy to the treatment of diabetic neuropathy underpins the therapeutic approaches to the disease. *Prevention* deals with potential risk factors for the development of neuropathy; *physiological management* corrects the altered physiological state that results from various neurological deficits accompanying diabetic neuropathy such as delayed gastric emptying; *prophylaxis* is designed to prevent some of the secondary complications of neurological impairment such as foot ulceration or Charcot's joints in diabetic distal symmetric polyneuropathy; *palliation* is designed only to alleviate specific symptoms but not the severity of underlying diabetic neuropathy; and definitive therapy is targeted against specific pathogenetic components of diabetic neuropathy. It is generally conceded that the development of effective *definitive* therapies to prevent and potentially reverse the neurological damage that underlies the clinical manifestations of diabetic neuropathy must await clearer understanding of the responsible pathogenetic mechanisms. Yet in today's clinical practice, available pharmacological, educational, hygienic and surgical interventions can effectively control the most severe and debilitating consequences of diabetic neuropathy if effectively and properly applied.

Prevention

As discussed above, several risk factors including hyperglycemia and alcohol consumption appear to be associated with the development of diabetic neuropathy. While prudent control of hyperglycemia and avoidance of other potential neurotoxins such as alcohol would likely prevent or delay the appearance of clinical neuropathy in some cases, prospective clinical trials to test these assertions are not available. Potential specific therapeutic intervention directed against elements of the pathogenetic sequence leading to the production of nerve damage and the appearance of clinical neuropathy in diabetes is discussed below in the section entitled "definitive therapy."

Prophylaxis

Prophylactic management of diabetic neuropathy depends upon its prompt recognition and diagnosis. Other than the generally mild subjective sensory symptoms and rare motor weakness, distal symmetric polyneuropathy would constitute only an incidental finding on clinical examination were it not for its secondary complicating disorders. These mechanical and traumatic consequences of sensory and/or motor denervation pose a significant risk to neuropathic patients, but are almost entirely preventable by standard diabetes patient-education, especially that dealing with foot care and hygiene. Prophylactic management of distal symmetric polyneuropathy is often complicated by the fact that the signs and symptoms as well as the electrophysiological characteristics vary depending on the classes of nerve fibers which are involved [5]. In mixed sensorimotor neuropathy, the most common variant, the fiber damage is diffuse, with a predominance of sensory over motor involvement [5]. Loss of large sensory fibers produces diminished position and light touch sensation, while small fiber damage produces diminished pain and temperature sensation and pain or paresthesiae; mixed neuropathy contains symptoms referable to both large and small fiber disease. In the large-fiber variant, subjective symptoms of pain and/or paresthesiae or numbness are usually absent, and, although the neuropathy may be detected by careful physical exam, unfortunately, it may not be noted until a late neuropathic complication such as a Charcot's joint or a neuropathic ulceration is present [5]. In a similar fashion, small fiber sensory neuropathy, which diminishes pain and temperature sensation, may not present until unfelt trauma of the extremities (burns of the fingers from cigarettes, or burns of the feet from stepping into hot bath water, acute abrasions and ulcerations of the feet from small objects retained inside the shoe which go undetected for prolong periods by the patient etc.) is noted by the patient. Most commonly, the patients with small-fiber involvement experience typical neuropathic distal paresthesias or dysesthesias [5]. At times, pain can become an overriding and disabling feature of small-fiber sensory diabetic neuropathy, yet conduction velocity may not be dramatically impaired, vibration sensation may be intact, motor weakness may be absent, and, if the patient's symptoms bring him to the physician's attention early in the course of the disease, sensory loss may not be striking, all because disease may be primarily confined to the small myelinated nerve fibers [168]. Most patients with diabetic neuropathy experience only slight subjective symptoms, and present to the physician with asymptomatic neurological deficits detected on physical examination, or with complications resulting from the asymptomatic sensory deficits that represent failure of prophylaxis [7]. Neuropathic foot ulceration occurs with great frequency in most sensory neuropathies including diabetic distal symmetrical polyneuropathy, and is thought to reflect traumatic damage to the skin and soft tissues of the foot, although diminished proprioception and muscle strength, and vascular factors may play contributing roles [169]. In the classic plantar ulcer, neurogenic atrophy of the intrinsic foot muscles that normally counterbalance the more proximal foot flexors and extensors produces chronic flexion of the metatarsal-phalangeal joints, thereby drawing the toes into a cocked-up position (claw toe deformity) [169]. Weight bearing is thereby redistributed to the now uncovered metatarsal heads, leading to thinning and atrophy of the normal fat pad, thick callus formation which further shifts weight bearing to the metatarsal heads, and subsequent breakdown of the callus with ulcer formation. This may remain unnoticed in the absence of pain sensation even when secondary infection develops. Prophylaxis of plantar foot ulceration requires careful examination of the feet to detect structural alterations in the foot and to determine the appropriateness of weight-bearing as reflected by the presence of telltale calluses. Adjustment of weight-bearing with orthotic devices should redistribute weight-bearing in a physiological fashion. Neuropathic foot ulceration at other than weight-bearing sites usually reflects incidental trauma that goes undetected by the neuropathic patient with diminished pain sensation and proprioception, and therefore becomes secondarily infected [8]. The generally thin dorsal dermis of the foot may be abraided within hours by ill-fitting foot wear or foreign bodies trapped within the shoe, requiring repeated self-examinations when wearing new foot wear or with prolonged weight bearing. Although ischemia has been invoked as a factor in diabetic foot ulceration, its role is controversial. Proximal occlusive vascular disease delays healing of neuropathic foot ulcers, but the neuropathic ulcerated foot is characteristically warm, with easily palpable dorsalis pedis pulses, militating against an important ischemic component [169]. Recent studies suggest that increased blood flow results from abnormal local arteriovenous shunting in the neuropathic foot that may paradoxically decrease oxygen delivery to the tissues [8], the relationship of this phenomenon to underlying neuropathy is not clear, however. Prophylaxis focuses on patient education, and recommendations regarding foot hygiene, self-examination and type of foot-wear. Treatment of diabetic foot ulcers requires avoidance of further traumatic insults that contributed to the ulcer formation by readjustment of weight bearing with appropriate orthopedic devices and callus debridement, or partial or complete elimination of weight-bearing through decreased ambulation, use of a cane, crutches, or a wheel chair, or enforced bed rest. Complicating infection should be treated vigorously, and, in refractory cases, removal of the offending metatarsal head, sometimes together with amputation of the toe, may be necessary [169].

Neuroarthropathy ("Charcot's joint") can occur in any neurological disease that leaves motor function relatively intact but impairs sensation [170]. Whereas syphillitic neuroarthropathy classically involves the large weight-bearing joints, diabetic neuroarthropathy primarily involves distal joints of the foot (tarsal-metatarsal or metatarsal-phalangeal) or ankle [170]. The pathophysiology involves diminished proprioception that magnifies the pressures sustained by the foot with each step and increases the likelihood of slips and falls, distal motor involvement that alters the normally shock-absorbing dynamic structure of the foot, and diminished or absent pain sensation that permits foot trauma to go unnoticed by the patient. Initial presentation of diabetic neuroarthropathy may be painless swelling and redness of the foot in the absence of fever or leukocytosis that is often mistaken for cellulitis or osteomyelitis depending upon the extent of radiographic bony destruction. Unhealed painless fractures are often visible radiographically, and a history of recent painless trauma is sometimes illicited [170]. Gross architectural distortion of the foot, with shortening and widening of the joint may occur with repeated injury. In its most advanced stage, multiple painless fractures are accompanied by extensive bone demineralization and reabsorption, so that the foot resembles "a bag of bones" [169]. Prophylaxis minimizes weight-bearing trauma with the use of cushioned shoes, a cane, restrictions in weight-bearing exercises, and avoidance of walking over rough terrain etc. Therapy for neuroarthropathy is also directed at removal of continued trauma by decreasing ambulation or redistributing weight bearing e. g. a cane, crutches or wheel chair. Prophylaxis is important in the management of some components of autonomic neuropathy as well. The blunted epinepherine response to hypoglycemia in chronic diabetes is generally ascribed to autonomic neuropathy of the adrenal medulla [163], though it may occasionally occur as an isolated finding [171]. Resultant hypoglycemic unawareness may significantly increase the risk of intensive insulin therapy, and can be diagnosed by reduced glucagon and epinepherine responses to a controlled insulin-induced hypoglycemia [172]. In diabetic autonomic sudomotor dysfunction, distal anhidrosis usually confined to the lower extremity diminishes thermoregulatory reserve [173, 174]. Symptoms include excessive compensatory truncal and facial sweating, and heat intolerance, with distal anhydrosis usually inapparent unless illicited by a careful history. Prophylactic management is aimed at the prevention of heat stroke and hyperthermia and consists primarily of heat stress avoidance.

Physiological treatment

Physiological treatment is particularly relevant to counteracting the altered physiological state induced by autonomic dysfunction in diabetic neuropathy. Diabetic autonomic neuropathy of the bladder initially affects the afferent limb blunting bladder sensation without impairing motor function [175, 176]; hence urologic symptoms are rarely volunteered at this point, although many patients report diminished urinary frequency and nocturia under direct questioning. Cystometric studies confirm impaired bladder sensation [175, 177]. With progression, autonomic efferent involvement leads to complaints of infrequent urination, incomplete or difficult bladder emptying, dribbling, and overflow incontinence. Urodynamic studies reveal bladder residual volumes exceeding 150 ml, predisposing to recurrent urinary tract infections. Physiologic management [178] includes voluntary voiding, colinergic stimulants, chronic catheterization (for patients with chronic recurring infection who cannot void otherwise), or resection of the internal sphincter (continence is usually retained since the external sphincter is left intact).

Diabetic autonomic postural hypotension is marked by a blunted or absent rise in circulating norepinephrine upon standing (orthostatic hypotension accompanied by supranormal norepinephrine responses in a subclass of diabetic patients is presently ascribed to subclinical vascular hypovolemia [179]. This is generally thought to reflect autonomic dysfunction but some observers have invoked primary baroreceptor dysfunction or inappropriate cardiac chronotrophic or ionotrophic response to catecholamines [180, 181].

Management involves volume repletion and control of glycosuria, elastic stocking, high salt intake, mineralocorticoids, military antigravity suits, and atrial pacing.

Retrograde ejaculation reflects uncoordinated closure of the internal vesicle sphincter and relaxation of the external vesicle sphincter by damaged efferent sympathetics. Erection, orgasm, and libido are normal, but ejaculate volume and fertility are reduced. Ejaculate azospermia plus recovery of live, mobile sperm in the post coital urine is diagnostic, but anatomic non-diabetic causes of retrograde ejaculation must be excluded. Sympathomimetics reportedly ameliorate retrograde ejaculation [176, 182, 183] but controlled studies are not available. Artificial insemination of sperm recovered from fresh urine samples may circumvent infertility resulting from retrograde ejaculation [184]. Diabetic autonomic gastropathy may cause both acid secretory and motility disorders, the former of which is invoked to explain the reduced frequency of duodenal ulceration in diabetics [185] while the latter has been associated with anorexia, nausea, vomiting, postprandial fullness, and early satiety, and may complicate diabetic control due to delayed postprandial caloric absorption [186]. Physiological management of the associated gastroparesis includes use of liquid diets, metachlopramide, or the placement of a feeding tube.

Palliative treatment

Current therapy for diabetic polyneuropathy is primarily symptomatic, palliative and supportive. Sensory deficits are usually asymptomatic unless complications develop; hence their management is primarily prophylactic patient education (see above). Paresthesias and dysesthesias are usually easily tolerated by most patients once informed that they may indicate reparative processes in the peripheral nervous system. Most observers have concluded that troubling painful symptoms generally improve spontaneously within a matter of months [5, 169], but some authors disagree with this conclusion [187].

A variety of pharmacological agents have been recommended for the treatment of painful diabetic neuropathy, including a variety of standard analgesics, phenytoin (Dilantin) in anticonvulsive doses, and amitriptyline (Elavil) in sub-antidepressive doses (50 – 150 mg po at bedtime) either alone or in combination with fluphenazine (Prolixin) 1 mg 3 times a day [5], but supporting well-controlled clinical trials are either nonexistent [188] or negative [189]. This is especially relevant in view of the dramatic analgesic placebo response which occurs with intensely perceived pain [190]. A single double-blind cross-over clinical trial of carbamazepine (Tegretol) in doses up to 600 mg/d in 30 patients with symptomatic sensory diabetic neuropathy produced

Table 7 Overall results for each carbamazepine and placebo period (from [190a])

Changes in symptoms		A	B	A	B	A	B
Disappearance	(5↓)	1	0	0	0	1	2
Improvement	(3↓ to 4↓)	6	2	8	0	9	2
Improvement	(1↓ to 2↓)	7	6	3	7	5	7
No change		0	0	1	4	1	0
Increase	(↑ to 5↑)	0	6	0	5	0	4
Not recorded				2			1

Table 8 Stepwise treatment protocol for pain relief in diabetic neuropathy (from [190b])

1.	IF	Neuropathic pain confirmed
	THEN	Simple analgesics (aspirin, paracetamol, mefenamic acid)
2.	IF	Simple analgesics fail
	THEN	Imipramine 50 mg nocte Increase stepwise to 150 mg nocte as required
3.	IF	Intolerant of imipramine (dry mouth, dizziness, hesitancy)
	THEN	Mianserin 30 mg nocte Increase stepwise to 90 mg nocte as required
4.	IF	Imipramine tolerated but insufficient
	THEN	Substitute amitriptyline 50–150 mg nocte ± chlorpromazine 50–100 mg per day or fluphenazine 1–6 mg per day
5.	IF	Severe 'restless legs' or 1–4 failed
	THEN	Clonazepam 0.5–3 mg
6.	AFTER	⩽6 months maximum response
	THEN	Try to withdraw treatment

diminished sensory symptoms somewhat more frequently than did placebo (Table 7, A = carbamazepine, B = placebo) [190a]. A comprehensive stepwise treatment protocol employing imipramine and related tricyclic antidepressants in patients with painful neuropathy (Table 8) appeared to relieve symptoms in the vast majority of patients with painful neuropathy (Fig. 12 and Table 9) [190b]. The observation that treatment of patients with intractable painful diabetic neuropathy with intravenous lidocaine [190c] led to a recent successful double-blind placebo-controlled clinical trial with mexiletine, an oral lidocaine analog, in patients with painful diabetic neuropathy [190d]. Mexiletine (in increasing doses from initially 150 mg daily to a maintenance

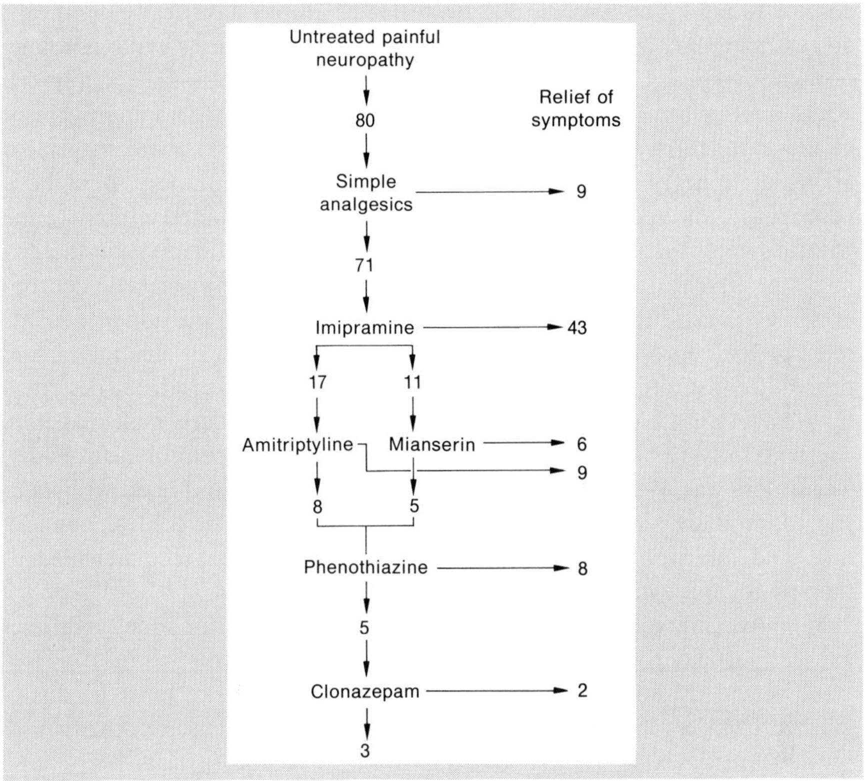

Fig. 12 Flow diagram of response to a therapeutic scheme (Table 8) in 80 consecutive patients with painful diabetic neuropathy.

Table 9 Pain severity before and during treatment. The number of patients in each category is shown. Patients content with simple analgesics alone (NPN 2; CPN 7) are not included. The key to the pain severity scale is in the text (from [190b])

Initial pain severity	Pain severity during treatment: New painful neuropathy					Chronic painful neuropathy					Painful mono-neuropathy				
	0	1	2	3	4	0	1	2	3	4	0	1	2	3	4
1	1	0	0	0	0	2	3	0	0	0	0	0	0	0	0
2	5	4	0	0	0	0	10	2	0	0	2	4	0	0	0
3	5	9	1	1	0	0	4	0	0	0	1	6	0	0	0
4	2	2	2	1	0	0	1	0	0	0	1	3	0	0	0

dose of 10 mg/kg bodyweight for 10 weeks) produced statistically significant decreases in pain, dysesthesia, paresthesia and total sensory symptomotology compared to placebo, with little in the way of side effects (nausea and tremor). These treatment modalities are palliative only, and produce no improvement in nerve function or in neurological deficits. Depression, with associated anorexia, appears to interact very strongly with painfulness in diabetic neuropathy, and seems to exceed that which can be attributed entirely to the painful symptoms alone, suggesting that simultaneous antidepressant therapy might be effacacious [169]. One study suggests that painful diabetic neuropathy may constitute a depressive equivalent in a large proportion of patients referred for neuropathic therapy [191]. An exaggeration of this interaction probably constitutes the syndrome of diabetic neuropathic cachexia described by Ellenberg in 1974 [192]. This syndrome, reported in elderly male diabetics, combined severe weight loss with mild diabetes and painful neuropathy; weight loss was of sufficient magnitude (up to 60% of total body weight) to suggest an underlying malignancy [192]. Improved diabetic control, counselling, and amitriptyline plus fluphenazine have all been recommended as therapy for this syndrome.

Palliative intervention is also helpful in some of the autonomic syndromes as well, particularly with erectile impotence, the commonest form of neurogenic sexual dysfunction. Diabetic neuropathic impotence must be distinguished from psychogenic impotence and organic impotence of other causes by a detailed sexual history and appropriate laboratory tests [193–196]. Medication-associated organic impotence is commonly managed by modification of treatment regimens. An endocrine cause for impotence is comparatively infrequent in diabetics, is usually accompanied by decreased libido and is unlikely in the face of a normal serum testosterone and prolactin [197–201]. Vascular insufficiency can cause penile erectile dysfunction in diabetic patients though usually only in the presence of atherosclerosis which is sufficiently generalized to reduce femoral pulses (although surgically-correctable selective penile artery insufficiency has been reported) [202–206]. Penile blood pressure may be measured directly by means of a doppler and penile blood pressure cuff [202, 203]. Penile prothesis (either semi-rigid and permanently erect or inflatable) may be efficacious following adequate family and psycho-social evaluation [207–214].

Preventative or definitive therapies

Improved control of hyperglycemia as treatment for clinically overt diabetic distal symmetrical polyneuropathy has been recommended by many [5, 18,

26, 136, 187] but proven efficacious by none. Hence, the diabetologist has no rational clinical basis on which to select among various alternatives of metabolic control for patients with distal symmetrical polyneuropathy. Prospective clinical trials, such as the Diabetes Control and Complications Trial, will hopefully resolve the role of intensive insulin regimens in the treatment or prevention of distal symmetrical polyneuropathy [192]. Furthermore, various specific metabolic interventions, based on specific metabolic pathogenetic hypotheses for diabetic neuropathy, have been attempted, with conflicting and/or marginal success, in part due to the difficulty in assessing clinical response in distal symmetrical polyneuropathy [26]. However, some of these agents are now undergoing or will shortly undergo carefully constructed large scale clinical trials to establish their potential efficacy in the treatment and/or prevention of diabetic neuropathy. Several sporadic attempts to administer oral *myo*-inositol supplements to small groups of diabetic subjects with or without clinically-overt diabetic neuropathy [26, 215–218] have yielded inconclusive results. Since patients with long-standing diabetes with or without superimposed clinical neuropathy were studied, the component of clinical neurological deficit or nerve conduction slowing that remained readily reversible within the time-frame of these short trials was not known, and the plasma *myo*-inositol elevations attained were modest compared to those in the rat studies [219]. Therefore, it is impossible to judge either the adequacy of the intervention or the power of the studies to detect a treatment effect if one were to have occurred. A well-designed, large-scale, prospective, comprehensive therapeutic trial of *myo*-inositol supplementation in diabetic neuropathy remains to be accomplished using carefully defined endpoints that are both sensitive to a treatment response and thought to be clinically relevant.

Although large-scale therapeutic trials of patented aldose reductase inhibitors using both clinical and electrophysiological endpoints are in progress, none have yet published their results. As with studies of *myo*-inositol supplementation, results from a handful of small, short-duration studies with aldose reductase inhibitors have appeared with somewhat conflicting results. For example, Fagius and Jameson [220] reported marginally improved symptom scores, sensory function, clinical examinations and nerve conduction in 30 patients in a placebo-controlled 12 week study with the aldose reductase inhibitor Alrestatin. However, Handelsman and Turtle [221] reported no benefit of the same drug in 9 neuropathic patients treated for over 1 year, and further studies with the drug were not undertaken because of significant hepatotoxicity [220–221]. Judzewitsch et al., using highly standardized and rigorous techniques to quantitate nerve conduction velocity in 39 well-defined patients with diabetes but without signs or symptoms of diabetic neuropathy, demonstrated that nine weeks of treatment with a different aldose reductase inhibitor, sorbinil 250 m/d, consistently and reproducibly raised median and peroneal motor and median sensory conduction velocity [222]. The magnitude of the increases were small, but of the same order of magnitude that the acute effect of blood glucose normalization produced by Troni [25] with the artificial pancreas; thus aldose reductase inhibition appeared to reproduce the effect of complete correction of insulin deficiency in restoring the rapidly-reversible component of nerve conduction slowing in non-neuropathic diabetic subjects. A more recent study, with a lower dose of sorbinil, and smaller number of patients, and different electrophysiological techniques, failed to find improved conduction velocity [223]. In an uncontrolled study in 11 patients with severely painful diabetic neuropathy, Jaspan et al [224] reported relief of pain and improved autonomic function in sub-groups of the patients, but possible "placebo" effects or the influence of sub-group analysis could not be excluded in this preliminary report. Young et al [225] reported improved pain, tendon reflex scores, and sural sensory potential amplitude but diminished scores of clinical sensory examinations in 15 neuropathic patients treated for 4 weeks with sorbinil in a double-blind crossover study, whereas similar studies with the same drug revealed no comparable improvement in 13 patients [226], or only an improvement in "overall subjective well-being" without confirmatory neurophysiological changes in 37 patients [226]. All of these studies were designed and carried out without knowing which clinical or electrophysiological parameters would be sensitive to improvement in the underlying pathology responsible for clinical signs and symptoms and neurological deficits in patients with overt clinical neuropathy, nor what duration of follow-up would be required. Indeed, except for the rapidly-reversible component of conduction slowing in asymptomatic diabetic subjects [14–16, 18, 20–24, 222], the extent to which diabetic neuropathy, and its largely anatomical basis is reversible in its clinically overt stage was still unresolved.

Therefore, attention turned to evaluation of underlying structural lesions in human peripheral nerve to explore the possible role of aldose reductase treatment in diabetic neuropathy. The effect of an aldose reductase inhibitor sorbinil on the underlying biochemical abnormalities and neuropathologicial lesions accompanying symptomatic diabetic peripheral polyneuropathy was explored in paired sural nerve fascicular biopsies obtained from 16 neuropathic subjects at entry and after completion of a 12-month randomized, placebo-controlled, double-masked clinical trial of the aldose reductase inhibitor sorbinil (250 mg/d). Sural nerve sorbitol levels declined in all but 1 patient over the 12-month study, and *myo*-inositol levels, which were decreased at baseline, were no longer statistically significantly different from control in the treated patients, but remained low in the placebo patients, where they tended to decrease (100). At the completion of the trial, sorbinil-treated patients exhibited a 4-fold increase in regenerating myelinated nerve fibers, a 33% increase in the number of myelinated fibers per unit cross sectional area of nerve, and evidence of repair of several myelinated-fiber lesions characteristic of diabetic neuropathy, such as axo-glial dysjunction and axonal atrophy [227]. The immediate clinical implications of this broad and active but early fiber regeneration and repair are uncertain. Accompanying electrophysiological and electromyographic evidence [228] suggest that these regenerating and remyelinating fibers are indeed functional. However, these young newly sprouting fibers of very small diameter would not be expected to have dramatic effects on composite nerve conduction velocity or amplitude. Their effects on painful and paresthetic symptoms, whose pathophysiological basis is controversial, are unknown. The extent to which these newly-regenerating fibers would produce a detectable decrease in sensory or motor deficits in distal symmetric diabetic neuropathy is equally uncertain. Thus this early stage of fiber regeneration and repair is more likely to herald rather than accompany any easily detectable clinical improvement. Thus, it is not surprising that short-term clinical responses to aldose reductase inhibitors would, as discussed above, reveal at best only marginal clinical improvement. On the other hand, the morphometric parameters improved by sorbinil, i. e fiber density and the frequency of teased fiber abnormalities, are just those parameters that distinguish diabetic subjects with and without clinical neuropathy [102]. Therefore, extrapolation of these early reparative and regenerative treatment responses to more prolonged administration of aldose reductase inhibitors would predict significant reversal of the characteristic morphometric and perhaps clinical components of diabetic neuropathy in patients afflicted with the disorder. These possibilities form the rationale for the longer-term prospective clinical trials with aldose reductase inhibitors that are currently underway. Other potential definitive forms of intervention e. g. thrombolytic, antiplatelet, or hemodynamic agonists have not yet been tested in clinical trials.

References

[1] Rollo J. Cases of Diabetes Mellitus. London: C Dilly, 1798.

[2] Johnson PC, Doll SC, Cromey DW. Pathogenesis of diabetic neuropathy. Ann Neurol 1986; 19: 450–457.

[3] Bernard C. Lecons sur le diabète et la glycogenèse animale. Paris: Baillière, 1877.

[4] Committee on Health Care Issues, American Neurological Association. Does improved control of glycemia prevent or ameliorate diabetic neuropathy? Ann Neurol 1986; 19: 288–290.

[5] Brown MJ, Greene DA. Diabetic Neuropathy: Pathophysiology and Management. In: Asbury AK, Gilliatt RW eds. Neurology, Peripheral Nerve Disorders: A Practical Approach. Boston: Butterworths, 1984; 126.
[6] Eng GD, Hung W, August GP et al. Nerve conduction velocity determinations in juvenile diabetes: Continuing study of 190 patients. Arch Phys Med Rehabil 1976; 57: 1.
[7] Pirart J. Diabetes mellitus and its degenerative complications: A prospective study of 4,400 patients observed between 1947 and 1973. Diabetes Care 1978; 1: 168–188, 252–263.
[8] Thomas PK, Ward JD, Watkins PJ. Diabetic Neuropathy. In: Keen H, Jarrett J, eds. Complications of Diabetes. London: Arnold, 1982; 109–136.
[9] Pirart J. Diabetic neuropathy: a metabolic or vascular disease? Diabetes 1965; 14: 1.
[10] Brown MJ, Asbury AK. Diabetic neuropathy. Ann Neurol 1984; 15: 2.
[11] Ward JD. Abnormal processes in the nerve. In: Brownlee M ed. Diabetes Mellitus. New York: Garland STPM Press, 1981; 87.
[12] Winegrad AI, Morrison AD, Greene DA. Late complication of diabetes. In: DeGroot LJ, Cahill G, Martini L et al eds. Endocrinology. New York: Grune & Stratton, Inc., 1979; 1045.
[13] MuCulloch DK, Campbell IW, Prescott RJ et al. Effect of alcohol intake on symptomatic peripheral neuropathy in diabetic men. Diabetes Care 1980; 3: 245.
[14] Gregerson G. Variations in motor conduction velocity produced by acute changes of the metabolic state in diabetic patients. Diabetologia 1968; 4: 273–277.
[15] Ward JD, Bowes CG, Fischer DJ et al. Improvement in nerve conduction following treatment in newly diagnosed diabetics. Lancet 1971; 1: 428–430.
[16] Terkidsen AB, Christensen NJ. Reversible nervous abnormalities in juvenile diabetics with recently diagnosed diabetes. Diabetologia 1971; 7: 113–117.
[17] Graf RJ, Halter JB, Halar E et al. Nerve conduction abnormalities in untreated maturity-onset diabetes: Relation to levels of fasting plasma glucose and glycosylated hemoglobin. Ann Intern Med 1979; 90: 298–303.
[18] Graf RJ, Halter JB, Pfeifer MD et al. Glycemic control and nerve conduction abnormalities in noninsulin-dependent diabetic subjects. Ann Intern Med 1981; 94: 307–311.
[19] Holman RR, White VM, Orde-Peckar C et al. Prevention of deterioration of renal and sensory-nerve function by more intensive management of insulin-dependent diabetic patients. A two-year randomized prospective study. Lancet 1983; 1: 204–208.
[20] Pietri A, Ehle A, Raskin P. Changes in nerve conduction velocity after six weeks of glycoregulation with portable insulin infusion pumps. Diabetes 1980; 29: 668–671.
[21] Service FJ, Rizza RA, Daube JR et al. Near normoglycaemia improved nerve conduction and vibration sensation in diabetic neuropathy. Diabetologia 1985; 28: 722–727.
[22] Steno Study Group. Effect of 6 months' strict metabolic control on eye and kidney function in insulin-dependent diabetes with background retinopathy. Lancet 1982; 1: 121–124.
[23] Gallai V, Agostini L, Rossi A et al. Evaluation of the motor and sensory conduction velocity (MCV, SCV) in diabetic patients before and after a three-day treatment with the artificial beta cell (Biostator). In: Canal N, Pozza G, eds. Peripheral Neuropathies. Amsterdam: Elsevier/North-Holland Biomedical Press, 1978; 287–289.
[24] Service FJ, Daube JR, O'Brien PC et al. Effect of artificial pancreas treatment on peripheral nerve function in diabetes. Neurology 1981; 31: 1375–1380.
[25] Troni W, Carta Q, Cantello R et al. Peripheral nerve function and metabolic control in diabetes mellitus. Ann Neurol 1984; 16: 178–183.
[26] Greene DA, Brown MJ, Braunstein SN et al. Comparison of clinical course and sequential electrophysiological tests in diabetics with symptomatic polyneuropathy and its implications for clinical trials. Diabetes 1981; 30: 139–147.
[27] Greene DA, Lattimer S, Ulbrecht J et al. Glucose-induced alterations in nerve metabolism: Current perspective on the pathogenesis of diabetic neuropathy and future directions for research and therapy. Diabetes Care 1985; 8: 290–299.

[28] Winegrad AI. Banting lecture 1986. Does a common mechanism induce the diverse complications of diabetes? Diabetes 1987; 36: 396–406.
[29] Greene DA, Lattimer SA, Sima AAF. Sorbitol, phosphoinositides, and sodium potassium-ATPase in the pathogenesis of diabetic complications. New Engl J Med 1987; 316: 599–606.
[30] Greene DA, Lattimer SA. Impaired rat sciatic nerve sodium-potassium adenosine triphosphatase in acute streptozotocin diabetes and its correction by dietary myo-inositol supplementation. J Clin Invest 1983; 72: 1058–1063.
[31] Greene DA. Metabolic abnormalities in diabetic peripheral nerve: relation to impaired function. Metabolism 1983; 32: 118–123.
[32] Greene DA, Yagihashi S, Lattimer SA et al. Nerve NA+-K+-ATPase, conduction and myoinositol in the insulin deficient BB-rat. Am J Physiol 1984; 247: E534–539.
[33] Greene DA, Lattimer SA. Impaired energy utilization and Na-K-ATPase in diabetic peripheral nerve. Am J Physiol 1984; 246: E311.
[34] Simmons DA, Winegrad AI, Martin DB. Significance in tissue myo-inositol concentrations in metabolic regulation in nerve. Science 1982; 217: 848.
[35] Greene DA, Lattimer SA. Protein kinase C agonists acutely normalize decreased ouabain-inhibitable respiration in diabetic rabbit nerve: implications for (Na,K)-ATPase regulation and diabetic complications. Diabetes 1986; 35: 242–245.
[36] Lattimer SA, Greene DA. Protein kinase C agonists rapidly correct impaired Na/K-ATPase in diabetic nerve in vitro. Diabetes 1987; 36: 75A.
[37] Sima AAF, Lattimer SA, Yagihashi S et al. Axoglial dysjunction: a novel structural lesion responsible for poorly-reversible nerve conduction slowing in the chronically diabetic BB-rat. J Clin Invest 1986; 77: 474–484.
[38] Mayhew JA, Gillon KRW, Hawthorne JN. Free and lipid inositol, sorbitol and sugars obtained post mortem from diabetic and control subjects. Diabetologia 1983; 24: 13–15.
[39] Dyck PJ, Sherman WR, Hallcher LM et al. Human diabetic endoneurial sorbitol, fructose and myo-inositol related to sural nerve morphometry. Ann Neurol 1980; 8: 590–596.
[40] Brismar T, Sima AAF. Changes in nodal function in nerve fibers of the spontaneously diabetic BB-Wistar rat. Potential clamp analysis. Acta Physiol Scand 1981; 113: 499–506.
[41] Greene DA, Lattimer SA, Sima AAF. Acute paranodal swelling and conduction-slowing in the insulin-deficient BB rat reflects myo-inositol depletion and Na/K-ATPase deficiency rather than sorbitol accumulation. Clin Res 1986; 34: 683A.
[42] Chakrabarti S, Sima AAF. Aldose reductase in the BB-rat: purification, immunological identification and localization in the retina and peripheral nerve. Diabetes 1986; 35: 406A.
[43] Greene DA, Lattimer SA, Finegold DN et al. Impaired Na-dependent amino acid uptake in diabetic peripheral nerve: correction by aldose reductase inhibition of myo-inositol supplementation. Clin Res 1985; 33: 431A.
[44] Streb H, Irvine RF, Berridge MJ et al. Release of Ca++ from a non-mitochondrial intracellular store in pancreatic acinar cells by inositol 1,4,5 triphosphate. Nature 1983; 306: 67–69.
[45] Nishizuka Y. Protein kinases in signal transduction. TIBS 1984; 9: 163–166.
[46] Asbury AK. Focal and multifocal neuropathies of diabetes. In: Dyck PF, Thomas PK, Winegrad AI et al., eds. Diabetic Neuropathy. Philadelphia: WB Saunders, 1987; 45–55.
[47] Dyck PJ, Lais A, Karnes JL et al. Fiber loss is primary and multifocal in sural nerves in diabetic polyneuropathy. Ann Neurol 1986; 19: 425–439.
[48] Williams E, Timperley WR, Ward JD et al. Electron microscopic studies of vessels in diabetic peripheral neuropathy. J Clin Pathol 1980; 33: 462–470.
[49] Fagerberg SE. Diabetic neuropathy, a clinical and histological study on the significance of vascular affection. Acta Med Scand 1959; 164: 1–97.
[50] Dyck PJ, Karnes JL, O'Brien P et al. The spatial distribution of fiber loss in diabetic polyneuropathy suggests ischemia. Ann Neurol 1986; 19: 440–449.

[51] Vracko R. A comparison of the microvascular lesions in diabetes mellitus with those of normal aging. J Am Geriatr Soc 1982; 30: 201–205.
[52] Yasuda H, Dyck PJ. Abnormalities of endoneurial microvessels and sural nerve pathology in diabetic neuropathy. Neurology 1987; 37: 20–28.
[53] Greene DA, Chakrabarti S, Lattimer SA et al. Role of sorbitol accumulation and myo-inositol depletion in paranodal swelling of large myelinated nerve fibers in the insulin-deficient spontaneously diabetic bio-breeding rat: Reversal by insulin replacement, an aldose reductase inhibitor and myo-inositol. J Clin Invest 1987; 79: 1479–1485.
[54] Sima AAF. Peripheral neuropathy in the spontaneously diabetic BB Wistar rat. Acta Neuropathol 1980; 51: 223–232.
[55] Sima AAF, Bouchier M, Christensen H. Axonal atrophy in sensory nerves of the diabetic BB-Wistar rat. A possible early correlate of human diabetic neuropathy. Ann Neurol 1983; 13: 264–272.
[56] Pryce TD. On diabetic neuritis with a clinical and pathologic description of diabetic pseudotabes. Brain 1983; 16: 416–424.
[57] Bischoff A. Ultrastructural pathology of peripheral nervous system in early diabetes. In: Camerini-Davalos RA, Cole HS eds. Vascular and Neurologic Changes in Early Diabetes. New York: Academic Press, 1973; 441–449.
[58] Reske-Nielsen E, Lundbaeck K. Pathological changes in the central and peripheral nervous system of young long-term diabetics. II. The spinal cord and peripheral nerves. Diabetologia 1968; 4: 34–43.
[59] Said G, Slama G, Selva J. Progression centripetal degeneration of axons in small fiber diabetic polyneuropathy. Brain 1983; 106: 791–807.
[60] Sima AAF, Larusso AC, Thibert P. Distal symmetric polyneuropathy in the spontaneously diabetic BB-Wistar rat. An ultrastructural and teased fiber study. Acta Neuropathol (Berlin) 1982; 58: 39–47.
[61] Low PA, Tuck RR, Takeuchi M. Nerve micro-environment in diabetic neuropathy. In: Dyck PJ, Thomas PK, Asbury AK et al, eds. Diabetic Neuropathy. Philadelphia: WB Saunders, 1987; 266–278.
[62] Tuck RR, Schmelzer JD, Low PA. Endoneurial blood flow and oxygen tension in the sciatic nerves of rats with experimental diabetic neuropathy. Brain 1984; 107: 935–950.
[63] Low PA, Ward K, Schmelzer JD et al. Ischemic conduction failure and energy metabolism in experimental diabetic neuropathy. Am J Physiol 1985; 248: E457–462.
[64] Greene DA, Winegrad AI. Effects of acute experimental diabetes on composite energy metabolism in peripheral nerve axons and Schwann cells. Diabetes 1981; 30: 967.
[65] Winegrad AI, Simmons DA. Energy metabolism in peripheral nerve. In: Dyck PJ, Thomas PK, Asbury AK et al, eds. Diabetic Neuropathy. New York: WB Saunders, 1987; 279–288.
[66] Low PA, Schmelzer JD, Ward KK. The effects of endoneurial hypoxia on peripheral nerve function. Neurology 1985; 35: 292 (abstract).
[67] Low PA, Schmelzer JD, Ward KK et al. Experimental chronic hypoxic neuropathy: relevance to diabetic neuropathy. Am J Physiol 1986; 250: E94–99.
[68] Low PA, Schmelzer JD, Ward KK et al. Effects of hyperbaric oxygenation on normal and chronic streptozotocin diabetic peripheral nerve. Neurology 1987; 37: 254 (abstract).
[69] Low PA, Tuck RR, Dyck PJ et al. Prevention of some electrophysiologic and biochemical abnormalities with oxygen supplementation in experimental diabetic neuropathy. Proc Natl Acad Sci USA 1984; 81: 6894–6898.
[70] Yao JK, Low PA. Improvement of endoneurial lipid abnormalities in experimental diabetic neuropathy by oxygen modification. Brain Res 1986; 362: 362–365.
[71] Newrick PG, Wilson AJ, Jakubowski J et al. Sural nerve oxygen tension in diabetes. Br Med J (Clin Res) 1986; 293: 1053–1054.
[72] Vlassara H, Brownlee M, Cerami A. Non-enzymatic glycosylation of 214. peripheral nerve protein in diabetes mellitus. Proc Natl Acad Sci USA 1981; 78: 5190–5192.

[73] Williams SK, Howarth NL, Devenny JJ et al. Structural and functional consequence of increased tubulin glycosylation in diabetes mellitus. Proc Natl Acad Sci USA 1982; 79: 6546–6550.

[74] Sharma AK, Duguid IGM, Blanchard DS et al. The effect of insulin treatment of myelinated nerve fiber maturation and integrity and on body growth in streptozotocin-diabetic rats. J Neurol Sci 1985; 67: 285.

[75] Sharma AK, Bajada S, Thomas PK. Influence of streptozotocin induced diabetes on myelinated nerve fiber maturation and on body growth in the rat. Acta Neuropath (Berl) 1981; 53: 257.

[76] Jakobsen J. Axonal dwindling in early experimental diabetes. I. A study of cross sectioned nerves. Diabetologia 1976; 12: 539.

[77] Robertson DM, Sima AAF. Diabetic neuropathy in the mutant mouse [C57/BL/Ks (db/db)]. A morphometric study. Diabetes 1980; 25: 60.

[78] Sima AAF, Robertson DM. Peripheral neuropathy in the diabetic mutant mouse [C57/BL/Ks (db/db)]. An ultrastructural study. Lab Invest 1979; 40: 627.

[79] Sima AAF, Zang WX, Tze WJ et al. Diabetic neuropathy in the streptozotocin diabetic rat and the effect of allegenetic islet cell transplantation. A morphometric analysis. Diabetologia (submitted).

[80] Sima AAF, Robertson DM. Peripheral neuropathy in mutant diabetic mouse [C57/BL/Ks (db/db)]. Acta Neuropath (Berl) 1978; 41: 85.

[81] Greene DA, Mackway AM. Decreased myo-inositol content and Na^+-K^+ATPase activity ain the superior cervical ganglion of STZ diabetic rat, and prevention by aldose reductase inhibition. Diabetes 1986; 35: 1106.

[82] Thomas PK, Wright DW, Tzeblikos E. Amino acid uptake by dorsal root ganglia from streptozotocin-diabetic rat. J Neurol Neurosurg Psychiatry 1984; 47: 912.

[83] Jakobsen J, Sidenius P. Decreased axonal transport of structural proteins in streptozotocin diabetic rats. J Clin Invest 1980; 66: 292.

[84] McLean WG, Meiri KF. Slow axonal transport of protein in sciatic motor nerves during early experimental diabetes. J Physiol 1980; 301: 57P.

[85] Medori R, Antilio-Gambetti L, Monaco S et al. Experimental diabetic neuropathy: impairment of slow transport with changes in axon cross-sectioned area. Proc Natl Acad Sci USA 1985; 82: 7716.

[86] Sima AAF. Neuropathic and ocular complications in the BB-Wistar rat. In: Shafrir E, Renold AE, eds. Lessons from Animal Diabetes. London: John Libbey: 1984; 447.

[87] Spences PS, Thomas PK. Ultrastructural studies on the dying-back process. II. The sequestration and removal by Schwann cells and oligodendrocytes of organelles from normal and diseased axons. J Neurocytol 1979: 3: 763.

[88] Sidenius P, Jakobsen J. Axonal transport in human and experimental diabetes. In: Dyck PJ, Thomas PK, Asbury AK et al, eds. Diabetic Neuropathy. Philadelphia: WB Saunders Co., 1987; 260.

[89] Masiori P, Vitadello M, Bianchi R et al. Impaired axonal transport of acetylcholinesterase in the sciatic nerve of alloxan-diabetic rats: Effect of ganglioside treatment. Diabetologia 1986; 29: 254.

[90] Mayer JH, Tomlinson DR. Axonal transport of cholinergic transmitter enzymes in vagus and sciatic nerves of rats with acute experimental diabetes mellitus: correlation with motor nerve conduction velocity and effects of insulin. Neuroscience 1983; 9: 951.

[91] Vitadello M, Couraud J-Y, Hassig R et al. Axonal transport of acetylcholinesterase in the diabetic mutant mouse. Exp Neurol 1983; 82: 143.

[92] Vitadello M, Filliatreau G, Dupont JL et al. Altered axonal transport of cytoskeletal proteins in the mutant diabetic mouse. J Neurochem 1985; 45: 860.

[93] Jakobsen J, Brimijoin S, Skan K et al. Retrograde axonal transport of transmitter enzymes, fucose-labeled protein and nerve growth factor in streptozotocin-diabetic rats. Diabetes 1981; 30: 797.

[94] Schmidt RE, Modert CW, Yip HK et al. Retrograde axonal transport of intravenously administered ^{125}I-nerve growth factor in rats with streptozotocin-induced diabetes. Diabetes 1983; 32: 654.
[95] Calker DV, Heumann R. Nerve growth factor potentiates the agonist-stimulated accumulation of inositol phosphates in PC-12 pheochromocytoma cells. European J Pharm 1987; 135: 259.
[96] Contreras ML, Guroff G. Calcium-dependent nerve growth factor-stimulated hydrolysis of phosphoinositides in PC12 cells. J Neurochem 1987; 48: 1466.
[97] Fisher SK, Agranoff BW. Receptor activation and inositol lipid hydrolysis in neural tissue. J Neurochem 1987; 48: 999.
[98] Ishii DN, Recio-Pinto E. Role of insulin, insulin-like growth factors, and nerve growth factor in neurite formation. In: Raizada MK, Phillips MI, Le Roith D, eds. Insulin, IFG's and Their Receptors in the Central Nervous System. New York: Plenum Pub, 1987; 315.
[99] Longo FM, Powell HC, Lebeau J et al. Delayed nerve regeneration in streptozotocin diabetic rats. Muscle and Nerve 1986; 9: 385.
[100] Chan K-FJ. Ganglioside-modulated protein phosphorylation in myelin. J Biol Chem 1987; 262: 2415.
[101] Dyck PJ, Karnes J, O'Brien PC. Diagnosis, staging, and classification of diabetic neuropathy and associations with other complications. In: Dyck PJ, Thomas PK, Winegrad AI et al, eds. Diabetic Neuropathy. Philadelphia: WB Saunders, 1987; 36.
[102] Eng GD, Nellinton H, August GP. Nerve conduction velocity determination in juvenile diabetes. Mod Probl Paediat 1975; 12: 213–219.
[103] Behse F, Buchthal F, Carlsen F. Nerve biopsy and conduction studies in diabetic neuropathy. J Neurol Neurosurg Psychiatry 1977; 40: 1072–1082.
[104] Woltman, HW, Wilder RM. Diabetes mellitus: pathologic changes in the spinal cord and peripheral nerves. Arch Intern Med 1929; 44: 575–603.
[105] Olsson Y, Säve-Söderbergh J, Sourander P et al. A pathoanatomical study of the central and peripheral nervous system in diabetes of early onset and long duration. Pathol Europ 3: 62–79.
[106] Budzilovich GN. Diabetic neuropathy complex. Virchow Arch Abt A Path Anat 1970; 350: 105–122.
[107] Thomas PK, Lascelles RG. Schwann-cell abnormalities in diabetic neuropathy. Lancet 1965; 1: 1355–1357.
[108] Thomas PK, Lascelles RG. The pathology of diabetic neuropathy. Q J Med 1966; 35: 489–509.
[109] Chopra JS, Fannin T. Pathology of diabetic neuropathy. J Path Bact 1971; 104: 175–184.
[110] Chopra JS, Hurwitz LJ, Montgomery DAD. The pathogenesis of sural nerve changes in diabetes mellitus. Brain 1969; 92: 391–418.
[111] Kimura J, Yamada T ad Stevland NP. Distal slowing of motor nerve conduction velocity in diabetic polyneuropathy. J Neurol Sci 1979; 42: 291–302.
[112] Hansen S, Ballanyne JP. Axonal dysfunction in the neuropathy of diabetes mellitus: A quantitative electrophysiological study. J Neurol Neurosurg Psychiatr 1977; 40: 555–564.
[113] Bischoff A. Diabetische Neuropathie. Dtsch Med Wochensch 1968; 93: 237–241.
[114] Bischoff A. Report at the Aarhus University 50 year Jubilee Symposium: Nervous system abnormalities and nervous disease in diabetes. Aarhus, Denmark, 1978.
[115] Yagihashi S, Matsumaja M. Ultrastructural pathology of peripheral nerves in patients with diabetic neuropathy. Tohoku J Exp Med 1979; 129: 357–366.
[116] Sima AAF, Nathaniel V, Bril V et al. Histopathological heterogeneity of neuropathy in insulin-dependent and non-insulin-dependent diabetes, and demonstration of axoglial dysjunction in human diabetic neuropathy. J Clin Invest 1988; 81: 349–364.
[117] Yue DK, Harwell MA, Satchell PM et al. The effect of aldose reductase inhibition on motor nerve conduction velocity in diabetic rats. Diabetes 1982; 31: 789–794.

[118] Sima AAF, Brismar T. Reversible diabetic nerve dysfunction: Structural correlates to electrophysiological abnormalities. Ann Neurol 1985; 18: 21–29.
[119] Greene DA, Bril V, Lattimer SA et al. Correction of myo-inositol depletion in diabetic human sural nerve by treatment with an aldose reductase inhibitor. Diabetes 1987; 36 (suppl 1): 86A.
[120] Asbury AK, Aldredge H, Herschberg R et al. Oculomotor palsy in diabetes mellitus: a clinicopathological study. Brain 1970; 93: 555.
[121] Dreyfus PM, Hakim S, Adams RD. Diabetic ophthalmoplegia. Arch Neurol Psychiatr 1957; 77: 337.
[122] Raff MC, Sangalang V, Asbury AK. Ischemic mononeuropathy multiplex associated with diabetes mellitus. Arch Neurol 1968; 18: 487.
[123] Appenzeller O, Ogin G. Myelinated fibers in human paravertebral sympathetic chain: white rami communicantes in alcoholic and diabetic patients. J Neurol Neurosurg Psychiat 1974; 37: 1155.
[124] Kristensson K, Nordborg C, Olsson Y et al. Changes in the vagus nerve in diabetes mellitus. Acta Pathol Microbiol Scand 1971; 79: 684.
[125] Smith B. Neuropathology of the oesophagous in diabetes mellitus. J Neurol Neurosurg Psychiat 1974; 37: 1151.
[126] Low PA, Walsh JC, Huang CY et al. The sympathetic nervous system in diabetic neuropathy – a clinical and pathological study. Brain 1975; 98: 357.
[127] Faerman I, Glacer L, Celener D et al. Autonomic nervous system and diabetes: histological and histochemical study of the autonomic nerve fibers of the urinary bladder in diabetic patients. Diabetes 1973; 22: 225.
[128] Appenzeller O, Richardson EP, Jr. The sympathetic chain in patients with diabetic and alcoholic polyneuropathy. Neurology 1966; 16: 1205.
[129] Duchen LW, Anjorin A, Watkins PJ et al. Pathology of autonomic neuropathy in diabetes. Ann Intern Med 1980: 92: 301.
[130] Consensus statement. Report and recommendations of the San Antonio Conference on Diabetic Neuropathy. Diabetes 1988: 37: 1000–1004.
[130a] Matschinsky FM et al. Design and application of quantitative histochemical and tissue culture approaches to test the myoinositol depletion hypotheses explaining the complications of diabetes. In: Shafrir E, Renold AE, eds. Frontiers in Diabetes Research. Lessons from Animal Diabetes II. John Libbey & Company Ltd., Chapt VIII.9 1988; 500–504.
[131] Melton LJ, Dyck PJ. Epidemiology. In: Dyck PJ, Thomas PK, Winegrad AI et al, eds. Diabetic Neuropathy. Philadelphia: WB Saunders, 1987; 27.
[132] Thomas PK, Brown MJ. Diabetic polyneuropathy. In: Dyck PJ, Thomas PK, Winegrad AI, Porte D eds. Diabetic Neuropathy. Philadelphia: WB Saunders, 1987; 56.
[133] Greene DA, Pfeifer M. Diabetic neuropathy. In: Olefsky JM, Sherwin R eds. New Concepts in Treatment and Complications of Diabetes, Contemporary Issues in Endocrinology and Metabolism. Churchill Livingstone Inc., Vol I, 1985; 223.
[134] Dyck PJ, Zimmerman BR, Vilen TH et al. Nerve glucose, fructose, sorbitol, myo-inositol, and fiber degeneration and regeneration in diabetic neuropathy. N Engl J Med 1988; 319: 542–548.
[135] Sima AAF, Bril V, Nathaniel V et al. Regeneration and repair of myelinated fibers in sural-nerve biopsy specimens from patients with diabetic neuropathy treated with sorbinil. N Engl J Med 1988; 319: 548–555.
[136] Gregersen G. Diabetic neuropathy: Influence of age, sex, metabolic control and duration of diabetes on motor conduction velocity. Neurology 1967; 17: 972–980.
[137] The DCCT Research Group. Factors in development of diabetic neuropathy: baseline analysis of neuropathy in feasibility phase of diabetes control and complications trial [DCCT]. Diabetes 1988; 37: 476–481.
[138] Gadia MT, Natori N, Ramos LB et al. Influence of height on quantitative sensory, nerve conduction, and clinical indices of diabetic peripheral neuropathy. Diabetes Care 1987; 10: 613–616.

[139] Wager EW, Buerger AA. A linear relationship between H-reflex latency and sensory conduction velocity in diabetic neuropathy. Neurology 1974; 24: 711–714.
[140] Dorfman LH, Cummins KL, Reaven GM et al. Studies of diabetic polyneuropathy using conduction velocity distribution (DCV) analysis. Neurology 1983; 33: 773–779.
[141] Horowitz SH, Ginsberg-Fellner F. Ischemia and sensory nerve conduction in diabetes mellitus. Neurology 1979; 29: 695–704.
[142] Gilliatt RW, Willison RG. Peripheral nerve conduction in diabetic neuropathy. J Neurol Neurosurg Psychiatry 1962; 25: 11–18.
[143] Odusote K, Ohwovoriole H, Roberts O. Electrophysiological quantification of distal polyneuropathy in diabetes. Neurology 1985; 35: 1432–1437.
[144] Dyck PJ, Karnes J, O'Brian PC. Detection thresholds of cutaneous sensation. In: Dyck PJ, Thomas PK, Asbury AK et al, eds. Diabetic Neuropathy. Philadelphia: WB Saunders, 1987; 107–121.
[145] Williamson RT. The vibrating sensation in affections of the nervous system and in diabetes. Lancet 1905; 1: 855.
[146] Williamson RT. The vibrating sensation in diseases of the nervous system. Am J Med Sci 1922; 164: 715.
[147] Barach JH. Test for quantitative vibratory sensation in diabetes, pernicious anemia, and tabes dorsalis. Arch Intern Med 1947; 79: 602.
[148] Collins WS, Zilinsky JD, Boas LC. Impaired vibratory sense in diabetes. Am J Med 1946; 1: 638.
[149] Nielsen VK, Lund FS. Diabetic polyneuropathy. Corneal sensitivity, vibratory perception and Achilles tendon reflex in diabetics. Acta Neurol Scand 1979; 59: 15.
[150] Chochinow RH, Ullyot LE, Moorhouse JA. Sensory perception thresholds in patients with juvenile diabetes and their close relatives. N Engl J Med 1972; 286: 1233.
[151] Goldberg JM, Lindblom U. Standardized method of determining vibratory perception thresholds for diagnosis and screening in neurological investigation. J Neurol Neurosurg Psychiatr 1979; 42: 793–803.
[152] Arezzo JC, Schaumburg HH, Laudadio C. Thermal sensitivity tester: device for quantitative assessment of diabetic neuropathy. Diabetes 1986; 35: 590.
[153] Arezzo JC, Schaumburg HH, Petersen CA. Rapid screening for peripheral neuropathy: a field study with the Optacon. Neurology 1983; 33: 626.
[154] Conomy JP, Barnes KL, Conomy JM. Cutaneous sensory function in diabetes mellitus. J Neurol Neurosurg Psychiatry 1979; 42: 656.
[155] Pfeifer MA, Winberg CR, Cook DL et al. Autonomic neural dysfunction in recently diagnosed diabetic subjects. Diabetes Care 1984; 7: 447–453.
[156] Hilsted J, Jensen SB. A simple test for autonomic neuropathy in juvenile diabetics. Acta Med Scand 1979; 205: 385–387.
[157] Genovely H, Pfeifer MA. RR-variation: the autonomic test of choice in diabetes. Diab/Metab Revs 1988; 4: 255–271.
[158] Ewing DJ, Campbell IW, Burt AA, Clarke BF. Vascular reflexes in diabetic autonomic neuropathy. The Lancet 1973; 2: 1354–1356.
[159] Hilsted J. Testing for autonomic neuropathy. Ann Clin Res 1984: 16: 128–135.
[160] Law PA, Fealey RD. Sudomotor neuropathy. In: Dyck PJ, Thomas PK, Asbury Ak et al, eds. Diabetic Neuropathy. Philadelphia: WB Saunders Co, 1988; 140–145.
[161] Pfeifer MA, Cook D, Brodsky J et al. Quantitative evaluation of sympathetic and parasympathetic control of iris function. Diabetes Care 1982; 5: 518–528.
[162] Smith SH, Smith SE. Assessment of pupillary function in diabetic neuropathy. In: Dyck PJ, Thomas PK, Asbury AK, eds. Diabetic Neuropathy. Philadelphia: WB Saunders Co, 1988; 134–139.
[163] Hilsted J, Madsbad S, Krarup T. et al. Hormonal, metabolic and cardiovascular responses to hypoglycemia in diabetic autonomic neuropathy. Diabetes 1981; 30: 626–633.
[164] Hilsted J. Testing for autonomic neuropathy. Ann Clin Res 1984; 16: 128–135.

[165] McCulloch DK, Campbell IW, Prescott RJ et al. Effect of alcohol intake on symptomatic peripheral neuropathy in diabetic men. Diabetes Care 1980; 3: 245–247.
[166] Sosenko JM, Gadia MT, Fournier AM et al. Body stature as a risk factor for diabetic sensory neuropathy. Amer J Med 1986; 80: 1031–1034.
[167] Gadia MT, Natori N, Ramos LB et al. Influence of height on quantitative sensory, nerve conduction and clinical indices of diabetic peripheral neuropathy. Diabetes Care 1987; 10: 613–616.
[168] Brown MJ, Martin JR, Asbury AK. Painful diabetic neuropathy. A morphometric study. Arch Neurol 1976; 33: 164–171.
[169] Ellenberg M. Diabetic neuropathy: clinical aspects. Metabolism 1976; 25: 1627–1655.
[170] Sinha S, Munichoodappa CS, Kozak GP. Neuroarthropathy (Charcot joints) in diabetes mellitus: clinical study of 101 cases. Medicine 1972; 51: 191–220.
[171] Boden G., Reichard GA Jr, Hoeldtke RD et al. Severe insulin-induced hypoglycemia associated with deficiencies in the release of counter-regulatory hormones. N Engl J Med 1981; 305: 1200–1205.
[172] Cryer PE, Silverberg AB, Santiage JV et al. Plasma catecholamines in diabetes. The syndromes of hypoadrenergic and hyperadrenergic postural hypotension. Am J Med 1978; 64: 407–416.
[173] Odel HM, Roth GM, Keating FR. Autonomic neuropathy stimulating the effects of sympathectomy as a complication of diabetes. Diabetes 1955; 4: 92–98.
[174] Goodman JI. Diabetic anhidrosis. Am J Med 1966; 41: 831–835.
[175] Buck AC, Reed PI, Siddiq YK et al. Bladder dysfunction and neuropathy in diabetes. Diabetologia 1976; 12: 251–258.
[176] Hosking DJ, Bennett T, Hampton JR. Diabetic autonomic neuropathy. Diabetes 1978; 27: 1043–1054.
[177] Frimodt-Moller C. Diabetic cystopathy. I. A clinical study of the frequency of bladder dysfunction in diabetics. Dan Med Bull 1976; 23: 267–278.
[178] Balfour J, Ankerman GJ. Atonic neurogenic bladder as a manifestation of diabetic neuropathy. J Urol 1956; 76: 746–752.
[179] Tohmeh JF, Shah SD, Cryer PE. The pathogenesis of hyperadrenergic postural hypotension in diabetic patients. Am J Med 1979; 67: 772.
[180] Olshan AR, O'Connor DT, Cohen IM et al. Baroreflex dysfunction in patients with adult-onset diabetes and hypertension. Am J Med 1983; 74: 233.
[181] Sundkvist G, Lilja B, Almer LO. Abnormal diastolic blood pressure and heart rate reactions to tilting in diabetes mellitus. Diabetologia 1980; 19: 433.
[182] Andaloro VA, Dube A. Treatment of retrograde ejaculation with brompheniramine. Urology 1975; 5: 520–522.
[183] Budd HA. Brompheniramine in treatment of retrograde ejaculation. Urology 1975; 6: 131.
[184] Walters D, Kaufman MS. Sterility due to retrograde ejaculation of semen: report of pregnancy achieved by autoinsemination. Am J Obstet Gynecol 1959; 78: 274–275.
[185] Clarke BF, Ewing DJ, Campbell IW. Diabetic autonomic neuropathy. Diabetologia 1979; 17: 195.
[186] Pinder RM, Brogden RN, Sawyer PR et al. Metoclopramide: a review of its pharmacological properties and clinical use. Drugs 1976; 12: 81.
[187] Boulton AJM, Drury J, Clarke B et al. Continuous subcutaneous insulin infusion in the management of painful diabetic neuropathy. Diabetes Care 1982; 5: 386–390.
[188] Davis JL, Lewis SB, Gerich JE et al. Peripheral diabetic neuropathy treated with amitriptyline and fluphenazine. JAMA 1977; 238: 2291–2292.
[189] Saudek CD, Werns S, Reidenberg MM. Phenytoin in the treatment of diabetic symmetrical polyneuropathy. Clin Pharm Therapeut 1977; 22: 196–199.
[190] Levine JD, Gordon NC, Bornstein JC et al. Role of pain in placebo analgesia. Proc Natl Acad Sci 1979; 76: 3528–3531.

[190a] Rull JA, Quibrera R, Gonzalez-Millan H et al. Symptomatic treatment of peripheral diabetic neuropathy with carbamazine (Tegretol): double blind crossover trial. Diabetologia 1969; 5: 215–218.
[190b] Young RJ, Clarke BF. Pain relief in diabetic neuropathy: the effectiveness of imipramine and related drugs. Diabetic Medicine 1985; 2: 363–366.
[190c] Kastrup J, Petersen P, Dejgard A et al. Treatment of chronic painful diabetic neuropathy with intravenous lidocaine. Br Med J 1986; 292: 173–175.
[190d] Dejgard A, Petersen P, Kastrup J. Mexiletine for treatment of chronic painful diabetic neuropathy. Lancet 1988; 1: 9–11.
[191] Turkington RW. Depression masquerading as diabetic neuropathy. JAMA 1980; 243: 1147–1150.
[192] Ellenberg M. Diabetic neuropathic chachexia. Diabetes 1974; 23: 5–9.
[193] Karacan I, Salis PJ, Williams RL. The roles of the sleep laboratory in the diagnosis and treatment of impotence. In: Williams RL, Laracan I eds. Sleep Disorders: Diagnosis and Treatment. John Wiley and Sons, 1978; 353–382.
[194] Karacan I, Salis PJ, Ware JC et al. Nocturnal penile tumescence and diagnosis in diabetic impotence. Am J Psychiatry 1978; 135: 191–197.
[195] Aners EK, Bradley WE, Krane RL. Snap-guage band: new concept in measuring penile rigidity. Urology 1983; 21: 63.
[196] Schiavi RC. Physiological treatment of erectile disorders in diabetic patients. Ann Intern Med 1980; 92: 337–339.
[197] Kent JR. Gonodal function in impotent diabetic males. Diabetes 1966; 15: 537.
[198] Faerman I, Vilar O, Rivaiola MA et al. Impotence and diabetes. Studies of androgenic function in diabetic impotent males. Diabetes 1972; 21: 23–30.
[199] Wright AD, London DR, Holder G et al. Lutenizing release hormone tests in impotent diabetic males. Diabetes 1976; 25: 975–977.
[200] Karacan I. Diagnosis of erectile impotence in diabetes mellitus. Ann Intern Med 1980; 92: 334–337.
[201] Barike A. Sexual dysfunction associated with hyperprolactinemia. Med Aspects Hum Sexual 1979; 13: 117–119.
[202] Abelson D. Diagnostic value of the penile pulse and blood pressure: a doppler study of impotence in diabetes. J Urol 1975; 113: 636–639.
[203] Gaskall P. The importance of penile blood pressure in cases of impotence. Can Med Assoc J 1971; 105: 1047–1051.
[204] Jevtich MJ, Edson M, Jarman WB et al. Vascular factor in erectile failure among diabetics. Urology 1982; 19: 163–168.
[205] Jevtich MJ. Importance of penile arterial pulse sound examination in impotence. J Urol 1980; 124: 820–824.
[206] Michal V, Kramer R, Pospichal J et al. Direct arterial anastomosis to the cavernous body in the treatment of erectile impotence. Rozhl Chir 1973; 52: 587–589.
[207] Small MP. Small-carrion penile prosthesis: a new implant for management of impotence. Mayo Clin Proc 1976; 51: 336–338.
[208] Scott FB, Fisman IJ, Light JK. An inflatable penile prosthesis for treatment of diabetic impotence. Ann Intern Med 1980; 92: 340–342.
[209] Malloy TR, Voneschenbach AC. Surgical treatment of erectile impotence with inflatable penile prosthesis. J Urol 1977; 118: 677–679.
[210] Scott FB, Byrd GJ, Karacan I et al. Erectile impotence treated with an implantable inflatable prothesis: five years of clinical experience. JAMA 1979; 241: 2609–2612.
[211] Gerstenberger DL, Osborne D, Furlow WL. Inflatable penile prosthesis. Follow-up study of patient–partner satisfaction. Urology 1979; 14: 583–587.
[212] Kamarsky-Binkhorst S. Female partner perception of small-carrion implant. Urology 1978; 7: 545–548.

[213] Beaser RS, Vanderhock C, Jacobson AM et al. Experience with penile prosthesis in the treatment of impotence in diabetic men. JAMA 1982; 248: 943–948.

[214] Pfeifer MA, Reenan A, Berger R et al. Penile prosthesis and quality of life. Diabetes 1983; 33 (suppl 1): 307.

[215] Clements RS, Vourganti B, Kuba T et al. Dietary myo-inositol intake and peripheral nerve function in diabetic neuropathy. Metabolism 1979; 28 (suppl 1): 477.

[216] Gregersen G, Bertelsen B, Harbo H et al. Oral supplementation of myo-inositol: Effects on peripheral nerve function in human diabetics and on the concentration in plasma, erythrocytes, urine, and muscle tissue in human diabetics and normals. Acta Neurol Scand 1983; 67: 164.

[217] Gregersen G. Børsting H, Theil P et al. Myo-inositol and function of peripheral nerves in human diabetics. A controlled clinical trial. Acta Neurol 1978; 58: 241.

[218] Salway JG, Finnegan JA, Barnett D et al. Effect of myo-inositol on peripheral-nerve function in diabetes. Lancet 1978; 2: 1282.

[219] Gregersen G. Myo-inositol supplementation. In: Dyck PJ, Asbury AK, Winegrad AI et al, eds. Diabetic Neuropathy. Philadelphia: WB Saunders, 1987; 188.

[220] Fagius J, Jameson S. Effects of aldose reductase inhibitor treatment in diabetic polyneuropathy – a clinical and neurophysiological study. J Neurol Neurosurg Psychiatr 1981; 44: 991.

[221] Handelsman DJ, Turtle JR. Clinical trial of an aldose reductase inhibitor in diabetic neuropathy. Diabetes 1981; 30: 459.

[222] Judzewitsch RG, Jaspan JB, Polonsky KS et al. Aldose reductase inhibition improves nerve conduction velocity in diabetic patients. N Engl J Med 1983; 308: 119.

[223] Martyn CN, Reid W, Young RJ et al. Six-month treatment with sorbinil in asymptomatic diabetic neuropathy: failure to improve abnormal nerve function. Diabetes 1987; 36: 987.

[224] Jaspan J, Maselli, R, Herold K et al. Treatment of severely painful diabetic neuropathy with an aldose reductase inhibitor: relief of pain and improved somatic and autonomic nerve function. Lancet 1983; 2: 758.

[225] Young RJ, Ewing DJ, Clarke BF. A controlled trial of sorbinil, an aldose reductase inhibitor, in chronic painful diabetic neuropathy. Diabetes 1983; 32: 938.

[226] Lewin IG, O'Brien IAD, Morgan MH et al. Clinical and neurophysiological studies with the aldose reductase inhibitor sorbinil in symptomatic diabetic neuropathy. Diabetologia 1984; 26: 445.

[227] Greene DA, Bril V, Sima AAF. Aldose reductase inhibitors promote sural nerve fiber regeneration and repair in patients with diabetic neuropathy. Clin Res. 1987; 35(3): 623A.

[228] Bril V, Werb MR, Greene DA et al. SFEMG response to sorbinil therapy. Sixth International Symposium in Single Fiber EMG, Vienna, Austria, June 1986.

Diabetes and heart disease

K. Pyörälä

Introduction

Heart disease is a major cause of mortality and morbidity among diabetic patients. Diabetes enhances the development of atherosclerosis, and coronary heart disease (CHD), an atherosclerotic vascular disease, is the most important form of heart disease in diabetic patients. Hypertension is commoner in diabetics than in non-diabetics and this may contribute to the occurrence of heart disease in diabetic patients. Independent of the excessive occurrence of CHD and hypertension in diabetic patients, diabetes itself is known to cause a specific heart muscle disease which may lead to left ventricular dysfunction and cardiac failure.

In the majority of earlier studies on diabetes and heart disease the two major types of diabetes, insulin-dependent diabetes mellitus (IDDM) and non-insulin-dependent diabetes mellitus (NIDDM), were not considered separately. More recent studies have made this distinction and these studies have revealed several new aspects of the occurrence and pathogenesis of various forms of heart disease in diabetes. This paper will review diabetes and heart disease from a clinical-epidemiological point-of-view, concentrating mainly on CHD in diabetes and only briefly commenting on the contribution of hypertension to heart disease in diabetes and on diabetic heart muscle disease. (For a detailed review on CHD and other forms of atherosclerotic vascular disease in diabetes see [1, 2].)

Diabetes and coronary heart disease

Autopsy studies and clinical angiographic studies on coronary atherosclerosis in diabetics versus non-diabetics

The so-called International Atherosclerosis Project [3] still remains the most important source of information concerning the extent of coronary atherosclerosis in diabetic patients as compared with that in non-diabetic subjects.

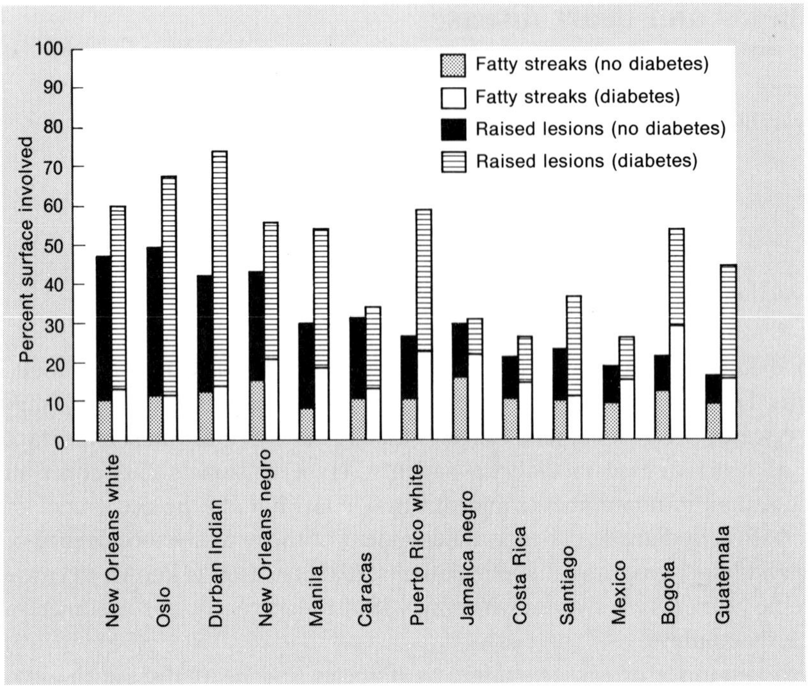

Fig. 1 Mean extent of atherosclerotic lesions in coronary arteries of non-diabetic and diabetic men aged 45–54 years in the study populations of the International Atherosclerosis Project [3].

In this autopsy study coronary arteries were collected and examined using a standardized protocol. As shown in Figure 1, in 13 populations representing a wide range of the occurrence of coronary atherosclerosis, in most instances the average extent of atherosclerotic lesions in the coronary arteries was markedly greater in diabetics than in non-diabetics. There was some increase in the extent of fatty streaks in diabetics, but the extent of raised lesions was especially increased. In this study distinction was not made between IDDM and NIDDM, but since the autopsy series mainly comprised middle-aged and elderly subjects, the majority of diabetics must have had NIDDM. In the International Atherosclerosis Project the variation between populations in the extent of coronary atherosclerosis in diabetics in general followed the same pattern as in non-diabetics, i. e., in populations with low mean extent of coronary atherosclerosis in non-diabetics, the extent of coronary atherosclerosis tended to be low also in diabetics and vice versa. However, even in populations with generally low levels of coronary atherosclerosis, the extent of atherosclerosis was usually higher in diabetics than in non-diabetics.

Another large autopsy study, the WHO-coordinated autopsy study carried out in five European towns [4, 5], confirmed the findings of the International Atherosclerosis Project concerning the increased extent of coronary atherosclerosis in diabetics. This study also dealt mainly with subjects dying above the age of 50 years and did not give information about the occurrence of coronary atherosclerosis in young patients with IDDM. More recently two smaller autopsy studies applying modern quantitative methods have demonstrated the increased extent and severity of coronary atherosclerosis in diabetics as compared to non-diabetics [6, 7]. One of them [6] showed that the extent of stenosing atherosclerotic lesions of the coronary arteries is markedly already increased in young adult patients with IDDM as compared to non-diabetic subjects of the same age.

Clinical angiographic studies carried out in patients with symptomatic CHD have serious limitations for the comparison of the severity of coronary atherosclerosis in diabetics and non-diabetics, because patients with equally severe symptoms may be expected to show, on the average, the same severity of atherosclerotic lesions, irrespective of the presence or absence of diabetes. In three angiographic studies [8–10] the severity of coronary atherosclerosis in diabetics was either equal to or somewhat greater than in non-diabetics. There was no clear indication in these studies that there is a more diffuse and peripheral distribution of atherosclerotic lesions in diabetics than in non-diabetics.

Frequency of coronary heart disease in diabetics versus non-diabetics

Although it has long been known that patients who develop IDDM at a young age often develop premature CHD, reliable quantitative data on the magnitude of the excess risk have not been available. Investigators from the Joslin Diabetes Center, Boston, Massachusetts, have, however, recently published a follow-up study of a cohort of 300 patients with juvenile-onset IDDM [11]. This study compared CHD mortality among these diabetics with that observed in the general population over a period of 20 to 40 years [11]. As shown in Figure 2, male and female patients with IDDM had a markedly increased risk of CHD death as compared to non-diabetic age-matched cohorts from the Framingham Study population. The earliest CHD deaths among the diabetics and control subjects occurred in early thirties, and after the age of 30 the excess CHD mortality of diabetics increased markedly. The cumulative CHD mortality of diabetics at the age of 55 years was about 35%. As shown in Figure 3, the excess CHD mortality in patients with IDDM was not related to the age at the onset of diabetes. It was, however, strongly

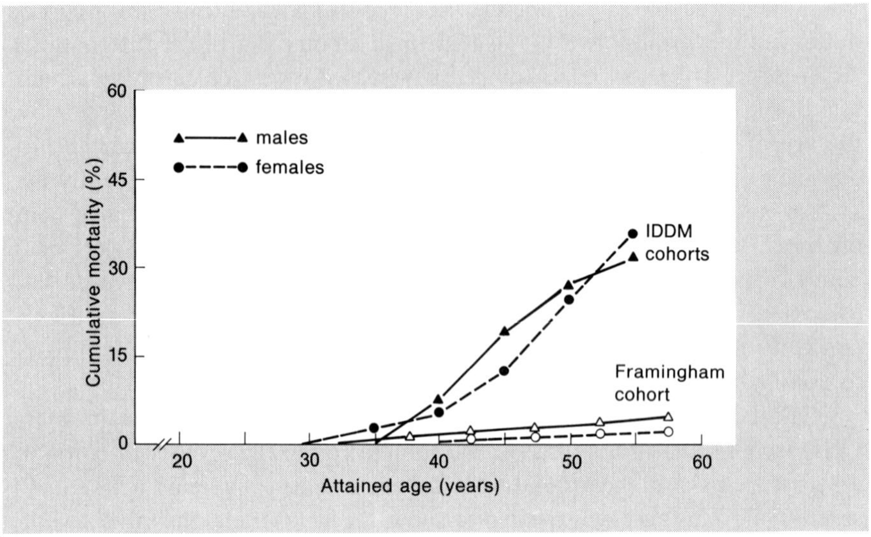

Fig. 2 Cumulative coronary heart disease mortality up to the age of 55 years in patients with insulin-dependent diabetes mellitus (IDDM) and in the Framingham Study population [11].

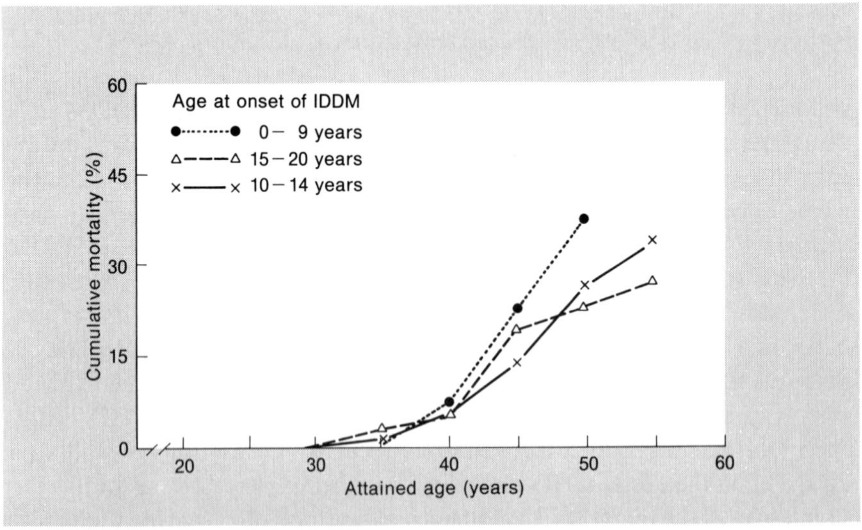

Fig. 3 Cumulative coronary heart disease mortality up to the age of 55 years in patients with insulin-dependent diabetes mellitus (IDDM) according to the age of onset of diabetes [11].

related to antecedent nephropathy, and the findings from this study suggested that in the absence of nephropathy the age-specific CHD mortality rate of patients with IDDM would be cut in half. Even so, the age-specific CHD mortality rates for patients with IDDM without proteinuria were still much higher than CHD mortality rates for non-diabetic subjects. The Joslin Diabetes Center investigators also addressed the question as to whether the particularly high CHD mortality in patients with diabetic nephropathy could be explained by hypertension or microvascular disease, both of which usually accompany diabetic nephropathy but may also occur without it. A case-control study carried out in the Joslin Diabetes Center series of diabetics indicated that, although hypertension without nephropathy caused a 6-fold increase in the CHD risk, this increase was markedly smaller than the 15-fold increase in the presence of nephropathy. Proliferative retinopathy without nephropathy was not associated with an increased CHD risk.

Several large population studies originally designed to investigate the incidence of CHD and its risk factors have included representative groups of middle-aged or elderly diabetics. The majority of these diabetics evidently had NIDDM, although distinction between the two main types of diabetes was not made. These studies, including the Framingham Study [12–15], the Isreal Ischaemic Heart Disease Study [16], the Whitehall Study [17, 18], and the Finnish Social Insurance Institution Study [19], have shown that the incidence of both total and non-fatal CHD events is from 1.5 to more than 3 times higher in middle-aged or elderly diabetic patients than in non-diabetic subjects of the same age. Figure 4 shows the incidence of all types of CHD events, myocardial infarction, angina pectoris, and sudden death in diabetic and non-diabetic men and women of the Framingham Study population. The excess risk of CHD associated with diabetes was more marked in women than in men, a finding confirmed by other studies including both men and women (e.g., [19]).

Since 1979 our own research group at the University of Kuopio has been carrying out population-based, prospective cohort studies of middle-aged patients with NIDDM and randomly selected, comparable control subjects with the main focus on the occurrence of CHD and other atherosclerotic vascular diseases and their risk factors [20, 21]. A striking finding in the cross-sectional baseline results of these studies was that the prevalence of previous definite myocardial infarction and angina pectoris was, within each sex, almost the same in patients with newly diagnosed NIDDM and in patients with previously known NIDDM of varying duration (Table 1). The CHD mortality rates of middle-aged previously known diabetics, newly diagnosed diabetics, and non-diabetic subjects were compared in the Finnish Social Insurance

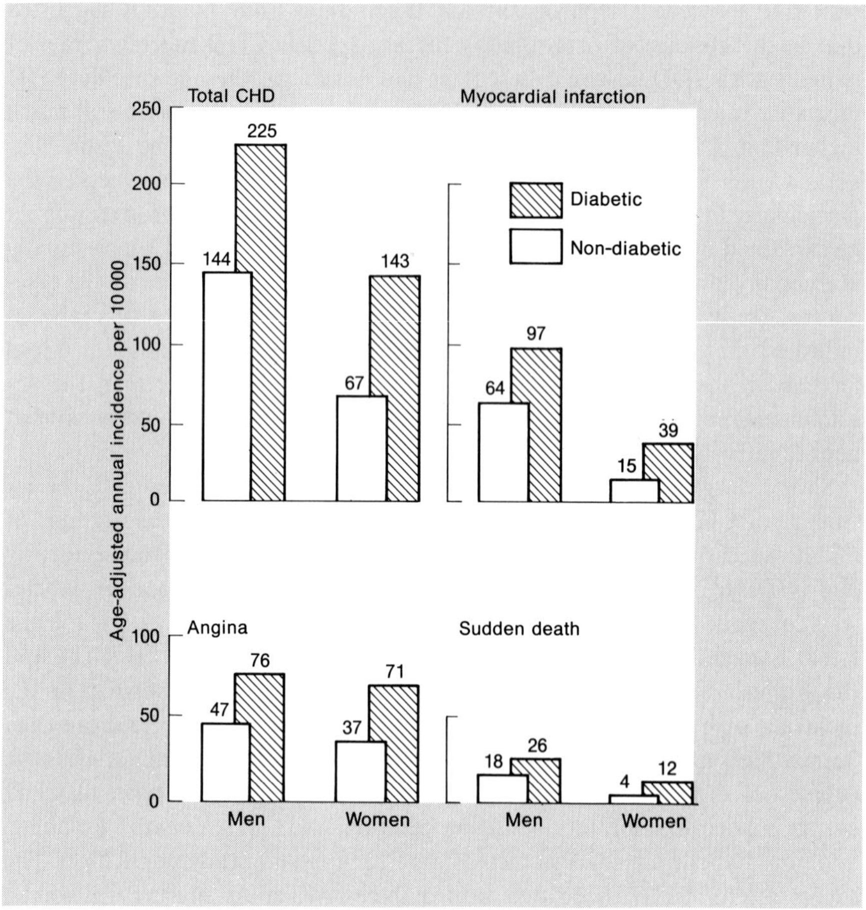

Fig. 4 The age-adjusted incidence of clinical manifestations of coronary heart disease in diabetic and non-diabetic men and women aged 45 – 74 years; 18-year follow-up results from the Framingham Study [13].

Institution Study population based on an average follow-up period of 11 years (Reunanen et al, unpublished results). The age-adjusted relative risks of CHD death in diabetes as compared to non-diabetics were as follows: among newly diagnosed diabetics 2.0 for men and 4.1 for women; among previously known diabetics 2.6 for men and 3.6 for women.

It is important to note in this context that CHD already occurs at an increased rate in the precursor stage of NIDDM, that is, in subjects showing impaired glucose tolerance (IGT) in an oral glucose tolerance test. This has

Table 1 Age-adjusted prevalence (%) of previous definite myocardial infarction and angina pectoris in men and women with newly diagnosed and previously known NIDDM aged 45–64 years and corresponding non-diabetic control subjects living in the Kuopio University Central Hospital district, East Finland (Uusitupa et al 1985, Laakso 1986)

	Men		
	Patients with newly diagnosed NIDDM (n = 70)	Patients with previously known NIDDM (n = 253)	Non-diabetic control subjects (n = 313)
Previous definite myocardial infarction¹)	16.5	20.3	8.3
Angina pectoris²)	44.0	44.2	19.9
	Women		
	Patients with newly diagnosed NIDDM (n = 63)	Patients with previously known NIDDM (n = 257)	Non-diabetic control subjects (n = 336)
Previous definite myocardial infarction¹)	17.7	7.9	2.1
Angina pectoris²)	43.3	35.7	19.8

¹) Minnesota Code 1.1–2 Q/QS-abnormalities or myocardial infarction verified at hospital
²) The Rose cardiovascular questionnaire

been shown in many studies (for a recent review see [2]), most convincingly in the Whitehall Study [17], the Paris Prospective Study [22] and the Helsinki Policemen Study [23]. These studies have shown that there is a positive, non-linear relationship between blood glucose levels after oral glucose load and CHD mortality and morbidity, with a sharp increase of CHD rate at the upper end of blood glucose distribution.

Possible mechanisms leading to the excessive occurrence of coronary heart disease in diabetics

Possible mechanisms which could explain the excessive occurrence of CHD in diabetic patients may be considered from two angles:

1. The effects of diabetes on the levels of general cardiovascular risk factors known to be causally linked to the occurrence of CHD in non-diabetic subjects.

2. Direct effects of hyperglycaemia or factors associated with diabetes itself on atherogenesis and/or thrombogenesis.

Table 2 attempts to give a summary of the various abnormalities in general cardiovascular risk factors in IDDM without and with nephropathy, in IGT and in NIDDM (for a recent review see [2]).

Elevation of blood pressure is not a common finding in uncomplicated IDDM, but already in early stages of diabetic nephropathy, blood pressure tends to become elevated. As to the levels of plasma lipids and lipoproteins, total and LDL cholesterol levels are not consistently elevated in IDDM if metabolic control is good. HDL cholesterol level is normal or even increased in IDDM and plasma total and VLDL triglyceride levels are usually not increased. However, when diabetic nephropathy ensues, even in its early microalbuminuric stage, multiple atherogenic plasma lipid abnormalities appear.

The frequency of hypertension is increased in NIDDM already at the time of diagnosis and even during its precursor stage, IGT. Plasma lipid and lipoprotein abnormalities in uncomplicated NIDDM are more marked than those occurring in uncomplicated IDDM. NIDDM dyslipoproteinemia is characterized by elevated plasma total, and elevated VLDL triglyceride levels and decreased HDL cholesterol. NIDDM dyslipoproteinemia responds to some extent to improved metabolic control of diabetes, although often less readily than IDDM dyslipoproteinemia. Plasma lipid and lipoprotein abnor-

Table 2 Coronary heart disease risk factor levels in insulin-dependent diabetes (IDDM) without or with nephropathy, in impaired glucose tolerance (IGT), and in non-insulin-dependent diabetes (NIDDM)

Risk factor	IDDM		IGT	NIDDM
	Without nephropathy	With nephropathy		
Plasma total cholesterol	=↑	↑	=↑	=↑
Plasma LDL cholesterol	=↑	↑	=↑	=↑
Plasma HDL cholesterol	=↑	⇩	⇩	⇩
Plasma triglycerides	=↑	⇧	⇧	⇧
Plasma insulin	⇧*	⇧*	⇧	⇧
Blood pressure	=↑	⇧	⇧	⇧
Body mass index	=	=	⇧	⇧
Smoking	=	=	=	=

* During insulin treatment

malities in subjects with IGT are similar to those in clinically manifest NIDDM and, on the average, more marked in women than in men. These plasma lipid and lipoprotein abnormalities associated with IGT may be present for a prolonged period of time before the clinical manifestation of diabetes. This may, in part, explain the high prevalence of CHD in patients with newly diagnosed NIDDM.

Current research is uncovering abnormalities in lipid and lipoprotein metabolism associated with diabetes which are not reflected in the plasma lipid and lipoprotein abnormalities usually measured. Such abnormalities with potential significance for enhanced atherogenesis in diabetes include: (1) increased turnover and "putthrough" of LDL-apo-B; (2) glucosylation of LDL and other lipoproteins leading to impairment of their binding to specific receptors; (3) changes in the composition of VLDL, IDL, and LDL particles and an increased production of atherogenic VLDL remnants; and (4) alterations in the fatty acid composition of plasma and tissue lipids.

Plasma insulin has been included in the list of risk factors, because prospective epidemiological studies on non-diabetic subjects have shown that high plasma insulin level is a CHD risk factor independent of other risk factors [22–26]. In IDDM treated with exogenous insulin, the circulating free plasma insulin levels are markedly elevated during most times of the day. In NIDDM and IGT fasting plasma insulin levels and usually also postprandial plasma insulin levels are elevated. Obesity is common in NIDDM and IGT and evidently forms an important link to elevated blood pressure, plasma lipid and lipoprotein abnormalities, and hyperinsulinaemia. As to smoking habits, diabetics of both types and subjects with IGT do not, of course, differ from non-diabetics.

Thus, diabetes is associated with changes in general cardiovascular risk factors and these changes are, to some extent, different in the two main types of diabetes. Very little information is available about the impact of these risk factors on the occurrence of CHD in juvenile-onset IDDM, since it is difficult to accomplish such studies for practical reasons. As to NIDDM, data is available from three population studies, the Framingham Study [13], the Whitehall Study [17], and the Finnish Social Insurance Institution Study [19], on the impact of the major general cardiovascular risk factors in subjects with this type of diabetes as compared to that observed in non-diabetic subjects. Answers are also being obtained to the question as to the extent to which the adverse effects of diabetes on risk factors explains the large excess of CHD in diabetics. The Framingham Study and the Finnish Social Insurance Institution Study populations included both men and women and both of these studies show that the excess CHD risk of diabetics as compared to non-diabetics did change essentially in men when statistical adjustment was made for the effect of plasma cholesterol, blood pressure, and smoking, whereas in women this adjustment reduced the excess CHD risk of diabetics by about 10–20%. In accordance with the results from these two studies, the 10-year follow-up data on the male population of the Whitehall Study showed that the adverse effects of diabetes on general cardiovascular risk factors explained only a very small proportion of the excess CHD risk in diabetic men. Thus, the results of these three studies indicate that the major part of the excess CHD risk in diabetic patients must be explained by the independent effects of diabetes itself and other metabolic abnormalities associated with it. It is, however, important to note in this context that data from the Framingham Study, Finnish Social Insurance Institution Study and Whitehall Study indicate that, in general, the predictive value of the three major cardiovascular risk factors, plasma cholesterol, blood pressure, and smoking, is similar in diabetics as in non-diabetics with respect to future risk of CHD events. Thus at increasing levels of these risk factors or their combinations the risk of CHD increases at the same rate in diabetics and non-diabetics, but at every risk factor level diabetics have much higher CHD risk due to independent effect of diabetes itself and associated factors. These findings are of major importance with respect to prevention of CHD in diabetic patients, since they indicate that diabetics, like non-diabetics, are susceptible to general, modifiable, major CHD risk factors. Therefore, not only effective control of hyperglycaemia, but also control of cardiovascular risk factors has great importance in the prevention of CHD and other clinical manifestations of atherosclerotic vascular disease in diabetics.

Hyperglycaemia or diabetes itself may influence atherogenesis and/or thrombogenesis by several mechanisms (for review see [27]). Hyperglycaemia may have direct effects on the cells and other components of the arterial wall. Cell culture studies have shown that high concentrations of glucose may inhibit the replication of endothelial cells, and this suggests the possibility that the repair of endothelial injuries may be impaired in diabetes. Hyperglycaemia may also lead to glucosylation of collagen and other tissue proteins which may cause changes in the physical properties of the arterial wall.

Insulin may be one of the factors participating in the enhanced atherogenesis in diabetes, as mentioned above. Insulin is known to have multiple effects on the cellular components and biochemical phenomena in the arterial wall, including stimulation of the proliferation of smooth muscle cells and synthesis of cholesterol and other lipids. In addition, hyperinsulinaemia (and/or associated insulin resistance) is known to have effects on the metabolism of very low density and high density lipoproteins in the entire body. It is also known to have links to blood pressure regulation. Thus, hyperinsulinaemia may be involved in the pathophysiologic mechanisms leading to the development of dyslipoproteinemia and hypertension in NIDDM and IGT.

Haemostatic abnormalities may contribute to the precipitation of acute events of CHD and other forms of atherosclerotic vascular disease by accelerating thrombus formation. They may also contribute more primarily to the atherosclerotic process per se. Since several abnormalities of haemostasis are known to occur in diabetes, the possible role of these abnormalities in the enhanced atherogenesis and increased occurrence of clinical manifestations of atheroscleotic vascular disease in diabetic patients has become an area of considerable research interest. Diabetes has been shown to cause abnormalities in the function of endothelial cells, including decreased production of prostacyclin and plasminogen activator and increased release of von Willebrand Factor (VIII:WF). Increased in vitro adhesiveness and aggregation of platelets, increased plasma levels of beta-thromboglobulin and platelet factor 4, and decreased platelet survival have been observed in diabetics. Elevated plasma fibrinogen is the most constant finding in studies on plasma fluid-phase clotting factor abnormalities in diabetics, but increased plasma levels of factors V, VII, and VIII have also been observed in some studies. There is also some evidence that the fibrinolytic system may be impaired in diabetes. Thus, as a whole, there is much circumstantial evidence suggesting that multiple haemostatic abnormalities may have an important role in the excessive occurrence of CHD and other clinical atherosclerotic vascular disease events in diabetic patients.

The Joslin Diabetes Center investigators [11] have proposed that the diabetic state may act mainly as a promoter of the progression of already existing atherosclerotic lesions rather than as their initiator. In the "western" populations living in an "atherogenic milieu", mainly determined by the habitual diets and life-styles of these populations, early atherosclerotic lesions in the coronary arteries of non-diabetic subjects already begin to appear in the male sex, on an average, by the end of the second decade of life and in the female sex about ten years later [4]. There is a great inter-individual variation in the appearance and progresion of these lesions, but already in middle-age the majority of subjects in these populations have definite atherosclerotic lesions in the coronary arteries and other parts of the arterial system, and in many subjects complicated, stenosing lesions are present. Seen against this background, IDDM, which usually develops in childhood or young adult life, leads to an acceleration of the progression of atherosclerotic lesions in subjects who are otherwise prone to develop them. This could explain why patients with IDDM have an increased risk of premature CHD, even in the absence of diabetic nephropathy which is accompanied with a particularly enhanced atherogenesis through several mechanisms.

NIDDM usually becomes manifest in middle-age or later in life – at a time when a large proportion of subjects in the "western" populations, even without the additional effect of diabetes, already have advanced atherosclerotic lesions in their coronary arteries and in other arteries. This type of diabetes is usually preceded by a long period of IGT, and this precursor stage of NIDDM is already associated with multiple metabolic and other abnormalities which have a powerful capacity to enhance the progression of atherosclerotic arterial lesions. This may explain the puzzling finding that subjects with IGT and patients with newly diagnosed NIDDM have almost the same prevalence of CHD as do patients with longer duration of diagnosed NIDDM.

Special features related to myocardial infarction in diabetic patients

Acute myocardial infarction (AMI) in diabetic patients is associated with several special features. The case-fatality of AMI is higher in diabetics than in non-diabetics, and atrioventricular and intraventricular conduction disturbances in connection with AMI are more common in diabetics than non-diabetics [28]. A painless or unrecognized AMI also appears to be more common in diabetic than in non-diabetic patients [29, 30]. This may be due to diabetic autonomic neuropathy [31].

Several studies have shown that the longterm prognosis of after AMI is worse in diabetics than in non-diabetics [32–34]. Accelerated progression of coronary atherosclerosis and enhanced thrombogenesis associated with diabetes may explain the less favourable prognosis of diabetic patients after AMI.

Contribution of hypertension to heart disease in diabetes

The prevalence of hypertension is higher in patients with IDDM and NIDDM than in comparable non-diabetic subjects (for reviews see [35, 36]). Diabetic nephropathy is the most important cause of hypertension in patients with IDDM, and blood pressure levels may already become elevated during the early phase of diabetic nephropathy characterized by microalbuminuria. Hypertension in NIDDM is clinically similar to essential hypertension in non-diabetic subjects, and the increased occurrence of hypertension in this type of diabetes may be largely explained by the high frequency of obesity in

NIDDM. Other factors may, however, also be involved in the pathogenesis of hypertension in NIDDM, e. g., the interaction of hyperinsulinaemia or insulin resistance with blood pressure homeostasis.

Since hypertension is a major risk factor for atherosclerotic vascular disease, the increased occurrence of hypertension in diabetic patients contributes importantly to their excessive CHD risk. Left ventricular hypertrophy and cardiac failure caused by hypertension could be expected to be commoner in diabetics than in non-diabetics. In fact, cross-sectional data from the Framingham Study from the era before widespread antihypertensive drug therapy showed that ECG signs of left ventricular hypertrophy were more frequent in diabetics than in non-diabetics [14]. During the longterm follow-up of the Framingham Study population the incidence of cardiac failure was markedly higher in diabetics than in non-diabetics, although in addition to hypertension, other causative factors, especially CHD, but also specific diabetic heart muscle disease were apparently involved [13]. Widespread use of antihypertensive drugs, and particularly a more aggressive drug treatment of hypertension in diabetic than in non-diabetic patients, has tended to mask the occurrence of hypertensive heart disease during the last two decades. Yet, hypertension, often jointly with CHD, evidently continues to be an important cause of cardiac failure in diabetic patients.

Diabetic heart muscle disease

It is now well established that diabetes may cause a specific heart muscle disease which is independent of CHD and hypertension (for reviews see [37–39]). Evidence for this concept has accumulated from epidemiological, clinical, morphological, and metabolic studies, although many unsolved questions still remain concerning the pathogenesis of diabetic heart muscle disease.

The Framingham Study [13] showed that the incidence of cardiac failure at all ages and in both sexes was markedly higher in diabetics than in non-diabetics (Fig. 5). The risk of cardiac failure in men was 2.4 times higher and in women 5.3 times higher in diabetics than in non-diabetics. When persons with previous CHD were excluded, the excess risk of cardiac failure was 3.8 times higher in male diabetics and 5.5 times higher in female diabetics. Multivariate analyses gave support to the view that it is unlikely that diabetes promotes the development of cardiac failure mainly through elevated CHD risk factor levels, including hypertension.

In our own cross-sectional studies of middle-aged patients with newly diagnosed and previously known NIDDM and comparable non-diabetic control subjects, we have found evidence for a marked increase in the

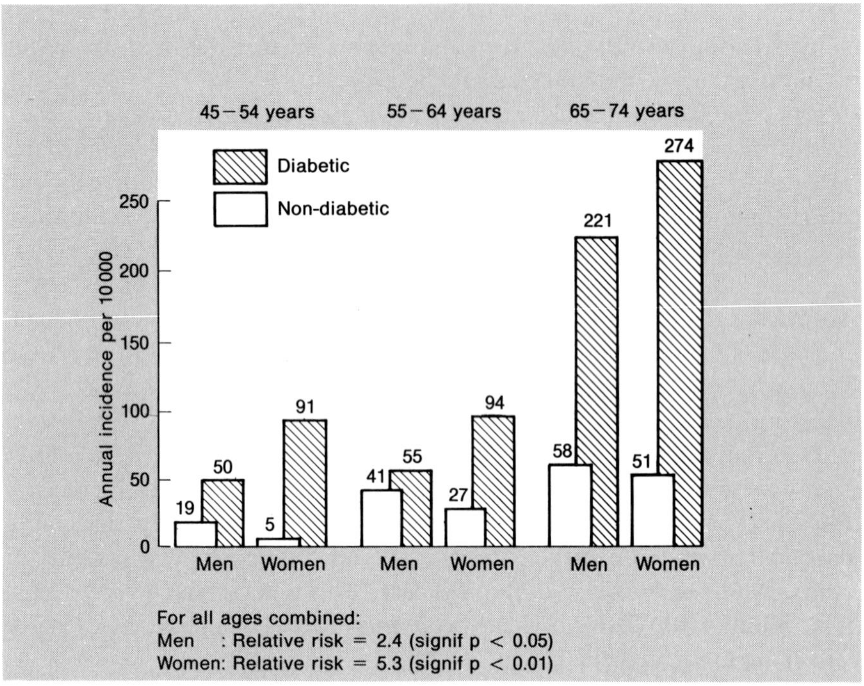

Fig. 5 The annual incidence of cardiac failure in diabetic and non-diabetic men and women aged 45 – 74 years by age; 18-year follow-up results from the Framingham Study [13].

prevalence of cardiac failure in diabetic patients based on the use of digitalis [20, 21]. Among patients with newly diagnosed NIDDM the prevalence of digitalis therapy was 3.3 times higher in male diabetics and 3.9 times higher in female diabetics than in non-diabetic subjects. Among patients with previously known NIDDM the excess of digitalis therapy as compared to that in non-diabetic subjects was even more marked; 5.9-fold in male diabetics and 8.2-fold in female diabetics.

Clinical studies, based on haemodynamic measurements or non-invasive techniques for the assessment of left ventricular function (systolic and diastolic time intervals, echocardiography, radionuclide angiography), have shown that subtle signs of impaired systolic and diastolic left ventricular function are frequently found in diabetic patients in the absence of any clinically detectable cardiac failure. Impairment of the diastolic function of the left ventricle appears to be the earliest detectable abnormality in diabetic heart muscle disease. In young patients with IDDM the occurrence and extent of abnormalities of left ventricular function has been found to show some relation to the duration of diabetes and the presence of proliferative retinopathy and nephropathy. Subtle abnormalities of left ventricular diastolic function may, however, already be detectable after relatively short duration of diabetes and in the absence of other diabetic complications. In patients with NIDDM, abnormalities of left ventricular function may be already present at the time of diagnosis and in the absence of CHD and hypertension. Diabetic autonomic neuropathy may have some role in the pathophysiology of left ventricular dysfunction in diabetic patients, but it is not the major underlying factor of this disorder.

Morphological changes of different types such as microvascular abnormalities, perivascular and interstitial fibrosis, and accumulation of glycoproteins and lipids have been observed in autopsy studies of the heart in diabetic patients, but the frequency and clinical significance of these morphological abnormalities and their relationship to metabolic abnormalities of diabetes and to the development of abnormalities of left ventricular function still are poorly understood. Studies on patients with NIDDM have shown that the impaired left ventricular function may improve considerably when hyperglycaemia is corrected by diet or oral hypoglycaemic drugs [40]. Thus it seems apparent that diabetic heart muscle disease may be caused, in part, by metabolic factors associated with poor control of diabetes.

Besides being a cause of cardiac failure in itself, diabetic heart muscle disease may contribute to the development of cardiac failure jointly with other causes, in particular CHD and hypertension. Furthermore, diabetic heart muscle disease may contribute to the increased case-fatality of acute CHD events in diabetic patients and also to the poorer longterm prognosis after such events as compared to non-diabetic subjects.

Summary

The incidence of coronary heart disease (CHD) is increased in both insulin-dependent diabetes mellitus (IDDM) and non-insulin-dependent diabetes mellitus (NIDDM) as one result of enhanced atherosclerosis in diabetes. In juvenile-onset IDDM increased occurrence of clinically manifest CHD begins to emerge after the age of 30 years and the excessive CHD risk is particularly marked in patients with diabetic nephropathy. Premenopausal female patients with IDDM develop CHD almost as often as male diabetics with IDDM of the same age – a situation in sharp contrast to that in non-diabetics with a large excess of CHD in men. In NIDDM the incidence of all clinical manifestations of CHD is markedly increased as compared to that in non-diabetic subjects, and more markedly in women than in men. In NIDDM the frequency of CHD shows very little relation to the known duration of diabetes. The risk of CHD is already increased in subjects with impaired glucose tolerance, precursor stage of NIDDM.

Diabetes, in particular NIDDM, is associated with changes in general CHD risk factors, including abnormalities in the levels and composition of plasma lipids and lipoproteins and increased frequency of hypertension. The major part of the excess risk of CHD in diabetics, however, is not explained by the effects of diabetes on general CHD risk factors, but must be due an independent effect of diabetes itself through mechanisms which are not completely understood. On the other hand, the impact of general, major CHD risk factors on the future risk of CHD events is similar in diabetics and non-diabetics. Thus at increasing levels of these risk factors or their combinations the risk of CHD shows the same increase in diabetics and non-diabetics, but at every risk factor level diabetics have much higher CHD risk due to the independent effect of diabetes itself and to associated factors.

Special features related to myocardial infarction in diabetic patients as compared to non-diabetic subjects include an increased case-fatality, poorer longterm prognosis and more frequent occurrence of painless of unrecognized myocardial infarction.

Increased frequency of hypertension in both IDDM and NIDDM contributes to the increased occurrence of cardiac failure in diabetic patients, although other causative factors, in particular CHD, are often involved.

Diabetes may lead to a specific diabetic heart muscle disease. Besides being a cause of cardiac failure in itself, diabetic heart muscle disease may contribute to the development of cardiac failure jointly with other causes (CHD, hypertension) and have an adverse influence on the prognosis of CHD events in diabetic patients.

References

[1] Pyörälä K, Laakso M. Macrovascular disease in diabetes mellitus. In: Mann JI, Pyörälä K, Teuscher A, eds. Diabetes in epidemiological perspective. Edinburgh: Churchill Livingstone, 1983; 183–247.

[2] Pyörälä K, Laakso M, Uusitupa M. Diabetes and atherosclerosis: An epidemiologic view. Diabetes/Metab Rev 1987; 3: 463–524.

[3] Robertson WB, Strong JP. Atherosclerosis in persons with hypertension and diabetes mellitus. Lab Invest 1968; 18: 538–551.

[4] Kagan AR, Uemura K, Sternby NH et al. Atherosclerosis of the aorta and coronary arteries in five towns. Bull WHO 1976; 53: 485–638.

[5] Zdanov VS, Vihert AM. Atherosclerosis and diabetes mellitus. Bull WHO 1976; 53: 547–553.

[6] Crall FV, Roberts WC. The extramural and intramural coronary arteries in juvenile diabetes mellitus. Analysis of nine necropsy patients aged 19 to 38 years with onset of diabetes before age 15 year. Am J Med 1978; 64: 221–230.
[7] Vigorita VJ, Moore GW, Hutchins GM. Absence of correlation between coronary arterial atherosclerosis and severity or duration of diabetes mellitus of adult onset. Am J Cardiol 1980; 46: 535–542.
[8] Verska JJ, Walker WJ. Aortocoronary bypass in the diabetic patient. Am J Cardiol 1975; 35: 774–777.
[9] Hamby RI, Sherman L, Mehta J et al. Reappraisal of the role of the diabetic state in coronary artery disease. Chest 1976; 70: 251–257.
[10] Dortimer AC, Shenoy PN, Shiroff RA et al. Diffuse coronary artery disease in diabetic patients. Fact or fiction? Circulation 1978; 57: 133–136.
[11] Krolewski AS, Kosinski EJ, Warram JH et al. Magnitude and determinants of coronary artery disease in juvenile-onset insulin-dependent diabetes mellitus. Am J Cardiol 1987; 59: 750–755.
[12] Garcia MJ, McNamara PM, Gordon T et al. Morbidity and mortality in diabetics in the Framingham population. Sixteen year follow-up study. Diabetes 1974; 23: 105–111.
[13] Kannel WB. Role of diabetes in cardiac disease: conclusions from population studies. In: Zoneraich S, ed. Diabetes and heart. Springfield, Charles C. Thomas, 1978; 97–122.
[14] Kannel WB, McGee DL. Diabetes and cardiovascular risk factors: the Framingham Study. Circulation 1979; 59: 8–13.
[15] Kannel WB, McGee DL. Diabetes and glucose tolerance as risk factors for cardiovascular disease: the Framingham Study. Diabetes Care 1979; 2: 120–126.
[16] Herman JB, Medalie JH, Goldbourt U. Differences in cardiovascular morbidity and mortality between previously known and newly diagnosed adult diabetics. Diabetologia 1977; 13: 229–234.
[17] Fuller JH, Shipley MJ, Rose G et al. Mortality from coronary heart disease and stroke in relation to degree of glycaemia: the Whitehall Study. Br Med J 1983; 287: 867–870.
[18] Jarrett RJ, Shipley MJ. The Whitehall Study: comparative mortality rates and indices of risk in diabetics. Acta Endocrinol 1985; 110 (suppl 272): 21–26.
[19] Reunanen A, Laakso, Pyörälä K. Cardiovascular and coronary heart disease mortality of diabetics and non-diabetics; impact of risk factors. J Am Coll Cardiol 1983; 1(2): 600 (Abstract).
[20] Uusitupa M, Siitonen O, Aro A et al. Prevalence of coronary heart disease, left ventricular failure and hypertension in middle-aged, newly diagnosed type 2 (non-insulin-dependent) diabetic subjects. Diabetologia 1985; 28: 22–27.
[21] Laakso M. Atherosclerotic vascular disease and its risk factors in non-insulin-dependent diabetics in East Finland. Thesis. Publications of the University of Kuopio. Original reports 5/1986.
[22] Eschwege E, Ducimetiere P, Thibult N et al. Coronary heart disease mortality in relation with diabetes, blood glucose and plasma insulin levels. The Paris prospective study, ten years later. Horm Metab Res 1985; 15 (suppl) 41–45.
[23] Pyörälä K, Savolainen E, Kaukola S et al. Plasma insulin as coronary heart disease risk factor: relationship to other risk factors and predictive value during the 9 1/2-year follow-up of the Helsinki Policemen Study population. Acta Med Scand 1985; (suppl 701): 38–52.
[24] Pyörälä K. Relationship of glucose tolerance and plasma insulin to the incidence of coronary heart disease: results from two population studies in Finland. Diabetes Care 1979; 2: 131–141.
[25] Welborn TA, Wearne K. Coronary heart disease incidence and cardiovascular mortality in Busselton with reference to glucose and insuline concentration. Diabetes Care 1979; 2: 154–160.
[26] Ducimetiere P, Eschwege E, Papoz L et al. Relationship of plasma insulin levels to the incidence of myocardial infarction and coronary heart disease mortality in a middle-aged population. Diabetologia 1980; 19: 205–210.

[27] Uusitupa M, Pyörälä K, Laakso M. Metabolic control and macrovascular disease. In: Alberti KGMM, Defronzo RA, Keen H et al, eds. The international textbook of diabetes mellitus. Chichester: John Wiley & Sons Ltd (In press).
[28] Czyzyk A, Krolewski AS, Szablowska S et al. Clinical course of myocardial infarction among diabetic patients. Diabetes Cares 1980; 3: 526–529.
[29] Partamian JO, Bradley RF. Acute myocardial infarction in 258 cases of diabetes. N Engl J Med 1965; 273: 455–461.
[30] Margolis JR, Kannel WP, Feinleib D et al. Clinical features of unrecognized myocardial infarction – silent and symptomatic. Eighteen-year follow-up: the Framingham study. Am J Cardiol 1973; 32: 1–7.
[31] Faerman I, Faccio E, Milei J et al. Autonomic neuropathy and painless myocardial infarction in diabetic patients. Histological evidence of their relationship. Diabetes 1977; 26: 1147–1158.
[32] Smith JW, Marcus FI, Serokman R. Prognosis of patients with diabetes mellitus after myocardial infarction. Am J Cardiol 1984; 54: 718–721.
[33] Ulfvenstam G, Åberg A, Bergstrand R et al. Long term prognosis after myocardial infarction in men with diabetes. Diabetes 1985; 34: 787–792.
[34] Mølstad P, Nustad M. Acute myocardial infarction in diabetic patients. Acta Med Scand 1987; 222: 433–437.
[35] Pacy PJ. Hypertension and diabetes mellitus. In: Taylor KG, ed. Diabetes and the heart. Tunbridge Wells, Kent: Castle Publications Ltd, 1987; 42–60.
[36] Pyörälä K, Uusitupa M, Laakso M. Hypertension and diabetes: a poorly understood relationship. In: Andreani D, Crepaldi G, Di Mario U et al, eds. Chichester: John Wiley & Sons Ltd, 1987; 43–51.
[37] Shapiro LM. Functional aspects of diabetic heart disease. In: Jarrett RJ, ed. Diabetes and heart disease. Amsterdam: Elsevier Science Publishers B. V., 1984; 81–98.
[38] Fein S, Sonnenblick EH. Diabetic cardiomyopathy. Progr Cardiovasc Dis 1985; 27: 255–270.
[39] Watson RDS, Waldron S. Heart disease and diabetes mellitus. In: Taylor KG, ed. Diabetes and the heart. Tunbridge Wells, Kent: Castle Publications Ltd, 1987; 19–41.
[40] Uusitupa M, Siitonen O, Aro A et al. Effect of correction of hyperglycaemia on left ventricular function in non-insulin-dependent (type 2) diabetics. Acta med Scand 1983; 213: 363–368.

Cerebral and peripheral vascular disease

(with special emphasis on the diabetic foot)

E. Standl, H. Stiegler, H.U. Janka, H. Mehnert

Coronary, cerebral, and peripheral vascular disease are the major macrovascular complications of diabetic patients in the western world, irrespective of the subtype of diabetes, and determine largely the prognosis of those patients. Although coronary heart disease and related complications are undoubtedly the leading cause of mortality in subjects with diabetes mellitus, macrovascular involvement of cerebral or limb arteries is by no means of minor importance. Cerebral vascular disease occurs approximately twice as commonly in diabetics than in the age-matched general population and also contributes considerably to mortality of diabetics [1 – 10].

The at least five-fold increase of peripheral artery disease in diabetes results in a 20- to 50-fold elevation of gangrene [1 – 4, 7 – 13]. The diabetic foot is particularly complex pathophysiologically and aetiologically and a serious socio-economic burden. An American study showed that 50% of all patients undergoing amputation were diabetics [14, 15] and one out of 10 diabetic patients was faced with this problem at some time during his life [11, 12]. It is not surprising, therefore, that 25% of the money spent on inpatient care of diabetic patients was devoted to the treatment of the diabetic foot according to a recent survey[16].

Pathophysiology and pathology

There is still no evidence for either a diabetes-specific macrovascular lesion or for a specific entity of diabetic arteriosclerotic disease. Diabetes does, however, markedly accelerate the atherosclerotic process normally occurring with aging in a given population [17]. This influence seems to be already apparent at the stage of impaired glucose tolerance [18]. Conversely, several cardiovascular risk markers other than diabetes obviously favor the manifestation of diabetes by their own through enhancing insulin resistance. This is particularly pertinent for hyperlipoproteinemia and – probably – hypertension [19, 19a, 20]. The atherosclerotic risk profile in many diabetic patients appears to be embedded in a prediabetic background. As a consequence, it is not uncommon for an individual with non-insulin-dependent diabetes to present with advanced macrovascular disease at the time of clinical diagnosis of diabetes [21], whereas insulin-dependent patients develop excessive macroangiopathy in general only long after diagnosis of diabetes. In fact, it has been suggested that the development of premature and abundant macroangiopathy is in this latter group mainly a matter of attained age rather than duration of diabetes [22]. Around age 35 to 40, when first signs of atherosclerotic disease usually become detectable in nondiabetics, macroangiopathy of cerebral and leg arteries – besides the coronaries – tends to begin to create serious clinical problems in insulin-dependent diabetic patients [22, 23, 24].

The enormous complexity of diabetes-related and unrelated atherogenic risk factors or markers has also complicated the understanding of how diabetes itself stimulates the formation of arteriosclerosis. Furthermore, different mechanisms may be operating in different subgroups of diabetic patients. In populations in which the overall prevalence of macrovascular disease is low, diabetes does not seem to markedly increase arteriosclerotic morbidity. At the same time such populations have lower cholesterol and triglyceride levels than western man. On the other hand, the impact of diabetes on atherogenesis is most striking in hypertensive, hypertriglyceridemic patients [4, 9, 10, 13].

The processes involved in the development of atheromatous plaques in both diabetics and non-diabetics include injury to or alteration of the endothelium, proliferation of smooth muscle cells and their migration from the media into the intima, uptake of lipids and lipoproteins by smooth muscle cells and macrophages in the arterial wall, and changes in connective tissue and clotting mechanisms, particularly those mediated by platelets. At the present time, however, no precise sequence of biochemical events in the pathogenesis of macrovascular disease in either diabetics or non-diabetics has been established [25, 26].

The effect of hyperglycemia

Chronic hyperglycemia may act either directly by increased effects on the arterial wall or indirectly by increased nonenzymatic protein glycosylation and sorbitol formation. In tissue culture hyperglycemia damages or alters the endothelial barrier which might allow platelets, lipoproteins, or other factors access to the inner part of the arterial wall. Higher glucose concentrations competitively inhibit the transport of myo-inositol into endothelial cells which, in turn, might affect the phosphatidyl-inositol pathway and Na/K-ATPase activity. Hemoconcentration secondary to hyperglycemia generates a higher risk of thrombus formation at irregularities of the arterial vessel lining [26, 27].

Increased glycosylation

Advanced glycosylation endproducts (AGE) accumulate in the vessel wall of diabetic patients [28] and might be a target for the attack of macrophages. These percursors of the foam cells in atheromatous plaques have been shown to exhibit specific AGE-receptors and to remove glucose modifications forming on long-lived proteins [28, 28a]. Increased nonenzymatic glycosylation due to an excess of glucose in the surrounding milieu has been found for virtually all proteins [29, 30]; Table 1 lists glycosylation of a number of blood and tissue proteins with possible pathophysiological relevance to macroangiopathy in diabetes. Glycosylation at the N-terminal of the hemoglobin β-chain interferes with the action of 2,3-diphosphoglycerate and oxygen release. The function of red blood cells is profoundly altered in terms of a marked decrease in deformability as well as a marked increase of adhesion and erythrocyte aggregation, although the evidence for a linkage with glycosylation is still indirect [31]. The same is true in the context of an increased uptake of arachidonic acid into platelets – the precursor for prostaglandin synthesis [27]. Furthermore, antithrombin III activity, but not concentration, appears

Table 1 Nonenzymatic glycosylation of proteins and possible pathophysiological relevance in diabetes mellitus

Blood	
Hemoglobin	↑ O_2 affinity; tissue hypoxia?
RBC membrane proteins	change in permeability; ↓ deformability? ↑ adhesion
Platelets	↑ uptake of arachidonic acid?
Albumin	↑ transcapillary permeation? ↑ deposition in basement membrane?
Globulins	↓ activities of immunoglobulins?
Fibrin	?
AT III	↓ activity?
Lipoproteins	loss of receptor specificity
Tissue proteins	
Basement membrane collagen	↑ permeability?
Connective tissue collagen	↑ platelet adhesion; ↑ LDL binding; ↑ stiffening
Lens, crystallins	opacity, cataract formation?
Myelins	impaired nerve function? ↑ uptake by macrophages
Tubulin	impaired polymerization

to be reduced [32] and lipoproteins might loose their receptor specificity with the result of scavenger clearing and accumulation in the vessel wall [17].

Increased sorbitol production

Increased sorbitol production, again secondary to an excess of glucose, is another important pathophysiological event in many tissues [30, 33, 34]. Sorbitol-derived osmotic damage, with the exception of that to the lens, is probably not a predominant problem, but rather changes in the NADPH and glutathione system, in the sodium-potassium ATPase activity, and – finally – in the phosphoinositide metabolism (Table 2). Much of the evidence for metabolic consequences of elevated sorbitol formation is still indirect and partially derived by the use of aldose reductase inhibitors. This applies also for the derangements of glycosaminoglycan (GAG) metabolism. Among other effects GAGs are connected with the retention of LDL in the vessel wall [35].

Table 2 Sorbitol production and possible pathophysiological relevance in diabetes mellitus

Metabolic consequences	
↓ Myo-inositol	↑ GMB collagen synthesis
↓ Na,K-ATPase	↓ GMB collagen turnover
↓ GSH	↓ GAG synthesis
↑ Platelet TXB_2 synthesis	↓ blood retinal barrier

Increased content observed in: RBC, isolated glomeruli, retina, lens, Schwann cells, pericytes, aortic vessel wall, granulation tissue?

Endothelial dysfunction

Partially in the context of glucose mediated effects, as already indicated by the above mentioned examples, but probably also independent of these, there is strong evidence for endothelial dysfunction and an imbalance of blood clotting in patients with diabetes mellitus [27, 30, 36, 37]. Dysfunction of the endothelial cells is suggested by increased factor VIII-related antigen (von Willebrand Factor) circulating in blood, decreased prostacyclin formation, and lowered concentrations of plasminogen activator. Increased blood concentrations of factor VIII-related antigen have been found very early in the course of diabetes and certainly preceding vascular disease as detectable by angiography or sonografic techniques, although it is significantly higher in patients with vascular complications. Factor VIII-related antigen stimulates platelet adhesion and is released by endothelial cells. Increased blood concentrations may indicate endothelial damage. Prostacyclin is also generated from endothelial cells and leads to vasodilatation and platelet disaggregation. In animal studies, low prostacyclin concentrations of the aortic vessel wall in uncontrolled diabetes could be restored to normal after insulin treatment and near normoglycemia [38].

Imbalance of blood clotting

In contrast to decreased prostacyclin generation, there is an increased platelet thromboxane formation in young diabetic patients. This has been observed by several groups, especially in subjects with high HbA_1 [27, 39, 40]. Thromboxane induces vasoconstriction and platelet aggregation; it can be reduced by improvement of metabolic control. Furthermore, a close correlation has been described between a reduced, probably sorbitol-mediated, glutathione content and an increased platelet thromboxane synthesis and release [40].

There is now an impressively long list of derangements in blood clotting occurring in diabetes mellitus [25, 27, 32, 36–46] (Table 3]. All these disturbances apparently tend to shift the delicate steady state among the various clotting factors towards aggregation and coagulation. This imbalance has also been seen by testing platelet aggregation in vitro. It has been shown that platelet aggregation is already increased prior to the detection of vasculopathy, but not at the onset of diabetes. Platelet aggregation is most marked in proliferative retinopathy and advanced large vessel disease. Although there seems to be no direct effect of either glucose or insulin on platelets in vitro, a correlation between platelet aggregation and fasting blood glucose has been described.

Table 3 Some effects on parameters of blood clotting in diabetes mellitus

↑ Factor VIII: Ag (platelet adhesion)
↑ Uptake of arachidonic acid in platelets
↓ Phospholipase A_2 activity
↓ α-Adrenergic binding sites of platelets
↑ TXB_2 formation
↑ ADP-adrenaline-induced platelet aggregation
↑ β-Thromboglobulin and platelet factor 4 formation
↓ Platelet survival time
↑ Fibrinopeptide generation
↓ Antithrombin III activity
↓ Prostacyclin formation
↓ Protein C levels
↑ Fibrinolysis
↓ Endothelial plasminogen activator
↑ Plasminogen activator inhibitor

Other areas of interest might be abnormalities of red and white blood cells, especially in terms of deformability and filterability, and increased plasma concentrations of fibrinogen and a_2-macroglobulin. Fibrinogen is the major determinant of plasma viscosity and its split products seem to be involved in proliferative processes of the vessel wall [30].

Hyperinsulinemia

Insulin among other hormones, e. g. growth hormone, has been hypothesised to act directly on the arterial wall or to induce changes in the artery by acting on other substances such as lipids and lipoproteins [10, 13, 26, 35, 47]. Since many diabetics are hyperinsulinemic to some extent and also since the classical cardiovascular risk factors hyperlipoproteinemia and hypertension seem to be associated with the hyperinsulinemia/insulin resistance syndrome [13, 19–21, 26], such a connection could be of great importance in the context of macrovascular disease in diabetes mellitus. There is evidence in favor of both above-mentioned mechanisms, although a definite chain of events has not been established.

Insulin seems to have no effect on endothelial cells of large arteries; it does have an effect on endothelial cells of microvessels, e. g., those of cerebral origin [48]. In physiological hormone concentrations insulin stimulates proliferation and migration of arterial smooth muscle cells, cholesterol synthesis in smooth muscle cells and macrophages, and, finally, perhaps the release of certain growth factors like IGF_1, or of plasminogen activator inhibitor [26, 44, 49, 50]. The latter would hamper fibrinolyctic capacity. Insulin's effect on the vessel wall has probably to be seen in the context of endothelial injury and effects of platelets and lipoproteins on smooth muscle cells, as outlined in a recent review article [26] (Fig. 1), whereby insulin by itself stimulates hepatic VLDL synthesis and chronic over-insulinization decreases lipoprotein lipase activity. Serum insulin concentration is, therefore, particularly closely correlated with serum triglycerides and, inversely, with HDL-cholesterol. In all, in spite of the still existing uncertainties in terms of pathobiochemistry, epidemiological evidence that hyperinsulinemia is a major cardiovascular risk marker is quite impressive and convincing (see below).

Morphology

The lesions of atherosclerosis in the diabetic are morphologically identical to those in nondiabetics [17], as has already been outlined. Besides being more frequent and severe, however, they show a distinct pattern of distribution.

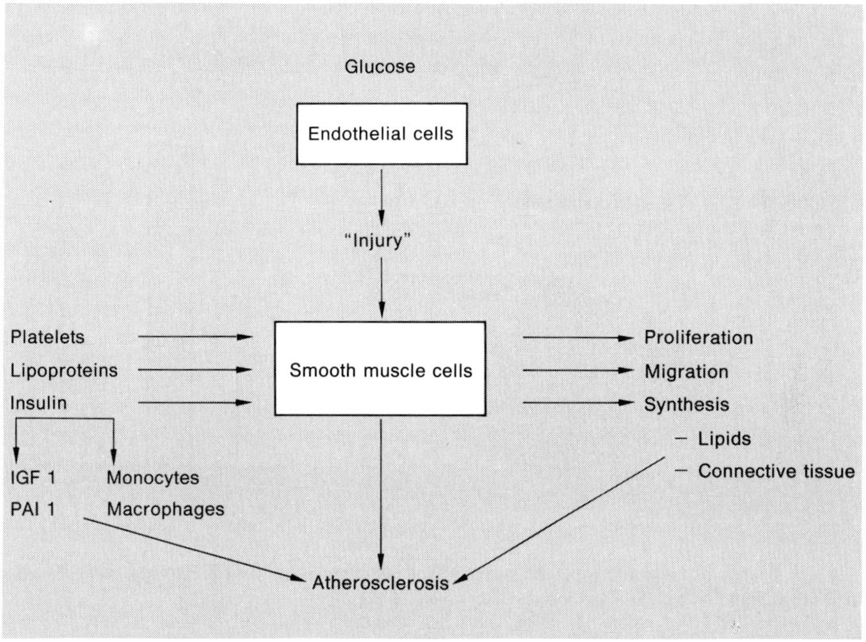

Fig. 1 Effects of insulin and glucose on atherogenesis (adapted from Stout [26])

The atherosclerotic process appears to be more diffuse and there is pronounced predilection for the involvement of more peripheral arterial segments, i.e., medium and small arteries. This holds true for all major targets of macrovascular disease in diabetes. Intracranial pathology of the cerebral arterial system is much more prominent and contributes considerably to neurological deficits and strokes [5]. Frequency of involvement of leg arteries below the knee is likewise very striking (Fig. 2) as is frequency of deep femoral artery disease [11, 12, 51, 52]. Prediliction for peripheral involvement seems to be responsible in part for the fact that the amputation rate in patients with foot ulcers is much higher in diabetics.

Another typical feature consists in the occurrence of mediasclerosis of the Mönckeberg type. Unlike the patchy calcification of the vessel intima within the framework of atherosclerosis in nondiabetics, Mönckeberg sclerosis is characterised by a linear dystrophic calcification of the tunica media (Fig. 3) and subsequent smooth muscle atrophy and collagen fibre proliferation. The pathologic significance, however, of these metaplastic changes which are usually associated with neuropathy is unclear as they do not appear to

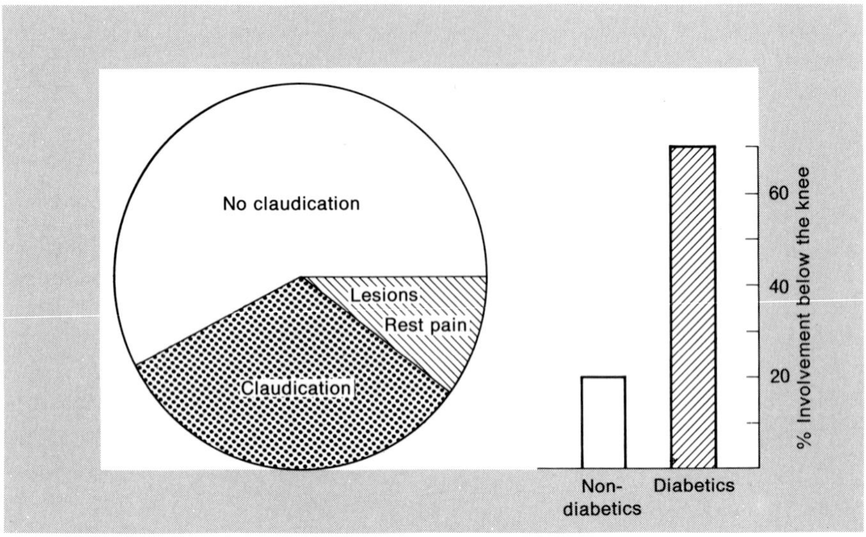

Fig. 2 Arterial vascular disease of the lower limb in 240 consecutive diabetic patients: clinical stages and involvement below the knee compared to nondiabetics

contribute to arterial occlusion. In some studies they are indeed accompanied by occlusive disease in almost every other case [53, 54]. Arterial medial sclerosis may be clinically important because existing obliterative angiopathy might be masked by erroneously high Doppler-measured blood pressure values. Furthermore, due to the decreased function of vasoconstriction, mediasclerosis and vasomotor neuropathy may favor blood flow through shunt vessels so that the actual tissue blood supply falls short.

One final aspect of macroangiopathy in diabetes is the apparently increased risk of females. The strong male preponderance of atherosclerotic disease seen in nondiabetic populations is virtually abolished, if not reversed [1–4, 8–10].

Microangiopathy

Obviously, concomitant diabetic microangiopathy and neuropathy both may affect considerably to the symptoms and clinical outcome of macrovascular disease in diabetes, especially diabetic foot disease (Fig. 4). Profound changes are seen in the function of capillaries of the foot, as demonstrated for nail fold capillaries by Bollinger et al. using a fluorescein technique [55]. After 10 years of diabetes almost every diabetic patient will show a striking loss of

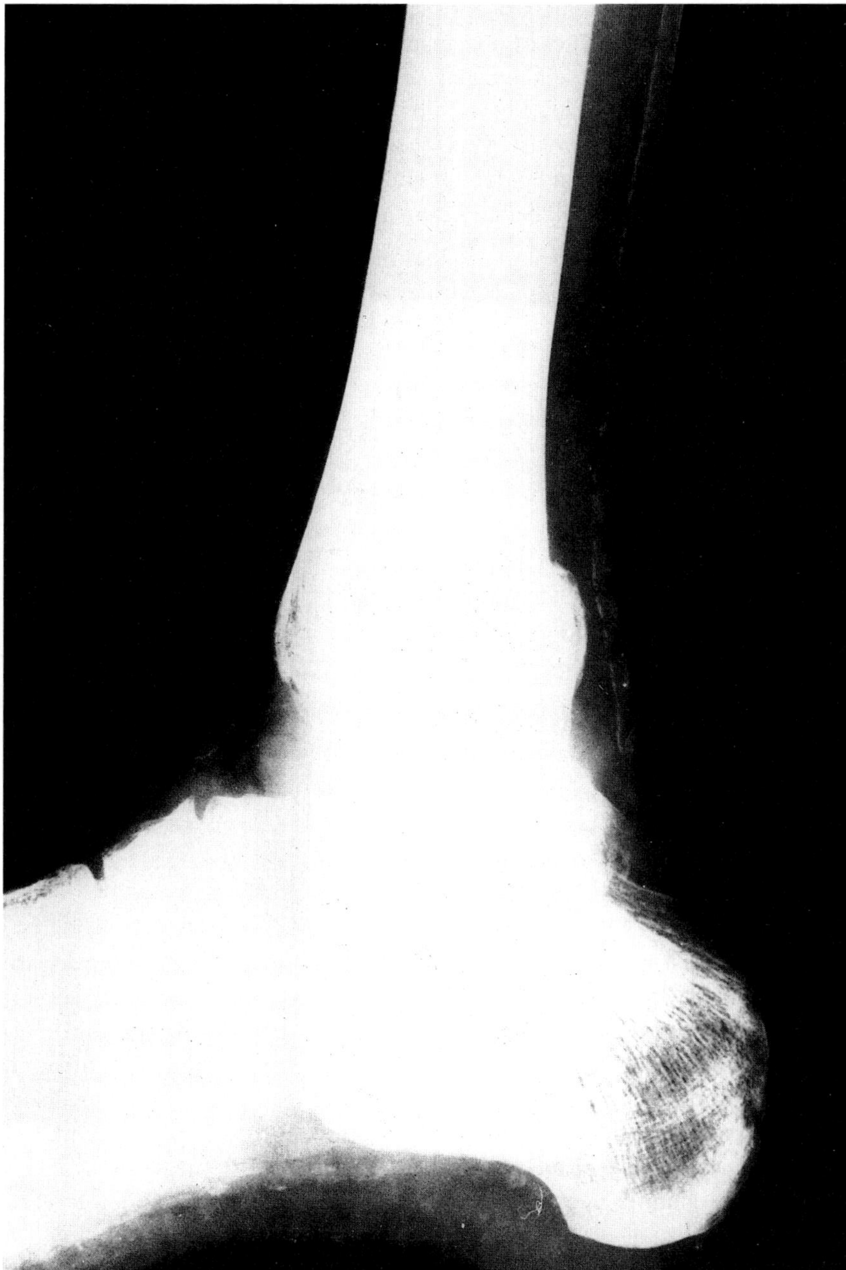

Fig. 3 Mediasclerosis of the posterior tibial artery

barrier function and leakiness of foot capillaries. Magnification angiograms have indicated avascular zones and reactive hypervascularities of the microvasculature in longterm diabetics. Endothelial proliferation, pericapillary structural changes, disordered blood flow, and clotting can lead to capillary occlusion and tissue necrosis. Microscopic traumas can form blister-like structures of the superficial epidermal layer which, after desiccation, form a necrosis; these are called diabetic blisters [11, 14].

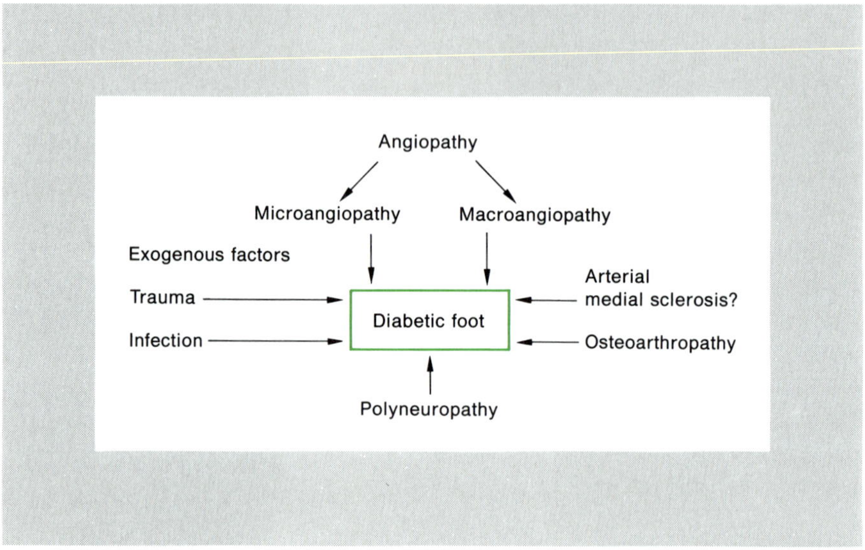

Fig. 4 Etiology and pathogenesis of the diabetic foot

Neuropathy

Diabetic polyneuropathy affects 50% of all diabetics who have had the disease for 15 years or more [56]. The neuropathic foot (Fig. 5) involves several factors: sensory and motor polyneuropathy with diminished pain and temperature sensation, loss of pressure sensation with pseudotabes and impaired autonomic peripheral nervous system. The latter leads, because of its disordered sympathetic innervation, to vasodilatation (Rubeosis plantarium) and anhidrosis, which makes the skin dry, dystrophic, and prone to fissures [11, 12]. Trophic changes occur in the skin, nails, ligaments, and joints. The inability to feel pain or heat renders the foot vulnerable to injuries, which may not be noticed for weeks.

Horny skin may form because of pressure from footwear on contact areas such as the first and fifth metatarsal heads and the heel. The impaired pain

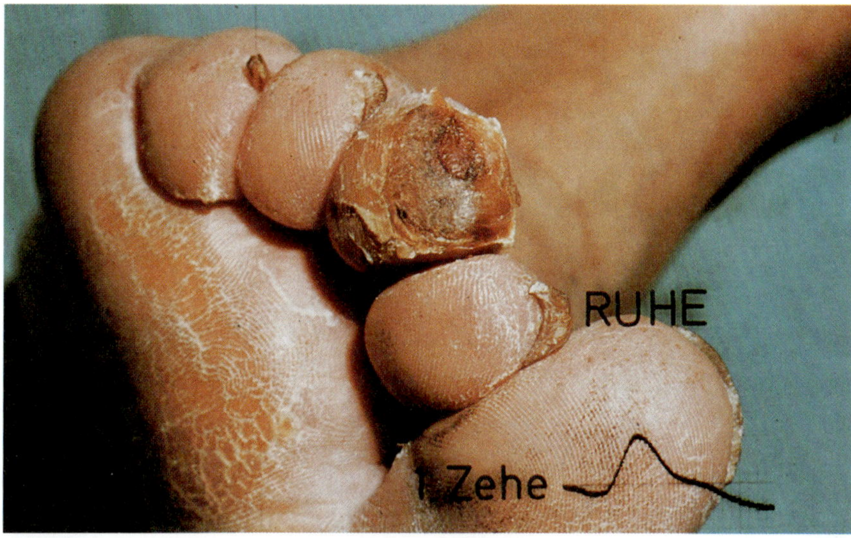

Fig. 5 Neuropathic foot

sensation and denervation-induced skin changes may lead to ulceration in these areas.

Further pressure necrosis may result from the altered mechanics of the foot, in which there are changes in the equilibrium between the extensors and flexors, resulting in secondary deformity. There is patchy or diffuse osteoporosis in neuropathic osteoarthropathy, which, in severe cases, can extend to destruction and dislocation, or even to total osteolysis of the phalanges (Fig. 6). In such cases, even a slight injury can destroy the whole skeletal architecture of the foot.

Early detection and classification

Both cerebral and peripheral vascular disease may be rather asymptomatic in diabetic patients, yet they influence the prognosis considerably. All diabetic patients should, therefore, be regularly screened for macrovascular disease and the associated risk profile. Besides a routine search for the risk factors, patients with manifestation of macroangiopathy at one site, e.g., of the coronary artery system, need to be checked specifically for disease of the other main arterial systems. The use of a check list is recommended (Table 4). Such a list already allows, to some extent, a differential diagnosis as to co-existing microangio- and neuropathy. Of course, examination should include

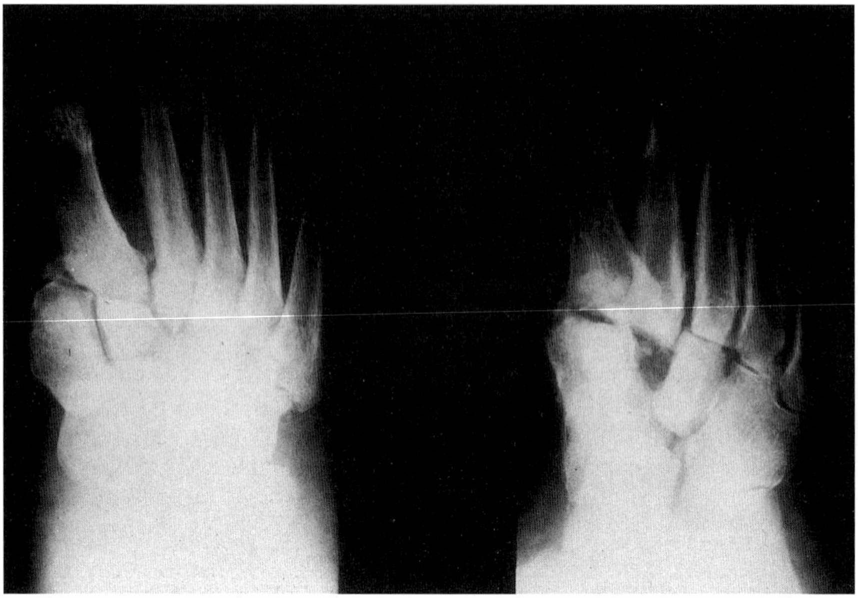

Fig. 6 X-ray of Charcot foot

a pertinent history, physical examination, and further examinations in case of disease. Table 5 summarizes possible diagnostic measures.

A history of painless ulcers may indicate neuropathy. The feet should be carefully inspected, with special attention to local infection between the toes, pressure points from foot wear, neuropathic deformities, and ingrown toenails.

Although only 39% of all angiographically confirmed stenoses and occlusions can be identified from the case history and palpation, the detection rate can be increased to 80% by auscultation at rest and on exercise [14]. Vessel wall stenoses which reduce the lumen by more than 30% can cause turbulence, detectable as a bruit. This does not always apply to areas where vessels branch, e. g., the inguinal region, where considerable turbulence may occur, particularly, when anemia or hyperthyroidism are also present. The angiological status may be further investigated using electronic oscillometry and Doppler and Duplex Ultrasound techniques.

The degree of arterial occlusive disease can be determined from the shape and height of the oscillographic curve. This method is also suitable for identifying peripheral circulatory disorders, since pulse-volume curves can be plotted for individual toes. In diabetic neuropathy, these curves may be excessively high due to digital vessel distension.

Table 4 Screening for the risk profile and presence of macrovascular disease in diabetes mellitus

Annually
– Lipid profile (cholesterol, triglycerides, HDL-chol.) – Fundoscopy – Kidney checkup (urinalysis, microalbuminuria, serum creatinine)
Every other year, especially if patient is older than age 35
– Vascular checkup including ECG, BP estimation, physical and Ultrasound-Doppler examination of cerebral and leg arteries – Examination of the peripheral nerve system ? – Assessment of clotting equilibrium?

Table 5 Diagnostic measures for cerebral and peripheral vascular disease and diabetic foot problems

- History of the duration and control of diabetes; identification of cardiovascular risk factors, previous or existing TIA, RIND or stroke, claudication, rest pain, foot ulcers, neuropathy, infections or trauma
- Examination for neurologic deficits, "hemi"-symptomatology etc. and for trophic changes, deformities, local inflammation, pressure points of the feet
- Palpation of pulses, temperature differences
- Auscultation of arteries in typical sites, eventually immediately following exercise
- Angiologic investigations (electronic oscillometry, Doppler ultrasound measurements, CW-Doppler tracings, duplex sonography, intracranial Doppler if warranted)
- Neurologic investigations (neurological status, electrophysiological measurements)
- Wound swab for bacteriological examination of ulcers etc.
- Pedografic tracing for identification of pressure points or changes in foot mechanics
- Identification of microangiopathy (fundus examination, microalbuminuria, capillary microscopy)
- Radiological investigations (x-rays of the feet for identification of osteomyelitis, osteoarthropathy, angiographic examinations if necessary)

Direct CW-Doppler tracings of arterial blood flow allow the detection of stenoses or occlusions of the subclavian, common carotid, external and internal carotid and vertebral arteries as well as of the leg arteries in the inguinal, adductor, and popliteal region. Duplex sonography may yield valuable information as to the morphology of the vessel intima, vessel calcifications, ulcerations, and thrombotic material of the extracranial carotid system; color-coded Dopplers add further details concerning flow direction, turbulences, etc. (Fig. 7). Duplex investigations and intracranial Doppler tracings may be warranted in cases of neurological deficit symptoms of the brain, yet normal CW-Doppler tracings of the extracranial cerebral arteries.

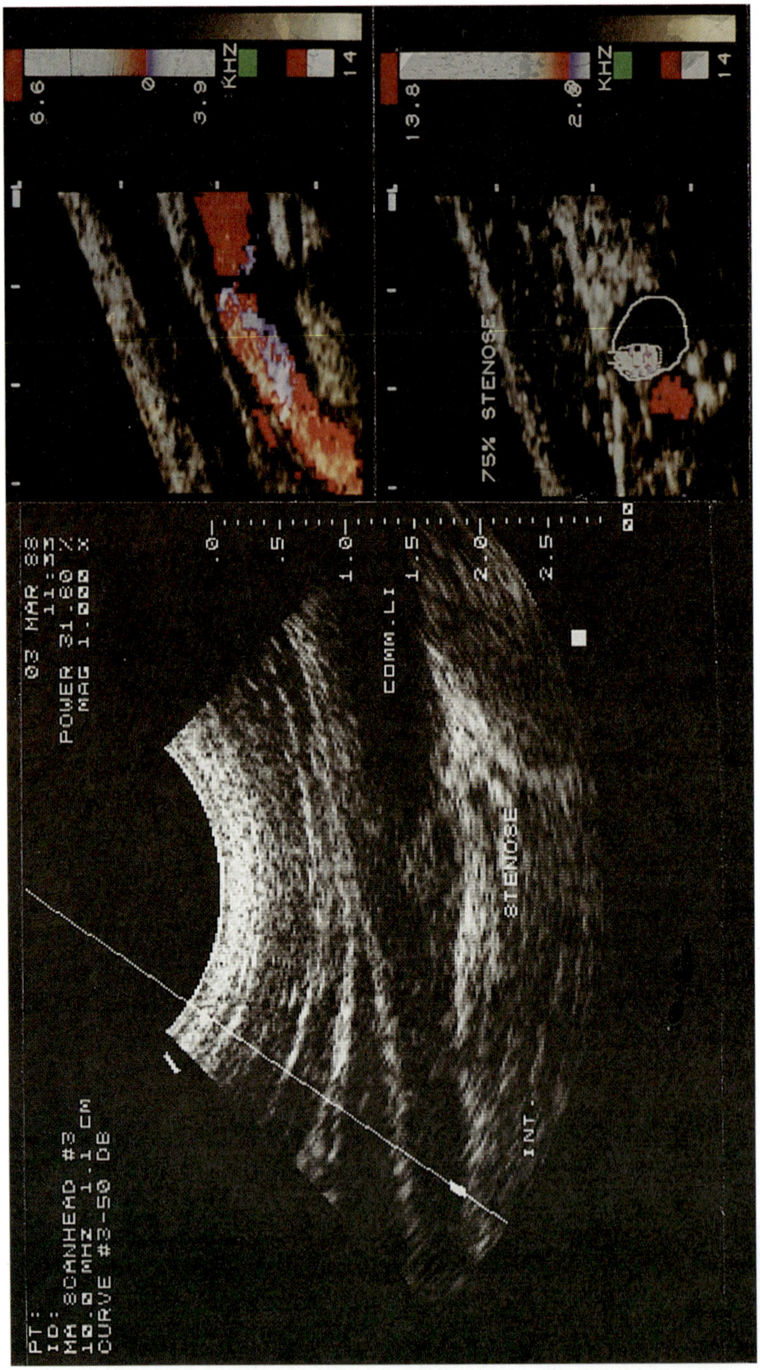

Fig. 7 Stenosis of an internal carotid artery as seen by regular Duplex and color-coded Duplex sonography

As far as Doppler examinations are concerned, the pressure index (PI) is very easy, but nevertheless very useful; it gives a reliable estimate of the leg circulation. This index is normally greater than 1:

$$PI = \frac{\text{Ankle blood pressure (systolic)}}{\text{Brachial blood pressure (systolic)}}$$

Ankle blood pressures which are 10 mmHg less than those in the arm almost always indicate occlusive arterial disease [57]. The body cannot compensate for ankle arterial blood pressures below 50 mmHg, with the result that rest pain and gangrene may develop. The validity of peripheral pressure measurements, however, is considerably reduced by the presence of arterial medial sclerosis, present in about 10% of unselected diabetics [53]. The increasing rigidity of the vessel wall leads to erroneously high pressures. Suspicion should always be aroused if there is discrepancy between the clinical findings and the pressures, particularly if the ankle pressure is 50 mmHg or more above the arm pressure. The foot should be X-rayed if arterial medial sclerosis is suspected or if there is peripheral ulceration (Fig. 3).

Angiography is invasive, and, therefore, always to be considered last when making an angiological diagnosis. It is useful for confirming decisions to untertake precutaneous transluminal angioplasty, local thrombolysis, and bypass surgery, as well as to determine amputation levels. An angiographic evaluation may also be necessary for the indication of carotid thrombendarterectomy, although when clear-cut results are gained from CW-Doppler and Duplex sonography by an experienced investigator, it can be omitted.

Neurological investigations

Detailed neurological examination is as essential as angiological investigation. It should include a careful history and testing of reflexes, with thermoreceptive measurement of the function of the small or nonmedullated fibres controlling temperature threshold and sensitivities to vibration, touch, and pain. This last technique is suitable for early recognition of peripheral neuropathy and correlates well with existing autonomic neuropathy. Measuring conduction velocity in sensory and motor nerves is less meaningful, as it mainly determines the status of the medullated and "fast" fibres [58].

Pedographic measurement of the dynamic distribution of pressure in the foot [59, 60] reveals increased loading on the forefoot and diminished toe function in diabetics (Fig. 8). The use of this technique allows the estimation of the risk of developing a neuropathic ulcer from the limiting pressure values.

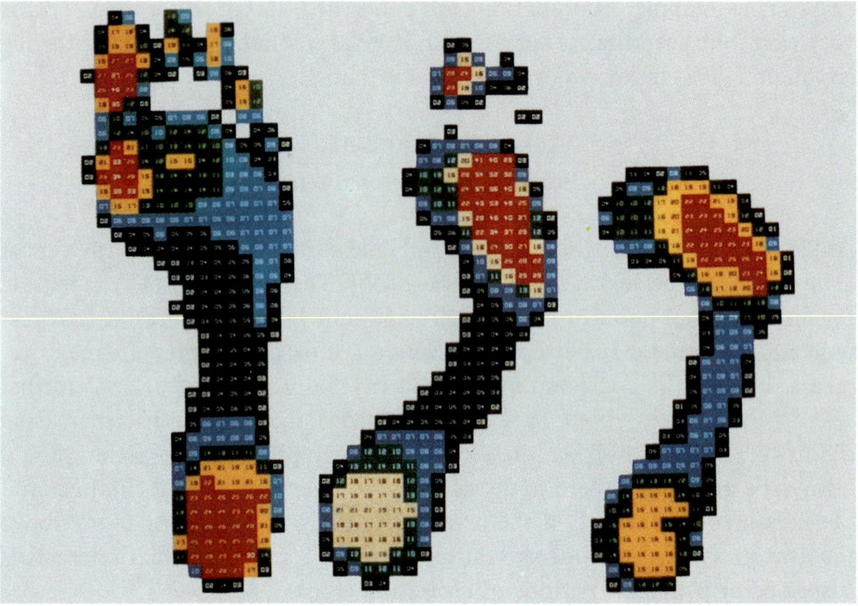

Fig. 8 Pedography: dynamic measurements of pressure distribution. The highest pressure values are shown in red color. Normal distribution of pressure in a healthy test subject with good function of the toes (left) and increasing loading of the forefoot region with loss of function of the toes in diabetic patients (middle and right panel)

Based on these examinations a clinically useful classification and staging of cerebral and peripheral vascular disease can be designed (Table 6).

Risk factors

Major progress has been made during recent years in more clearly defining the risk profile associated with the excess of macrovascular diseases in diabetic patients. A whole series of epidemiologic, mostly prospective, studies has accumulated a large body of informatioan. The risk profile was depicted in Table 7 summarized from studies like the Framingham Study, the WHO Study, the Schwabing Study, the DIS Study, the PARD Study, Finnish studies, the Pittsburg Study and the MR.FIT Project in the United States [1–4, 6–9, 13, 18, 21–26, 36, 37, 51, 61–76]. Although at first view many of these parameters seem to represent classical cardiovascular risk factors, diabetes mellitus itself is related to many of these, either in the sense of contributing to their occurrence or, vice versa, being accelerated by the preexistence of these conditions. Much of the excessive macrovascular risk of diabetic patients

Table 6 Classification and staging of cerebral and peripheral vascular disease

	Cerebral	Peripheral
Stage I (Silent)	Significant Doppler- or Duplex abnormalities; no symptoms	Significant changes seen at physical examination, decreased Doppler pressure, abnormal Doppler tracings; no symptoms
Stage II (Incipient)	TIA, RIND	Intermittent claudication
Stage III (Manifest)	Progressive stroke	Rest pain
End Stage IV (+ longterm complications)	Completed stroke, incapacitating cerebral deficit	Foot ulcer, gangrene, amputation

can be predicted on the basis of these parameters. Little is known, however, in terms of true risk factors as proven by intervention trials in diabetic populations, i. e., that a lower macrovascular complication rate results from elimination of a given risk factor. In this respect, e. g., with reference to cholesterol or hypertension, one has to rely upon results not obtained from diabetic patients alone [17].

Table 7 Risk profile of macrovascular disease in diabetes mellitus

- Age
- Hypertension (incl. systolic hypertension)
- Nephropathy (incl. early abnormalities of glomerular function, e.g. microalbuminuria)
- Dyslipoproteinemias (hypertriglyceridemia!)
- Insulin resistance/hyperinsulinemia
- Hemostasiological and hemorheological abnormalities
- Smoking

At what time during diabetes does this risk profile emerge? It has been suggested (Table 8) that in IDDM but not in NIDDM impaired kidney function sets the pace towards accelerated atherogenesis by giving rise to a whole host of the above-mentioned risk factors [17]. More recent studies of microalbuminuria, however, seem to indicate that this process is already initiated at the stage of microalbuminuria [17]. Mean blood pressure, at least, starts to rise at that stage. In NIDDM the cardiovascular risk profile may

Table 8 Prevalence of atherogenic risk markers in diabetes

Risk marker	Type 1 (IDDM)		Type II (NIDDM)
	Normal kidney function	Impaired kidney function	
Hypertension	0	+++	++
Hypercholesterolemia	0 – +	+++	+
Hypertriglyceridemia	0 – +	+++	+++
Decreased HDL cholesterol	0 – +	+++	++
BMI	0	0	+++
Risk of atherosclerosis	+?	+++	+++

Adapted from Ruderman and Haudenschild [17]

already exist at the diagnosis of diabetes; it may be literally overwhelming, diabetes just being the tip of the iceberg, as has been shown in the Schwabing Study (Table 9).

Table 9 The GP-program in the greater Munich area: risk profile in a random sample of NIDDM

	Prevalence %
HbA_{1c} (>8%)	49
Hypertension	65
Micro- and macroalbuminuria	42
Hypertriglyceridemia (>200 mg/dl)	64
Hypercholesterolemia (>250 mg/dl)	39
Fasting C-peptide (>1.4 pmol/ml)	18
BMI (male >24; female >25)	77
Factor VIII R : Ag (>130%)	73

In the Schwabing Study on macrovascular disease in diabetes, a representative cohort of more than 600 diabetic patients of all types and ages, who were seen in the outpatient clinic within a limited period of time, was followed since 1977 for up to 10 years. Based on the multiple logistic analysis, the strongest risk predictors at baseline in the whole group turned out to be "triglycerides, systolic blood pressure, and duration of diabetes, besides age" [9, 13]. Surprisingly, neither gender nor smoking, diabetes therapy, diastolic blood pressure, or cholesterol came out as significant risk predictors – which does not mean that they do not play an important role in the individual patient. In a more detailed multivariate analysis of the same data, in which men and women were considered separately, then exclusively NIDDM patients, again men vs. women, systolic blood pressure remained as the most powerful predictor of risk in all subgroups, whereas triglycerides indicated risk predominantly in females [9, 13]. It should be mentioned that cholesterol has been found to be significantly associated with macrovascular disease in diabetics in several population studies in which it was either the only lipid parameter measured or the overall background of increased cholesterol levels was high in the general population [1, 2, 4, 7].

Triglycerides are probably not a risk as such, but rather part of a syndrome, induced by poor blood glucose control, and including an atherogenic lipid profile with low HDL cholesterol, active VLDL remnants, etc. and associated with the problem of insulin resistance and hyperinsulinemia. Higher insulin levels alone have been found to be associated with, or even predictive of, macrovascular disease, both in non-diabetic and in diabetic populations [13, 47, 62–67, 71, 72, 75]. In the Schwabing Study, peripheral vascular disease was also anticipated by the use of a higher daily insulin dose at baseline in the subgroup of all insulin-treated patients, triglycerides and age being other risk predictors. Without doubt, diabetics with the most marked hyperinsulinemia carry a higher macrovascular risk, irrespective of whether hyperinsulinemia is exogenous or endogenous or caused by insulin resistance, although the pathophysiological linkage is still under debate.

Hemostasiological and hemorrheological abnormalities have been studied for many years in the context of macrovascular disease in diabetes mellitus. Recently, the PARD Study disclosed the results of a five-year prospective investigation in some 500 NIDDM patients [68]. The risk determined was mainly associated with male diabetics. Interestingly enough, higher values of spontaneous platelet aggregation, von Willebrand Factor, and fibrinogen were found to have a significant predictive power for new vascular occlusions and vascular death in diabetic men. Furthermore, a longterm intervention trial using aspirin was performed in diabetic patients of the Veterans Administration in the United States who exhibited advanced macroangiopathy and had to undergo leg amputation. Although the overall outcome of the intervention over 5 years was disappointing in terms of mortality or a second amputation, a significant reduction in the number of strokes was observed [78]. Microalbuminuria seems to be a hallmark for early cardiovascular death in NIDDM according to the results of Mogensen and Viberti [69, 70]. These observations have created a lot of interest and several groups have tried to assess the prevalence of this marker in relation to macrovascular disease in NIDDM. In a random sample of NIDDM in general practices mircoalbuminuria has been found to be very common [61], largely independent of gender, duration of diabetes, or age (Table 10). It was closely correlated with the existence of peripheral vascular disease and another parameter of glo-

Table 10 Urinary tract infection (UTI) and urine albumine excretion (UAE) in unselected NIDDM patients (percent for UAE ranges after exclusion of UTI)

Groups	n	UTI (n)	UAE (mg/l)			
			% normal	15–29	30–200	>200
All	284	44	57.7	17.1	19.6	6.7
males	101	10	50.5	18.7	19.8	11.0
females	183	34	60.4	16.1	19.5	4.0
age < = 64 y	125	13	58.9	17.8	18.8	4.5
age 65 – 75 y	159	31	54.9	16.4	20.3	8.6
♂ < = 64 y	53	3	52	20	20	8
♂ 65 – 75 y	48	7	48.8	17.1	19.5	14.6
♀ < = 64 y	72	10	64.5	16.1	17.7	1.6
♀ 65 – 75 y	111	24	57.5	16.1	20.7	5.7

merular kidney function, β_2-microglobulin in serum, as well as with other risk indicators like systolic blood pressure, triglycerides, etc. Since such a strong and complex interdependence with other risk variables is more or less true for every single parameter on the list of risks for macrovascular disease in diabetes mellitus (Table 7), specific "mono" intervention is nearly impossible.

As already touched upon several times, a risk profile of the various target areas of macrovascular disease in diabetic patients is now available. Table 11 summarizes these parameters for cerebral and peripheral vascular disease and both sexes. For cerebral vascular disease this list implicates, besides age and other macrovascular disease, mainly systolic blood pressure and clotting abnormalities, whereas for peripheral vascular disease a number of additional parameters are involved, especially in females. These parameters definitely include triglycerides, insulin dose, microalbuminuria, β_2-microglobulin in serum, von Willebrand factor, duration of diabetes, and smoking.

Prevention and treatment

If there is risk – as found by the use of a check list (Table 4) – it should probably be reduced. A lot of circumstantial evidence seems to be in favour of such a treatment approach, although intervention trials such as those carried out in nondiabetics, e. g., selectively on lipids, hypertension, aggregation, etc., are difficult, if not impossible to untertake as has been outlined in the previous chapter. The interdependence of weight and glycemia influ-

Table 11 Specific risk profile of cerebral and peripheral vascular disease in diabetes mellitus

	Vascular disease			
	Cerebral		Peripheral	
	♂	♀	♂	♀
Systolic BP	+	+	+	+
Triglycerides i.s.				+
Low HDL-cholesterol			+	+
Insulin dose			+	+
Microalbuminuria			+	+
β_2-microglobulin i.s.			+	+
Platelet aggregation	+			
v.-Willebrand factor				+
Duration of diabetes			+	+
HbA_1				+
Age	+	+	+	+
Other macroangiopathy	+	+	+	+
Smoking				+

ences insulin sensitivity, lipids, especially triglycerides and HDL cholesterol, some clotting parameters, perhaps early microalbuminuria; weight will affect blood pressure, microalbuminuria, etc., etc.. A very effective rheologic approach often consists in the avoidance of the marked hemoconcentration secondary to hyperglycemia. In all, it seems prudent to aim at good levels of glycemia, blood lipids, blood pressure, etc. at the lowest possible insulinemia, especially in insulin-treated patients.

This approach is supported by longterm survivors with diabetes. In the German Democratic Republic, where registration of all diabetics is obligatory, the "risk profile" of the total population of longterm survivors with diabetes of all types has been evaluated [79]. Three findings are particularly striking: the low prevalence of lipid disorders, the low daily insulin dose, the rather low relative body weight. Since these parmeters are connected with the potential to become a longterm survivor, shouldn't such a low risk profile be the goal for all diabetics?

More or less, such targets have been adopted by an European Consensus Conference on NIDDM and the Working Group on Hypertension in Diabetes [80, 81] (Table 12). The need for individual targets, however, has to be stressed, especially for very senior patients for whom relief of diabetes specific symptoms may be a more pertinent goal (Table 13).

At the same time one other implication becomes quite obvious: proper treatment of diabetes and prevention of vascular complications can not be

Table 12 Possible targets for patients requiring and/or aiming at "near-normoglycemia"

HbA_1 (%)	< 8
Total cholesterol (mg/dl)	<200
HDL cholesterol (mg/dl)	> 40
Fasting triglycerides (mg/dl)	<150
Blood pressure (mm/Hg)	<140/90
BMI (kg/m^2), male	< 25
female	< 24

"European Consensus Conference on NIDDM" 1987
"Working Group on Hypertension in Diabetes" 1985

Table 13 Possible targets for patients primarily seeking "relief of diabetes-specific symptoms"

HbA_1 (%)	< 9.5
Urine glucose (%)	0
Total cholesterol (mg/dl)	<250
HDL cholesterol (mg/dl)	> 35
Fasting triglycerides (mg/dl)	<200
Blood pressure (mm/Hg)	<160/95

"European Consensus Conference on NIDDM" 1987

achieved without adequate education and motivation of the patient. For example, general measures need to be taken to prevent diabetic foot problems (Table 14). It has been shown that the implementation of a sufficient education program can reduce the numbers of leg amputations by half, although macrovascular disease persists to the same degree [82]. Neurologic investigations, pedography, and pressure measurements under the sole in the shoe [83] allow shoes and insoles to be tailored to individual needs, and thereby prevent the development of neuropathic foot ulcers. A recent survey on both the state of knowledge in diabetic patients and the state of the feet, however, disclosed a profound deficit particularly in terms of appropriate foot care [10]! To make prophylaxis even more complicated: the full risk profile may be there years before the clinical diagnosis of diabetes.

Manifest disease, including hypertension, hyperlipidemia, and cardiac disease, needs to be treated, usually in the same way as in nondiabetics, although options in treatment may have distinct advantages, and disadvantages for diabetics. Metabolic control may be affected and hypoglycemia masked or prolonged by drugs with hyperglycemic potency, like β-blockers or diuretics. Interference with blood clotting and the risk of uncontrolled bleeding have to be considered carefully in patients with advanced microvascular as well as macrovascular disease. As a rule, an individual tailoring of the treatment is recommended for the diabetic with macrovascular disease. As far as prognosis or revascularisation is concerned, quite often the situation may not be the same as in nondiabetics. In particular the more peripheral vascular involvement and the combination with microangiopathy makes the problem more complex and the outcome poorer. A similar situation provided, however, results of treatment of diabetics do not seem to deviate grossly from the outcome in nondiabetics.

Table 14 Prophylactic measures to prevent diabetic foot

- Avoidance of walking in bare feet (danger of trauma)
- Avoidance of tight footwear
- Relief of pressure on deformed feet by use of orthopaedic shoes
- Correct trimming of toenails (by filing)
- Effective treatment of fungal infections and corns by the physician
- Use of foot powder for sweaty feet
- Use of lanolin ointment for dry skin
- Daily foot inspection
- Regular vascular exercise

Rheological measures

In cases of hemoconcentration and increased blood viscosity, venesection and fluid replacement to produce isovolemia or hypervolemia may be considered. A 10% hydroxyethyl starch infusion has been shown to be favourable [84]. While simple venesection without fluid replacement does not improve perfusion, the rheological improvements persist for several weeks when normovolaemia is restored after venesection [85]. Intra-arterial prostacyclin may also be tried, although the success rate is lower in diabetics than in nondiabetics, possibly because of the lower density of prostacyclin receptors in diabetics [86].

Another way to improve blood viscosity is to lower the fibrinogen level, which is often raised in diabetics [87]. Ancrod, a fibrinolytic agent, improves the microcirculation by raising tissue $p0_2$ and evening out the capillary blood flow [88].

In terms of foot problems, the success of measures depends on the maintenance of a minimum systolic pressure of about 50 mmHg in the ankle. A combination of multilevel occlusion and ankle arterial pressures below 50 mmHg is particularly unfavourable. Under such conditions, peripheral arterial ulcers do not heal, and percutaneous transluminal angioplasty, local thrombolysis, surgical vascular reconstruction, and, ultimately, amputation have to be considered.

Local measures for foot lesions

The lesion should be examined daily and necrotic layers removed and blisters drained. Swabs should be taken and cultured before antibacterials are prescribed. Local antiseptics and, in some cases, systemic, specific antibiotics are recommended. Bacterial sensitivity tests should be performed weekly, since both the resident and the infecting bacteria may change. Additional antibiotics may have to be given intra-arterially to achieve higher tissue levels.

Angioplasty and local thrombolysis

Both percutaneous transluminal angioplasty (PTA) and local thrombolysis have a low incidence of complications and produce results comparable to those of vascular surgery in both diabetics and non-diabetics [89, 90]. The longterm effects after PTA or local thrombolysis depend more on the type of peripheral occlusion in the diabetic than on the state of metabolism. There is a relationship between the patency rate and the peripheral blood flow (Fig. 9) [91].

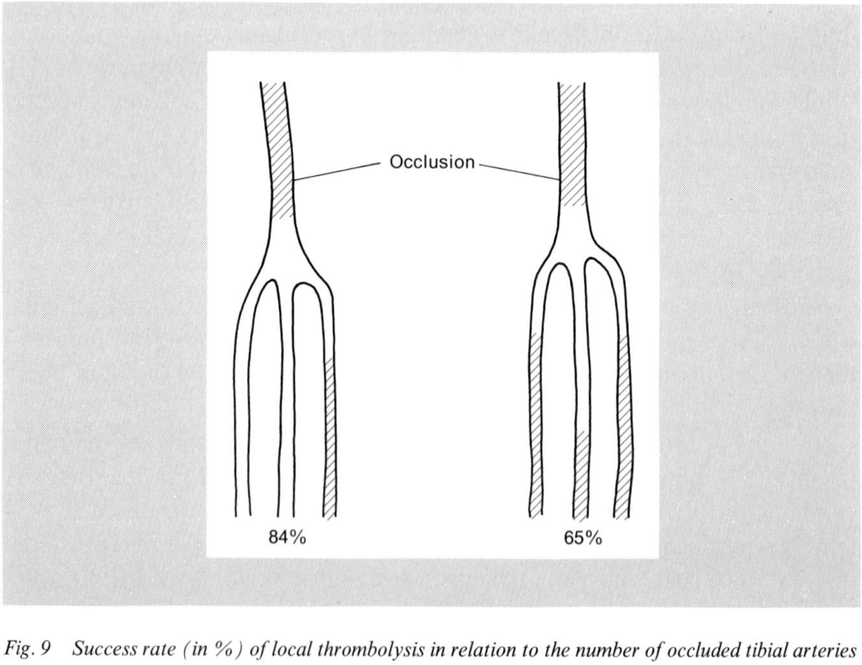

Fig. 9 Success rate (in %) of local thrombolysis in relation to the number of occluded tibial arteries

The incidence of early reocclusion is 11.5% in diabetics, compared with 3.5% in non-diabetics, and 54% of vessels in the femoro-popliteal region are still patent 5 years after PTA, compared with 79% in non-diabetics [92]. Longer occlusions may be accessible to local thrombolysis using small amounts of streptokinase, e. g. 40 000 units, or urokinase applied locally through a catheter [93]. The primary success rate of this procedure appears to be the same (85%) in diabetics and nondiabetics, and the longterm outcome is also equally good in both groups (approx. 65% patency after 30 months). Thus, there is no reason why diabetics should not undergo local thrombolysis or angioplasty, even though many are hyperaggregators. Longterm anti-platelet therapy is recommended in all patients.

Vascular surgery

Bypass surgery should be attempted in state III or IV of peripheral vascular disease if recanalisation by PTA or local thrombolysis is impossible due to the chronic nature of the occlusion. In a diabetic patient with combined femoral and popliteal occlusion, this means the implant of a femoro-crural bypass, which has a 5 year patency rate of 48 – 65% depending on the number of patent tibial arteries [94].

Reconstructive surgery can also be used to limit the extent of amputation. As the chances of success of a "limit-zone" amputation depend on the formation of a wall of granulation to limit the spread of gangrene, it should be preceded by measures to improve the peripheral circulation. In such cases, local and rheological measures can be integrated with surgical revascularization.

As far as vascular surgery of carotid artery disease is concerned, the situation has become rather ambivalent. Whereas noninvasive methods of detection have been greatly improved by the use of continuous wave Dopplers or by the advent of Duplex sonography or color coded Doppler in recent years (Fig. 7), surgical intervention i. e., carotid endarterectomy, has been questioned. It adds the risk of an operation, yet does not seem to improve overall mortality, which is quite marked (45% within 5 years) and mainly due to non-carotid related causes [95, 96]. Diabetic patients with poor metabolic control seem to do even worse than that, as do patients who object to the use of aggregation inhibitors [96]. For the time being, it seems reasonable to be even more reluctant and selective than usual in performing carotid endarterectomy in diabetics, especially if longterm glycemic control is unfavorable. Only patients with recurrent TIA or RIND (stage II) or with a rapidly progressive stenosis and a corresponding reversible neurologic deficit should be considered.

Conclusion

Most cases of acute complications of cerebral or peripheral vascular disease in diabetic patients are diagnosed in general practices, where the ultimate fate of the extremity or even of the patient is often decided. At this point, a diabetes center with experience in both the metabolic and the vascular aspects of diabetes needs to be consulted without delay. An appropriate approach to management should foresee a well functioning interaction between the general practice and a diabetes center. On that basis adequate control and care of diabetes from the beginning can bc provided aiming for prevention rather than intervention of vascular complications.

References

[1] Kannel WB, McGee DL. Diabetes and glucose tolerance as risk factor for cardiovascular disease: The Framingham Study. Diabetes Care 1979; 2: 120–126.

[1a] Kannel WB. Hypertension and other risk factors in coronary heart disease. Am Heart J 1987; 114: 918–925.

[2] Pyörälä K, Laakso M. Macrovascular disease in diabetes mellitus. In: Mann JI, Pyörälä K, Teuscher E, eds. Diabetes in epidemiological perspective. Edinburgh: Churchill Livingstone, 1983; 183–247.

[3] Krolewski AS, Warram JH, Christlieb AR. Onset, source, complications and prognosis of diabetes mellitus. In: Marble A, Krall LP, Bradley RF et al, eds. Joslin's Diabetes mellitus, 12th ed., Philadelphia: Lea & Febiger, 1985; 251–277.

[4] Prevalence of small and large vessel disease in diabetic patients from 14 centres. The WHO Multinational Study of Vascular Disease in Diabetics. Diabetologia 1985; 28 (suppl): 615–640.

[5] Steinke W, Al-Deeb S, Hennerici M. Prävalenz extrakranieller Gefäßprozesse und Risikoprofil bei Patienten mit peripherer und koronarer Arteriopathie. Vasa 1987; 16: 283–290.

[6] Panzram G, Pißarek D, Lundershausen R et al. Prospektive Verlaufsbeobachtungen beim Langzeitdiabetes. Ergebnisse der Erfurt-Studie. Dtsch med Wschr 1987; 112: 1283–1287.

[7] Laakso M, Rönnemaa T, Pyörälä K et al. Atherosclerotic vascular disease and its risk factors in non-insulin-dependent diabetic and nondiabetic subjects in Finland. Diabetes Care 1988; II: 449–463.

[8] Panzram G, Zabel-Langhenning R. Diabetes mellitus: Bedingte Gesundheit oder schicksalhafte Erkrankung. Med Klin 1984; 70: 282–289.

[9] Janka HU. Five year incidence of major macrovascular complications in diabetes mellitus. Horm Metabol Res 1985; 15 (suppl): 15–19.

[10] Standl E. Die Angiopathien des Typ II-Diabetes. Verh Dtsch Ges Inn Med 1986; 92: 579–586.

[11] Standl E. Der diabetische Fuß. Med Welt 1986; 37: 1018–1021.

[12] Stiegler H, Frey S, Standl E. Diagnostische und therapeutische Überlegungen beim "diabetischen Fuß". Med Klin 1988; 83: 263–269.

[13] Standl E, Stiegler H, Janka HU et al. Risk profile of macrovascular disease in diabetes mellitus. Diabete Metabolisme 1988; 14: 505–511.

[14] Levine ME, O'Neal IW. The diabetic foot. 3rd ed. St. Louis–Toronto–London: Mosby, 1983.

[15] National Health Interview Survey. Harris MI, Hamman RF, eds. Diabetes in America. US Government Printing Office, NIH Publication 1985; No 85–1468.
[16] Jönsson B, Persson U. Diabetes – eine gesundheitsökonomische Studie. Swedish Institute for Health Economics, Copenhagen 1981.
[17] Ruderman NB, Haudenschild C. Diabetes as an atherogenic factor. Progr Cardiovasc Dis 1984; 26: 373–412.
[18] Fuller JH, Shipley MJ, Rose G et al. Coronary heart disease and impaired glucose tolerance: The Whitehall study. Lancet 1980; I: 1373–1376.
[19] Reaven GM, Hoffman BB. A role for insulin in the aetiology and course of hypertension? Lancet 1987; II: 435–437.
[19a] Reaven GM. Abnormal lipoprotein metabolism in noninsulin-dependent diabetes mellitus. Am J Med 1987; 83 (suppl 3 A): 31–40.
[20] Ferrannini E, Buzzogoli G, Bonadonna R et al. Insulin resistance in essential hypertension. N Engl J Med 1987; 371: 350–357.
[21] Uusitupa M, Niskanen L, Siitonen O et al. Hyperinsulinemia and hypertension in patients with newly diagnosed non-insulin-dependent diabetes. Diabete Metabolisme 1987; 13: 369–374.
[22] Krolewski AS, Kosinski EJ, Warram JH et al. Magnitude and determinants of coronary artery disease in juvenile-onset, insulin-independent diabetes mellitus. Am J Cardiol 1987; 59: 750–755.
[23] Dorman JS, La Porte RE, Kuller LH et al. The Pittsburgh insulin-dependent diabetes mellitus (IDDM) morbidity and mortality study. Mortality results. Diabetes 1984; 33: 271–276.
[24] Borch-Johnsen K, Andersen PK, Deckert T. The effect of proteinuria on selective mortality in type I (insulin dependent) diabetes mellitus. Diabetologia 1985; 28: 590–596.
[25] Janka HU. Pathogenetische Faktoren für die Atherosklerose des Diabetikers. Akt Endokr Stoffw 1983; 4: 9–15.
[26] Stout RW. Insulin and atheroma – an update. Lancet 1987; I: 1077–1079.
[27] Standl E. Intravascular clotting factors. Diab Res Clin Pract 1988; 4 (suppl I): 11–14.
[28] Vlassara H, Brownlee M, Cerami A. Nonenzymativ glycosylation: role in the pathogenesis of diabetic complications. Clin Chem 1986; 32 B: 37–41.
[28a] Cerami A, Vlassara H, Brownlee M. Glucose and aging. Sci Am 1987; 256: 90–96.
[29] Gonen B, Go R, Quinn T. Nonenzymatic glycosylation of proteins: possible relevance to microangiopathy. Front diabetes. Basel: Karger, 1987; 8: 1–15.
[30] Williamson JR, Chang T, Tilton R et al. Etiopathogenesis of diabetic microangiopathy. An integrated view. Front Diabetes. Basel: Karger, 1987; 8: 58–66.
[31] Standl E. Diabetische Mikroangiopathien. Internist 1987; 28: 262–272.
[32] Ceriello A, Giugliano D, Dello Russo P et al. Metabolic control may alter antithrombin III activity but not its plasma concentration in diabetes: a possible role for nonenzymativ glycosylation. Diabetes Care 1986; 9: 32–35.
[33] Greene DA, Lattimer SA. Biochemical alterations and complications in diabetes. Clin Chem 1986; 32 B: 42–47.
[34] Robey C, Dasmakapatra A, Cohen MP et al. Sorbinil partially prevents decreased erythrocyte deformability in experimental diabetes mellitus. Diabetes 1987; 36: 1010–1013.
[35] Moore S. Pathogenesis of Atherosclerosis. Metabolism 1985; 34 (suppl I): 13–16.
[36] Janka HU, Standl E, Schramm W et al. Platelet enzyme activities in diabetes mellitus in relation to endothelial damage. Diabetes 1983; 32 (suppl 2): 47–51.
[37] Colwell JA, Winocour PD, Lopes-Virella M et al. New Concepts about the pathogenesis of atherosclerosis in diabetes mellitus. Amer J Med 1983; 75: 67–80.
[38] Harrison HE, Johnson M. Vascular prostacyclin release and metabolic derangement in diabetes. Horm Metab Res 1981; (suppl 11): 43–49.
[39] Mayfield RK, Halushka PV, Wohltmann HJ et al. Platelet function during continuous insulin infusion treatment in insulin-dependent diabetic patients. Diabetes 1985; 34: 951–954.

[40] Thomas G, Skrinska V, Lucas FV et al. Platelet glutathione and thromboxane synthesis in diabetes. Diabetes 1985; 34: 951–954.

[41] Jones RL. Fibrinopeptide A in diabetes mellitus. Relation to levels of blood glucose, fibrinogen disappearance and hemodynamic changes. Diabetes 1985; 34: 836–843.

[42] Jones DB, Davis TME, Bown E et al. Determinants of ADP-induced platelet aggregation in diabetes mellitus. Diabetologia 1986; 29: 291–294.

[43] Sugimoto H, Franks DJ, Lecavalier et al. Therapeutic modulation of growth promoting activity in platelets from diabetics. Diabetes 1987; 36: 667–672.

[44] Vague P, Juhan-Vague I, Ailand MF et al. Correlation between blood fibrinolytic activity, plasminogen activator inhibitor level, plasma insulin level, and relative body weight in normal and obese subjects. Metabolism 1986; 35: 250–253.

[45] Voisin PJ, Rousselle D, Streiff F et al. Reduction of beta-thromboglobulin levels in diabetics controlled by artificial pancreas. Metabolism 1983; 232: 138–141.

[46] Vukovich TC, Schernthaner G. Decreased protein C levels in patients with insulin-dependent type 1 diabetes mellitus. Diabetes 1986; 35: 617–619.

[47] Standl E, Vague P. Hyperinsulinemia as a possible risk factor of macrovascular disease in diabetes mellitus. Diabete Metabolisme 1987; 13: 277–394.

[48] Vinters HV, Berliner JA. The blood vessel wall as an insulin target tissue. Diabete Metabolisme 1987; 13: 294–300.

[49] Young IR, Stout RW, Effect of insulin and glucose on the cells of the arterial wall: interaction of insulin with dibutyryl cyclic AMP and low density lipoprotein in arterial cells. Diabete Metabolisme 1987; 13: 301–306.

[50] Pfeifle B, Hamann H, Fußgänger R et al. Insulin as a growth regulator of arterial smooth muscle cells: effect of insulin on IGF 1. Diabete Metabolisms 1987; 113: 326–330.

[51] Janka HU, Standl E, Mehnert H. Peripheral vascular disease in diabetes mellitus and its relation to cardiovascular risk factors: screening with the Doppler-ultrasound technique. Diabetes Care 1980; 3: 207–213.

[52] Hach W, Beule J. Funktionsfähigkeit des Profunda-Kreislaufs bei Patienten mit peripherer arterieller Verschlußkrankheit. Med Welt 1980; 31: 1814–1818.

[53] Janka HU, Bloss G, Oberparleiter F et al. Mediasklerose bei Diabetikern. Reihenuntersuchung ambulanter Patienten mit der Ultraschall-Doppler-Methode. In: Ehringer H, Betz E, Bollinger A et al, eds. Gefäßwand, Rezidivprophylaxe, Raynaud-Syndrom. Baden-Baden: Witzstrock, 1979; 573–575.

[54] Edmonds ME, Morrison N, Laws JW et al. Medial arterial calcification and diabetic micropathy. Br Med J 1982; 284: 928–930.

[55] Bollinger A, Frey J, Jäger K et al. Patterns of diffusion through skin capillaries in patients with longterm diabetes. New Engl J Med 1982; 307: 1305–1308.

[56] Cicmir J, Berger J, Gries FA. Die diabetische Polyneuropathie. Dtsch Ärztebl 1983; 80: 25–31.

[57] Köhler M, Roth FJ, El-Mammoun B. Untersuchungen über die Spezifität der peripheren systolischen Druckmessung mit der Ultraschall-Doppler-Technik an gesunden angiografierten Extremitäten. Z Kardiol 1982; 71: 156–159.

[58] Greene DA, Brown MD, Braunstein SN et al. Comparison of clinical course and sequential electrophysiological tests in diabetics with symptomatic polyneuropathy and its implication for clinical trials. Diabetes 1981; 30: 139–147.

[59] Kirsch D, Frey S, Schuh D et al. Dynamische Druckverteilungsmessung unter dem Fuß an Patienten mit diabetischen Ulcera. Akt Endokrin Stoffw 1985; 6: 133–142.

[60] Boulton AJM, Betts RP, Franks CI. Abnormalities of foot pressure in early diabetic neuropathy. Diab Medicine 1987; 4: 225–228.

[61] Standl E, Rebell B, Stiegler H et al. Prevalence and risk of incipient diabetic nephropathy in type 2 (non-insulin-dependent) diabetes mellitus. Diabetologia 1987; 30: 584–585.

[62] Welborn TA, Wearne K. Coronary heart disease incidence and cardiovascular mortality in Busselton with reference to glucose and insulin concentrations. Diabetes Care 1979; 2: 154–160.

[63] Pyörälä K, Savolainen E, Kankola S et al. Plasma insulin as coronary heart disease risk factor: relationship to other risk factors and predictive value during 9.5 years follow-up of the Helsinki Policemen Study population. Acta Med Scand 1985; 701 (suppl I): 38–52.
[64] Eschwege E, Richard JL, Thibault et al. Coronary heart disease mortality in relation with diabetes, blood glucose and plasma-insulin levels. The Paris Prospective Study, ten years later. Horm Metab Res 1985; 15 (suppl): 41–46.
[65] Hockaday TDR, Phil D. Serum insulin concentrations and anticipatory factors of cardiomyopathy in NIDDM. Diabete Metabolisme 1987; 13: 354–358.
[66] Standl E, Janka HU. High serum insulin concentrations in relation to other cardiovascular risk factors in macrovascular disease of type II diabetics. Horm Metab Res 1985; 15 (suppl): 46–51.
[67] Janka HU, Ziegler AG, Standl E et al. Daily insulin dose as a predictor of macrovascular disease in insulin treated non-insulin-dependent diabetics. Diabete Metabolisme 1987; 113: 359–364.
[68] Breddin HK, Krzywanek HJ, Althoff P et al. PARD Platelet aggregation as a risk factor in diabetics: Results of a prospective study. Horm Metabol Res 1985; 15 (suppl): 63–68.
[69] Mogensen CE. Microalbuminuria predicts clinical proteinuria and early mortality in maturity onset diabetes. N Engl J Med 1984; 310: 356–360.
[70] Viberti GC, Hill RD, Jarrett RJ. Microalbuminuria as a predictor of clinical nephropathy in insulin-dependent diabetes mellitus. Lancet 1982; I: 1430–1431.
[71] Pyörälä K, Uusitupa M, Laakso M et al. Macrovascular complications in relation to hyperinsulinemia in non-insulin-dependent diabetes mellitus. Diabete Metabolisme 1987; 13: 345–349.
[72] Fontbonne A, Eschwege E. Diabetes, hyperglycemia, hyperinsulinemia and atherosclerosis: epidemiological data. Diabete Metabolisme 1987; 13: 350–353.
[73] Jarrett RJ, McCartney P, Keen H. The Bedford survey. Ten year mortality in newly diagnosed diabetics and normoglycemic controls and risk indices for coronary heart disease in borderline diabetics. Diabetologia 1982; 22: 79–84.
[74] Beach KW, Bedford GR, Bergelin RO et al. Progression of lower-extremity arterial occlusive disease in type II diabetes mellitus. Diabetes Care 1988; 11: 464–472.
[75] Pyörälä K, Laakso M, Uusitupa M. Diabetes and atherosclerosis: an epidemiological view. Diabetes Metab Res 1987; 3: 463–524.
[76] Stamler J, Wentworth D, Neaton J et al. Diabetes and risk of coronary, cardiovascular, and all cause mortality. Findings of 356000 men screened by the multiple risk factor intervention trial. Circulation 1984; 70: 11– 16 IA.
[77] Wiseman W, Viberti G, Mackintosh D et al. Glycemia, arterial pressure and microalbuminuria in type 1 diabetes mellitus. Diabetologia 1984; 26: 401–405.
[78] Colwell JA, Bingham SF, Abraira C et al. Veterans Administration cooperative study on antiplatelet agents in diabetic patients after amputation for gangrene. II. Effect of aspirin and dipyridamole on atherosclerotic vascular disease rates. Diabetes Care 1986; 9: 140–148.
[79] Panzram G, Pißarek D. Long-term diabetes. Associated factors in survivorship and mortality. Horm Metab Res 1985; 15 (suppl): 10–15.
[80] Gries FA, Alberti KGMM for the European Consensus Group. Management of non-insulin-dependent diabetes mellitus in Europe: A consensus statement. IDF-Bulletin 1987; 32: 169–173.
[81] The Working Group on Hypertension in Diabetes. Statement on Hypertension in Diabetes mellitus. Final report. Arch Int Med 1987; 147: 830–842.
[82] Davidson JK, Alogna MT, Goldsmith MP et al. Assessment of program effectiveness at Grady Memorial Hospital. In: Lawrence P, Steiner G, eds. Educating of the diabetic patient. New York: Springer Publishing Co, 1981; 329–348.
[83] Schaff P, Kirsch D, Hauser W et al. Eine Geräteentwicklung zur Messung der Druckverteilung unter der Fußsohle im Schuh und deren Anwendbarkeit in der Diabetologie. Akt Endokr Stoffw 1987; 7: 129–135.

[84] Haaß A, Kroemer H, Jäger H et al. Dextran 40 or HAES 200/05? Dtsch Med Wschr 1986; 111: 1681–1686.
[85] Rudofsky G, Meyer P, Strohmeyer HG. Effect of hemodilution on resting flow and reactive hyperemia in lower limbs. Bibl Haemat 1982; 47: 157–161.
[86] Steurer G, Ettl K, Janovic B et al. Characterisation of (^{3}H) Iloprost receptors in human platelet membranes in comparison with smokers and diabetics. 4th Congr Soc Thrombos Haemostas (GTH) Düsseldorf 1986.
[87] Jensen T, Stender S, Deckert T. Abnormalities in plasma's concentrations of lipoproteins and fibrinogen in type 1 (insulin-dependent) diabetic patients with increased urinary albumin excretion. Diabetologia 1988; 31: 142–145.
[88] Ehrly AM, Köhler HJ, Ichvondet W et al. Sauerstoffdruckwerte im ischämischen Muskelgewebe von Patienten mit chronischen peripheren arteriellen Verschlußkrankheiten. Klin Wschr 1975; 53: 687–691.
[89] Stiegler H, Lander Th, Standl E. Angioplastie einschließlich lokaler Thrombolyse beim diabetischen Patienten. Akt Endokrin Stoffw 1987; 8: 40–43.
[90] Stiegler H, Standl E. Nichtchirurgische Maßnahmen zur Wiederherstellung der Strombahn bei peripher arterieller Verschlußkrankheit unter besonderer Berücksichtigung der lokalen Thrombolyse. Intern Welt 1985; 5: 135–141.
[91] Roth FJ, Krings W, Cappius G et al. Die lokale, niedrig dosierte fibrinolytische Therapie. Indikation, Technik und Resultat. Vasa 1984; 12: 52–56.
[92] Bollinger A, Schlumpf M. Grüntzig A et al. Perkutane transluminale Angioplastie (PTA) bei Diabetikern mit peripherer arterieller Verschlußkrankheit. Akt Endokr Stoffw 1983; 2: 62–65.
[93] Stiegler H, Hufen V, Weichenhain B et al. Ergebnisse der lokalen Thrombolyse unter besonderer Berücksichtigung einer diabetischen Stoffwechsellage. Dtsch med Wschr 1989 (In press).
[94] Raithel D. Die crurale Gefäßrekonstruktion als Alternative zur Amputation der ischämischen Extremität. In: Denk H, Hagmüller GW, Brunner U, eds. Arterielle Durchblutungsstörungen der unteren Extremitäten: "Grenzzonen der Therapieentscheidung". TM Oeynhausen 1982; 53–56.
[95] Winslow CM, Solomon DH, Chassin MR et al. The appropriateness of carotid endarterectomy. N Engl J Med 1988; 318: 721–727.
[96] Stiegler H, Forsmann T, Standl E et al. 5 Jahresverlauf nach Thromendarteriektomie der A.carotis. Dtsch med Wschr 1988; 113: 1987–1993.

General monitoring of risk factors and late complications

C.E. Mogensen, E. Standl

The prognosis and quality of life of diabetic patients depend largely on the chronic complications in the context of the disordered metabolism, together with associated disease. It is the main purpose of this entire publication to focus on the prevention and appropriate treatment of these diabetic late complications. Particular attention has, therefore, to be paid to the established precipitating factors and to the early detection and monitoring of emerging

Table 1 Baseline monitoring of risk factors and late complications in diabetic patients

Family history of
Hypertension
Arteriosclerotic disease
Individual history of
Hypertension
Dyslipoproteinemias
Smoking
Vascular and neuropathic complications
3 monthly assessment
Body weight
Glycated hemoglobin
Blood pressure
Annual assessment
Lipid profile (cholesterol, triglycerides, HDL-cholesterol)
Fundoscopy (dilated pupils)
Kidney check-up (urinalysis, microalbuminuria in an overnight urine sample, serum creatinine)
Foot inspection
Bi-annual assessment (especially in patients after 35 years of age)
Vascular check-up including ECG, chest x-ray, physical and Ultrasound-Doppler examination of cerebral and limb arteries
Autonomic nervous heart rate control
Examination of the peripheral nerve system
Hemostatic and hemorrheologic evaluation (e. g. F VIII R:AG, fibrinogen)

vascular and non vascular sequelae. More specifically, emphasis has to be put on the screening, treatment or elimination, respectively, of hypertension, dyslipoproteinemias, smoking, retinopathy, renal disease, neuropathy, foot problems, and coronary, cerebrovascular and other severe macrovascular disease. The following recommendations for screening are derived from the specific chapters in this book and differentiate between baseline screening and monitoring of patients with already incipient or more advanced disease (Tables 1 and 2). For details, the pertinent chapters of this book should be consulted.

Table 2 *Monitoring of risk factors and late complications in addition to baseline screening in diabetic patients with incipient or more advanced sequelae*

Monthly assessment
Blood pressure (supine and standing)

3 to 6 monthly assessment
Lipid profile (if abnormal)
Urine albumine (if elevated)
Fundoscopy (if retinopathy is present or in longterm diabetics; in addition fundus fotography and fluorescence angiography may be warranted) GFR, serum creatinine and electrolytes (if baseline kidney function parameters are abnormal)

Assessment in appropriate cases
Kidney ultrasound scan
Echocardiogram, thallium scan of the heart, eventually followed by coronary angiography
Longterm ECG
Duplex sonography of peripheral, cerebral, and renal arteries, eventually followed by the respective angiograms
Transcranial Doppler
Pedographic evaluation
Quantitative sensory testing
Electrodiagnostic evaluation of the peripheral nerve-muscle system
Autonomic function testing
Whole blood and plasma viscosity
Refined evaluation of the clotting equilibrium (e. g. platelet aggregation, β-thromboglobulin in serum, thromboxane excretion in urine)

In special cases
Kidney biopsy or sural nerve biopsy should be considered

Note! Referral of patient to a specialised diabetes center may be advisable if progress is unsatisfactory or diagnostic assessment and sequence of procedures appear to be doubtful.

Treatment in relation to risk factors

T. Jensen, T. Deckert

Life expectancy and quality of life are reduced in patients with both insulin-dependent and non-insulin-dependent diabetes mellitus. This reduction is due to metabolic catastrophies like hypoglycemia, ketoacidosis, and hyperosmolar hyperglycemia as well as to the development of late complications like micro- and macroangiopathy. The etiology and pathogenesis of late complications is complicated and not fully understood. Recent observations indicate that not only hyperglycemia but also several other factors can contribute to the onset and progression of late complications. Such factors are called risk factors. This chapter deals with the occurrence and importance of some of these risk factors. We will especially discuss whether intervention directed against risk factors results in prognostic benefits for the patient.

Hyperglycemia

Morphologic alterations

The influence of the metabolic abnormalities of diabetes on late complications are clearly seen in studies of discordant monozygotic twins and in patients with secondary diabetes. Thus, non-diabetic monozygotic twin mates had less *basement membrane thickening* of muscle capillaries than did their twin mates with insulin-dependent diabetes [1]. Also, the thickness of the glomerular basement membrane and the mesangial volume in all diabetic twins exceeded the values in the respective sibling ($p < 0.0035$), even when the result in the diabetic twin was within established normal ranges [2]. Significant basement membrane thickening of muscle capillaries has been demonstrated in patients without genetic diabetes who developed diabetes after ingestion of Vacor, a rat poison which results in hyperglycemia [3]. After only 6.2 years of diabetes duration, the muscle capillary basement membrane width (MCBMW) in these patients had increased to a level similar to that of patients with "genetic" insulin-dependent diabetes. Not less than 44% of the patients had retinopathy, and 28% proteinuria. The level of hyperglycemia seems to play a role in MCBMW, as demonstrated by Sosenko [4]. This investigator found that in post-pubertary diabetic patients the thickness of muscle capillary basement membrane is positively related to the level of glycemia as evaluated by serial determinations of glycated hemoglobin. In a prospective controlled study of 23 insulin-dependent (Type 1) diabetics who had had the disease for an average of 15 years [5], 13 received intensive treatment with insulin infusion, while the other 10 received conventional treatment. After two years the average width of the muscle capillary basement membranes was significantly reduced in the intensively treated group, whereas no significant change had occurred in the conventionally treated subjects. Similar results were obtained with patients suffering from Type 2 diabetes [6].

Transplantation of normal kidneys to hyperglycemic diabetic patients leads to increased glomerular basement membrane thickening and to *mesangial expansion* within two years. This is not the case in kidneys transplanted to non-diabetics [7]. These alterations do not appear in diabetics who were successfully treated with simultaneous pancreas transplantation and kidney transplantation [8]. Recently reversal of some of the renal lesions has also been observed after successful pancreas transplantation to 6 patients with IDDM [9] and after transplantation of one diabetic glomerulosclerotic kidney to a non-diabetic recipient [10]. Thus, the diabetic environment is a necessary condition for the development of basement membrane thickening and glomerular changes.

Retinopathy

The formation of *microaneurysms* seems to be also dependent on glycemic control. Thus, Weber et al. [11] found that the appearance of microaneurysms was delayed by 4.5 years in young insulin-dependent diabetics on good metabolic control as compared to similar patients on poor metabolic control. Doft et al [12] followed adolescents aged 14–17 years with diabetes of at least 8 years duration for a mean period of 3 years. There was a highly significant correlation between degree of metabolic control and presence of early retinopathy. However, these studies were not randomized and regular measurements of hemoglobin A_{1c} were not taken from the onset of diabetes. In a controlled prospective study (the Oslo study) [13] where patients were randomized to different treatment groups resulting in statistically significant differences of mean hemoglobin A_{1c} during a 2-year treatment period, patients treated with continuous subcutaneous insulin infusion (CSII) and multiple insulin injections (MIT) developed only 1.5 red retinal spots per patient, whereas the conventionally treated patiens developed 9.5 red spots per patient during the 2 year experimental period, the difference being significant (p <

0.05). However, after 4 years the difference between the groups was no longer significant [14]. In another prospective controlled study comprising 64 patients, the Kroc Study [15, 16], in which the randomized treatment groups also demonstrated significant differences in hemoglobin A_{1c} during a 2-year experimental period, no difference in the number of microaneurysms was seen at the end of the experimental period. In alloxan diabetic dogs [17], however, a 5-year, prospective, controlled study demonstrated clearly that the development of microaneurysms could be prevented by strict metabolic control. In Type 2 (non-insulin-dependent) diabetes mellitus the influence of glycemic control on the onset of retinopathy was less convincing. Thus, in the UGDP study [18] retinopathy could not be related to treatment regimen. In the Oxford Study [19] comprising 149 patients with Type 2 diabetes under the age of 66 and followed from diagnosis for about 7 years, a graded relationship between glycemic control and the prevalence of reinopathy as judged by fundus color photography could be demonstrated. In another study the prevalence of retinopathy was found to be linearly correlated to the level of hemoglobin A_{1c} over its entire range in 185 Type 2 diabetics between 55–75 years of age [21]. Taken together these studies indicate that the formation of early retinopathy can be prevented by strict metabolic control.

Although the onset of capillary basement membrane thickening, mesangial enlargement, and microaneurysms are dependent on hyperglycemia or its associates, the correlation to the level of glycemia is poor. This may indicate that factors other than hyperglycemia play a considerable role or that the difference in glycemic level which can be obtained between two experimental groups in a clinical setting are inadequate. This is also the problem in the few prospective, controlled, randomized trials which until now have been performed to investigate the influence of near normal glycemia on the progression of diabetic retinopathy.

Six centers have studied the *progression of retinopathy* [13, 16, 23, 24, 25]. Since dramatic effects were expected when the studies started, the number of patients studied in the various groups was small. The degree of retinopathy varied greatly in the different study groups, but cases with proliferative retinopathy were not included. The observation time was about 2 years in all experiments. In all studies except the last one a significant difference in hemoglobin A_{1c} between the experimental group and the control group was demonstrated during and at the end of the experimental period. The results were rather similar: in most of the patients progression could not be stopped, but was less in those groups of patients who were allocated to intensified insulin therapy and, therefore, had significantly better metabolic control. However, statistically significant differences in the retinal morphology changes during the observation period were only obtained in the extremely well matched Olso Study [13] and the study from Dallas [24], which was, however, non-randomized. None of the studies demonstrated significant statistical differences in the morphology of the retina between the experimental group and the controls at the end of the study. However, a significant correlation was seen between changes in retinal morphology and mean hemoglobin A_{1c} during the 2 years experimental period in the Steno Study, but the correlation coefficient was weak ($r = 0.32$, $p < 0.05$ (unpublished observation). Taken together these studies strongly indicate that strict metabolic control retards the progression of early retinopathy, though the differences obtained by ordinary moderate control versus so-called near normalization of blood glucose were by no means dramatic.

The only dramatic changes seen in three of the studies [13, 15, 26] were rapid but reversible deterioration of retina morphology within 3–12 months after the onset of the study in the near normal glycemic groups. Similar deterioration was seen by others [27]. Deterioration was most typically seen in the form of cotton wool exudates and was more frequent in patients with more advanced retinopathy at onset of the study [22]. Patients who deteriorated reversibly were characterized by steeper decrement of hemoglobin A_{1c} than patients who did not develop cotton wool exudates [13].

The influence of strict metabolic control on *advanced retinopathy* is difficult to assess. The Joslin Group studied the incidence of proliferative retinopathy in relation to diabetes control [28]. They found the incidence of proliferative retinopathy to be unrelated to diabetic control during the first 5 years of diabetes. However, 5–9 years and 10–14 years after the onset of diabetes, control was significantly correlated to the incidence of proliferative retinopathy [28]. Dornan [29] compared the mean of all postprandial blood glucose measurement at hospital clinics from the time of diagnosis of diabetes to detection of retinopathy in 37 insulin-dependent diabetics who had remained free from retinopathy despite diabetes of long duration (mean 30 years) with mean blood glucose of 44 patients of similar age at onset of diabetes who had developed proliferative retinopathy after 19 ± 5 years of diabetes. He found a highly significant difference between the two groups (9.9 ± 2.1 mmol/1 and 12.4 ± 2.1 mmol/1, respectively, $p < 0.0001$). However, blood pressure and serum creatinine were higher in patients with proliferative retinopathy and the disturbing factor of clinical nephropathy was not taken into consideration [30]. Similar results were found by Rand et al. [31] and Klein et al. [32]. In the Steno Study [22] the development of proliferative retinopathy during the 2 year prospective randomized trial was similar in the CSII and the control group (5/15 and 6/15, respectively).

Whether cure of diabetes by successful pancreas transplantation had any favourable influence on late stage retinopathy in patients with Type 1 diabetes was studied by the Minneapolis group [33]. The study groups consisted of 22 patients with functional grafts for a mean of 24 months. The control group consisted of 16 patients who were followed after a failed pancreas transplantation or while awaiting pancreas transplants. The number of eyes which progressed to a more severe stage of retinopathy was similar in the two groups, 44% and 32%, respectively, the difference being not significant.

The conclusion from these studies is that the level of hyperglycemia is of importance for the onset and progression of early retinopathy. Its influence on advanced retinopathy is, however, doubtful (Table 1). It has to be pointed out that Argon-laser treatment in patients with proliferative retinopathy or maculopathy seems to be far more effective than the strict metabolic control which today can be obtained in a clinical setting.

Table 1 Effect of strict metabolic control on diabetic retinopathy

Onset of retinopathy	+
Progression of background retinopathy	+
Progression of proliferative retinopathy	0

Neuropathy

Prospective controlled randomized studies of strict metabolic control on early nerve morphology have not yet been published. However, persistently decreased *nerve conduction velocity* (NCV) indicating distal axonal transport defects probably reflect morphologic changes in the long nerves. Positive correlation between nerve conduction velocity (NCV) and blood glucose control has been found in numerous studies of diabetic patients [34, 35]. In unstable hyperglycemic patients with Type 2 diabetes the degree of improvement in NCV was found to be proportional to the degree of glycemic lowering [34, review see 36]. Recently improvement of nerve conduction velocity has also been found in prospective controlled studies using CSII to establish strict metabolic control. Thus, conventionally treated patients with IDDM and normal NCV demonstrated a significant decrease of NCV during a 2 year observation period, a deterioration which was totally prevented by strict metabolic control in the pump-treated patients [37]. In the total group of patients a statistically significant negative correlation ($r = -0.40$, $p < 0.01$) was found between the change of NCV and the mean hemoglobin A_{1c} during the 2 year experimental period.

Service et al. [38] found significant improvement in several of 40 different parameters measured after 8 months of CSII. Gries [39] also found an improvement of NCV after 2 years of strict metabolic control (hemoglobin $A_{1c} < 8,6\%$) in a controlled prospective study including 70 patients with insulin-dependent diabetes. In the poorly regulated group of patients (hemoglobin $A_{1c} > 8,5\%$) improvement of NCV was seldom seen. In another 2 year randomized prospective trial, deterioration of sensory nerve function was effectively prevented by intensive management of insulin-dependent diabetes [40]. Young [41] found the progression of subclinical polyneuropathy in a representative group of 75 young patients with Type 1 diabetes to be significantly related to poor glycemic control over a 2.5 year period, but other influences were also important. In the Steno Study [22] autonomous neuropathy as measured by beat to beat variation significantly deteriorated in the control group treated by conventional insulin treatment, whereas beat to beat variation was stable in CSII treated patients. In the second Steno Study (Feldt-Rasmussen, unpublished results) a significant improvement in beat to beat variation was seen in 18 insulin-dependent patients with persistent microalbuminuria allocated to CSII treatment while deterioration was seen in the control group. An uncontrolled 2 year trial on 20 IDDM patients, however, failed to show improvement of autonomous neuropathy by improvement of glycemic control [42]. Advanced diabetic neuropathy does not seem to be favorably influenced by successful pancreas transplantations [43].

In general the results of prospective controlled treatment studies on nerve function seems to be more convincing than those on retinopathy [Table 2]. However, here too the overlap of glycemic levels during the treatment period between cases and controls makes it difficult to render clearcut results. As pointed out by Hanssen [44], however, the effects obtained by strict metabolic control seem to be much more consistent than those obtained by aldose reductase inhibitors.

Table 2 Effect of strict metabolic control on diabetic neuropathy

Motor nerve conduction velocity	+
Sensory nerve function	+
Autonomous neuropathy	+
Advanced neuropathy	0

Nephropathy

Persistently increased urinary albumin excretion rate (UalbV) is an early marker of clinical nephropathy (protein excretion > 0.5 g/24 h in several consecutive urine samples in diabetes without urinary infection, cardiac insufficiency, or other chronic renal diseases). The influence of strict metabolic control on UalbV has, therefore, been investigated by several groups. The importance of short term poor metabolic regulation for UalbV has been clearly demonstrated by Parving [45], who measured UalbV in 10 insulin-dependent diabetic patients of short duration (< 4 years), in both good and poor metabolic regulation. UalbV doubled after reduction of insulin therapy for a couple of days, however, GFR and β_2-microglobulin excretion also increased. In another study [46] a significant but weak correlation was seen between UalbV and hemoglobin A_{1c} among 256 normo-albuminuric patiens with IDDM ($r = 0.22$, $p < 0.001$). The increase of UalbV during periods of poor metabolic regulation is probably due to an increase of glomerular filtration rate (GFR) and a decrease in the tubular reabsorption of proteins; changes in glomerular pore size and pore charge are unlikely [47].

Due to the considerable day to day variation of UalbV the question of whether longterm strict metabolic control influences UalbV can only be answered if frequent urine sampling is performed in controlled, long-lasting, prospective studies. Such studies have demonstrated that in moderately well regulated normo-albuminuric patients with Type 1 diabetes (UalbV < 30 mg/24 h or <20 μg/min) UalbV does not seem to be influenced by longterm strict metabolic control [48, 49]. In the Oslo study [50] it was demonstrated that urinary albumin excretion decreased from 26 ± (mean ± SEM) to16 ± 4 mg/24 h after 2–4 years of CSII (2p = 0.03). In a similar group of patients who received 3–6 insulin injections/day, however, no decrease of UalbV was seen (17 ± 3 vs. 14 ± 3 mg/24 h). The decrease of UalbV in the CSII group might have been due to the differing proportions of patients with microalbuminuria in the various groups of this study. In fact, nine of the 13 CSII treated patients had UalbV > 20 mg/24 h and in especially these patients UalbV improved significantly. Thus, it seems that normal UalbV in fairly well regulated diabetics cannot be lowered by longterm strict metabolic control.

If patients with UalbV above the upper normal level were included in transsectional studies, significant but weak correlations were seen between UalbV and hemoglobin A_{1c} [51, 46]. The question whether the increase of normal UalbV into the microalbuminuric range (UalbV 30–300 mg/24 h) is caused by poor glycemic control is difficult to answer. In a case control study with 113 children with a mean observation of 46 months, longterm metabolic control as assessed by multiple HbA_{1c} measurement was significantly higher ($2p < 0.05$) in children with microalbuminuria compared to children without microalbuminuria [52]. Furthermore, in a prospective study over 5 years among 200 patients with IDDM characterized by persistent normo-albuminuria, patients who developed persistent microalbuminuria at the end of the experimental period had significantly higher hemoglobin A_{1c} levels during the observation period compared to patients who remained persistent normo-albuminuric (to be published). In transsectional studies higher hemoglobin A_{1c} concentrations were found in microalbuminuric patients, but the differences were not very significant [46, 51], and mean hemogobin A_{1c} in 49 consecutive patiens with UalbV 50 – 300 mg/24 h was not higher than hemoglobin A_{1c} in 95 patients with insulin-dependent diabetes of more than 40 years duration but normal UalbV [53]. In groups of patients with florid clinical nephropathy hemoglobin A_{1c} has nearly always been found to be higher compared to patients with normal UalbV [46, 54, 55], but this can be due to the special difficulties of diabetes regulation and the higher renal glucose threshold in these patients [55].

The above-mentioned studies indicate that diabetics with poor regulation bear a higher risk of developing albuminuria than well-regulated diabetic patients. This conclusion is in agreement with recent studies on the incidence of clinical nephropathy. Thus, among patients from the Joslin Clinic the incidence rate of clinical nephropathy per 1000 person years was found to be significantly related to metabolic control as characterized by an index of hyperglycemia [56]. In a study at the Steno Memorial Hospital [57] it was found that 57 patients who later developed clinical nephropathy (characterized by persistent proteinuria and decreasing GFR) had higher postprandial blood glucose concentration during the first 10 years of diabetes compared to 103 patients who survived 40 years of diabetes without clinical nephropathy, although multiregression analysis including other clinical data of importance failed to show significance ($p = 0.052$). The same research group [58] also found that 246 patients who attended the outpatient clinic regularly for diabetes control had significantly lower cumulative incidence of nephropathy than 395 similar patients who were not followed at the specialized unit. Hasslacher [59] found a negative correlation between median postprandial blood glucose and median duration of diabetes until onset of persistent proteinuria ($p < 0.01$). The most convincing evidence for the causal relation between glycemic control and nephropathy comes from the second Steno Study [60] which demonstrated that the development of persistent proteinuria could be prevented or retarded by strict metabolic control. 36 patients with persistent microalbuminuria were allocated to either CSII or CIT. Mean hemoglobin A_{1c} and other clinical data were similar at the onset of the study. The CSII treated patients had persistently lower hemoglobin A_{1c} during the 2 year follow-up period. None of the CSII treated patients developed persistent proteinuria at the end of the 2 year observation period, whereas 5 of the control patients did ($2p < 0.05$). Other researchers have found that glycemic control influences UalbV in patients with microalbuminuria. Thus, among the 20 patients of the Kroc Study [48] who had UalbV between 13 and 190 μg/min at onset of the study, the 10 CSII treated patients showed significant decreases during the 8 month period ($30 \pm 9 \rightarrow 10 \pm 4$, (mean $\pm$ SEM)), whereas the CIT group remained relative constant ($34 \pm 7 \rightarrow 26 \pm 14$). However, the decrease of UalbV in the CSII group was mostly related to the 2 patients with high UalbV (105 and 193 μg/min) who demonstrated a very impressive reduction of UalbV already after 4 months of treatment. Since repeated determination of UalbV at the onset of the study was not done, regression towards the mean could not be excluded [61]. In another controlled study among 12 Type 1 diabetic patients with intermittent proteinuria – a mixed group of patients – Bending [62] found a constant fractional albumin clearance in the CSII treated patients, but a slightly increasing fractional albumin clearance in the conventionally treated patients during the 12 month experimental period where hemoglobin A_{1c} differed significantly between the groups. When the data from the second Steno Study were combined with data from the first Steno Study [60, 62, 63] a highly significant influence of glycemic control was demonstrated not only on the progression of UalbV but also on the incidence of persistent proteinuria, the fractional albumin clearance, the fractional IgG clearance, and the increase of blood pressure [63]. Taken together these studies strongly indicate that good metabolic control can prevent or retard the onset and progression of albuminuria (Table 3). But again it must be pointed out that the correlation between mean hemoglobin A_{1c} during the experimental period and changes in UalbV was rather low [60, 64].

Table 3 Effect of strict metabolic control on diabetic nephropathy

Albuminuria	
Normoalbuminuria	(+)
Incipient nephropathy	+
Persistent proteinuria	0
Mesangial expansion	+
Glomerular basement membrane thickening	+

The influence of glycemic control on albuminuria in patients with *advanced clinical nephropathy* (decreased GFR) is difficult to evaluate, because blood pressure, which is elevated in these patients, has a remarkable influence on UalbV [65]. In a prospective randomized controlled study on 12 patients, 6 on CSII and 6 on CIT, Viberti [66] could not find any influence of glycemic control at the end of the 24 months treatment period, and Ciavarella [67] and Sandahl Christiansen [68] found similar results. In these studies blood pressure was constant during the experimental period.

Since UalbV is, in itself, symptomless as long as nephrotic syndrome does not develop, and since increased glomerular filtration of plasma proteins, in itself, is unlikely to have a deleterious influence on renal function, the influence of glycemic control on the decline rate of GFR is more interesting.

However, since it is no longer possible to conduct longterm prospective randomized controlled studies of several years duration because of the demand for antihypertensive therapy, which highly influences the decline rate of GFR, conclusions must be based on indirect evidence. The first evidence comes from an observation by Hasslacher [59], who found the delay until elevation of serum-creatinine to be negatively correlated with blood glucose in 52 patients with Type 1 diagbetes sequentially followed after onset of persistent proteinuria ($p < 0.01$). Still more convincing is a study from Nyberg et al. [69] who follwed 18 insulin-dependent diabetic patients with clinical nephropathy for nearly 2 years prospectively with multiple blood pressure and hemoglobin A_{1c} measurements. The mean hemoglobin A_{1c} during the observation period was the only factor which, by stepwise regression analysis, correlated significantly to decline of glomerular filtration rate ($p < 0.01$). The results of the Steno Studies (unpublished results) agree with this observation indicating that strict metabolic control influences the decline rate of GFR (mesangial expansion) in a favorable way. However, it must be pointed out that antihypertensive treatment seems to be more effective in these patients than minor improvements of metabolic control by one percentage of hemoglobin A_{1c} [65].

Macroangiopathy

It has not yet been demonstrated whether glycemic control has any influence on the incidence of cardiovascular events (Table 4). In the UGDP study [18], the percentage of patients who had new non-fatal cardiovascular events in the 9–11 year observation period was remarkably similar in the control group and the insulin group, two groups which differed statistically significantly in the level of glycemic control (only 1.5 mmol glucose/1). Similar

Table 4 Effect of strict metabolic control on macroangiopathy

Macroangiopathy	
in normoalbuminurics	0
in albuminurics	?

results were also found by others [41]. On the basis of a critical review of epidemiological studies, Jarrett [70] concluded that the supposition that hyperglycemia or its associates somehow causes the increased prevalence of macroangiopathy (atherosclerosis/coronary heart disease (CHD)) can be challenged. He pointed out that macroangiopathy seeems to be independent of diabetes duration among non-insulin-dependent diabetic patients. Also the level of glycemia seems to play a minor role since NIDDM and impaired glucose tolerance (IGT) appear to indicate a similar risk for CHD, but a totally different risk for microangiopathy. Furthermore, NIDDM seems to be found in groups of patients within the general population with higher than average frequency of risk factors for CHD [70]. In IDDM the epidemiologic data available support Jarrett's assumption since relative cardiovascular mortality in IDDM patients without proteinuria was demonstrated to be independent of diabetes duration [71]. Prospective randomized controlled studies which can elucidate this very important issue were not available. In spite of the fact that glycemic control seems to be of importance for the lethality of patiens with acute myocardial infarction and apoplexia [72], overall glycemic control has only a slight, if any influence on the survival of insulin dependent diabetics without proteinuria [53].

Conclusion

Hyperglycemia is causally related to the onset and progression of early microangiopathy and neuropathy. Strict metabolic control (near normalization of blood glucose), therefore, makes sense. However, the correlation between the level of glycemic control and microangiopathy is poor and advanced microangiopathy and neuropathy seem to be unaffected by strict metabolic control. Furthermore, macroangiopathy in patients with normal urinary albumin excretion seems to be unrelated to glycemic control. It seems, therefore, important to look for other factors of importance for the development and progression of late diabetic complications.

Lipoproteins

Introduction

In recent years, increasing attention has been focused on the role of lipoproteins in the pathogenesis of atherosclerosis [73, 74]. Increased blood cholesterol levels, or more specifically, increased levels of low density lipoprotein (LDL) cholesterol, are causally related to coronary heart disease. In addition, high density lipoprotein (HDL) cholesterol, is also independently related to coronary heart disease, but the relationship is inverse; low levels of HDL increase risk while high levels seem to protect [75]. The relationship between plasma triglyceride levels and cardiovascular disease is controversial [76, 77]. Although plasma triglyceride levels are positively associated with increased risk for cardiovascular disease, in most studies they are not independently predictive of coronary heart disease after adjustments for other risk factors. Thus, it seems probable that high plasma triglyceride levels are not a direct cause of atherosclerotic disease, but rather a reflection of the presence of certain atherogenic lipoproteins.

Lipoprotein abnormalities in diabetic patients

Lipid and lipoprotein abnormalities are common in diabetic patients. In poorly controlled insulin-dependent diabetic patients the clearance of very low density lipoprotein (VLDL) and of chylomicrons are decreased because the enzyme lipoprotein lipase depends on insulin. Optimized insulin therapy rapidly reverses this, and the degree of hypertriglyceridaemia in IDDM patients correlates well with diabetes control [78]. Also non-insulin-dependent diabetic patients often have increased plasma levels of VLDL and of triglyceride. The mechanism is disputed but the hyperinsulinemia in NIDDM patients may stimulate hepatic VLDL production, and the insulin resistance may reduce the activity of lipoprotein lipase which leads to slower clearance. NIDDM patients are more likely to have raised LDL levels than IDDM patients. Diabetes can affect LDL metabolism in several ways. The number of LDL receptors is dependent on insulin and glycosylation of LDL apoprotein B may reduce LDL/LDL receptor interaction [79]. There are major differences in the impact of IDDM and NIDDM on HDL metabolism. Plasma HDL cholesterol levels are decreased during poor metabolic control in both, but after adequate insulin therapy HDL levels increase in IDDM, whereas in NIDDM the levels often remain low when even hypertriglyceridaemia and hyperglycemia are corrected. There is also evidence of altered HDL composition in NIDDM [80], and reverse cholesterol transport from the arterial wall may be impaired. A number of drugs often used in diabetic patients raise lipid levels as a significant side effect. These include several antihypertensive drugs [81] (including thiazide diuretics and β-adrenergic blocking agents) and estrogenic hormones (including oral contraceptives).

Recent studies have demonstrated that diabetic patients developing proteinuria have lipoprotein abnormalities even from the earliest stage of diabetic nephropathy [82, 83]. The proteinuric patients characterized by an extremely high cardiovascular mortality had elevated plasma cholesterol, VLDL cholesterol, LDL cholesterol, and triglyceride. These abnormalities were associated with urinary albumin excretion but not with hypertension, hyperinsulinemia, or poor metabolic control.

Treatment of lipoprotein abnormalities

For clinical management of the diabetic patient, estimation of fasting plasma cholesterol, triglyceride, and HDL cholesterol is sufficient. LDL cholesterol can be calculated using the Friedewald Equation [84], and if abnormalities are found [74] then glycaemic and diet control should be considered. In IDDM patients, achievement of near-normoglycaemia is often sufficient to normalize lipid abnormalities secondary to a diabetic state. In NIDDM patients attention should also be given to improving metabolic control with nutrition counselling, hypoglycemic drugs, or insulin therapy. However, it is often difficult to obtain satisfactory plasma levels of triglyceride, HDL cholesterol, and LDL cholesterol in NIDDM. Attempts to correct obesity and other cardiovascular risk factors often seen in NIDDM patients (e.g. hypertension and smoking) should be made, and other causes of hyperlipidemia either primary (familial) or secondary (e.g. hypothyroidism, drugs, and alcohol) should be considered. The most important change in diet is a reduction in total fat content to 30%. There has been increasing interest in the type of fat that should be included in the diet. Monounsaturated fat is recommended in order to lower LDL since, unlike some polyunsaturated fatty acids, they have no depressive effect on HDL levels [85]. If the results are not satisfactory 3–6 months after achievement of improved metabolic control and dietary changes [74] then appropriate hypolipidemic drugs should be considered. In NIDDM patients the fibrates (which reduce triglyceride and increase HDL) are useful [86], while bile acid sequestrants are the drugs of first choice in hypercholesterolemia. A detailed account of the benefits of the individual drugs is beyond the scope of this chapter, but this topic has been discussed in a recent review [86].

In conclusion, the increasing evidence that intervention against hyperlipidemia in the non-diabetic population is associated with reduced risk of coronary heart disease [87, 88, 89], shows that it is important to diagnose and treat hyperlipidemia in the diabetic population. This involves improvement of glycemic control, nutritional counselling, and, in a small group, use of hypolipidemic drugs.

Platelet reactivity and the haemostatic system

Platelet hyperreactivity and changes in the coagulation and fibrinolytic system have led to the postulation of a "hypercoagulable state" in diabetic patients. Thus most studies have described increased plasma levels of coagulation factors, changes in the activity of coagulation inhibitors and a reduction in fibrinolytic activity. In most studies these changes, together with signs of platelet hyperreactivity have been found to be associated with metabolic control and vascular complications (for recent reviews see [90] and [91]). The literature on this subject is vast so that only certain points of therapeutical relevance can be emphasized in this chapter.

As to *platelet function* divergent results have been described [90, 91, 92]. However, despite methodological problems in studying platelet adhesion/aggregation, platelet interaction with plasma components such as fibrinogen and lipoproteins, and platelet arachidonic acid metabolism, there is general agreement in the literature that platelet hypersensitivity is seen in diabetic patients with vascular disease.

Therapy with fish oil supplements to the diet was followed in IDDM patients by a reduction in thromboxane B_2 production by platelets [93, 94]. However, in one study [93], this effect was accompanied by increases of LDL cholesterol and fibrinogen. Nevertheless, epidemiologic findings have indicated that it is possible that dietary fish could prevent coronary artery disease [95]. Longterm controlled studies are needed to clarify whether benefits of fish oil supplementation overweigh the risks in the diabetic population.

Studies of the effects of intensified insulin therapy and of antiplatelet agents (e.g. aspirin and dipyridamole) on platelet function and development of late diabetic complications are now being carried out. Data are still inconclusive [96] but the "platelet hypothesis" as a contribution to the understanding of diabetic vascular disease is still attractive. Clearly, additional intervention studies are needed.

Recent studies of the hemostatic system have shown that the plasma level of fibrinogen is a strong and independent risk factor for myocardial infarction [97, 98] (Table 5). The impact of the fibrinogen level was found to be com-

Table 5 Importance of plasma fibrinogen as a risk factor for coronary heart disease. Relative risk is the risk in the group considered divided by the risk in patients in the lowest tertile group [98]

Plasma fibrinogen	Relative risk
Lowest tertile	1
Middle tertile	1.4
Highest tertile	2.6

parable with established risk factors such as blood pressure and hypercholesterolemia. In diabetic patients, elevated plasma fibrinogen levels have been related to small vessel disease [83, 99] (Table 6). Although fibrinogen levels were lowered with treatment of hyperglycemia [99], until now no fibrinogen lowering agents have been developed. Epidemiological studies [97] have shown an association between smoking and plasma fibrinogen in non-diabetics. In summary, changes in the coagulation and fibrinolytic systems together with platelet hyperreactivity are of possible importance for development of both small and large vessel disease. However, the pathogenetic mechanisms are only poorly understood. There have been only few intervention studies and therapeutical guidelines have not been developed.

Table 6 Plasma concentration of fibrinogen (μmol/l) (median and range) in IDDM patients with varying levels of urinary albumin excretion [83]

Normal UalbV	(<30 mg/24 h)	7.66 (5.16–11.52)
Incipient nephropathy	(30–300 mg/24 h)	8.68 (5.24–12.85)
Clinical nephropathy	(>300 mg/24 h)	9.62 (6.04–13.73)

Hypertension

The progression of atherosclerosis and diabetic nephropathy is clearly associated with the presence of hypertension. This topic is discussed in detail in the chapters by Mogensen, Pyörälä and Standl, and will only be considered briefly in this section.

Treatment of hypertension in patients without nephropathy

Recommendations for treatment of hypertension in diabetes have recently been published [100]. As other cardiovascular risk factors (e.g. obesity, hypercholesterolemia, and smoking) are often present and act synergistically in hypertensive diabetic patients, initial nonpharmacologic approaches are important. These include dietary changes, weight reduction, exercise, and cessation of smoking. No antihypertensive agents seem to be contraindicated in diabetic patients, but knowledge of and careful control of side effects (e. g. changes in lipoproteins and hypoglycemia) are important.

Treatment of hypertension in patients with nephropathy

As outlined in detail in the chapter by Mogensen, early antihypertensive treatment reduces the progression of diabetic nephropathy [101]. Patients with this complication also have a high risk of early cardiovascular death [71]. Established risk factors such as abnormalities in lipoproteins and fibrinogen are often present [102]. Diagnosis of these abnormalities and control of antihypertensive drug side effects are, therefore, necessary in treating diabetic patients with nephropathy.

Large scale trials of antihypertensive treatment in non-diabetic patients have shown a reduction in the number of strokes but no effect in the number of coronary events in the treated groups [103]. In the treated non-smokers, however, a trend toward reduction in coronary events was observed, which shows the importance of smoking as a risk factor. The effect of early antihypertensive treatment on the longterm survival may be more pronounced in diabetic patients. Results from yet unpublished cohort studies at the Steno Memorial Hospital clearly show a dramatic reduction in mortality in proteinuric patients when antihypertensive treatment was started soon after onset of persistent proteinuria.

Hyperinsulinemia

Results form experimental and clinical studies have suggested that hyperinsulinemia may be linked with the development of atherosclerosis [104]. The majority of diabetic patients have systemic hyperinsulinemia that is the result of either exogenous insulin therapy or the chronic hyperinsulinemia seen in many NIDDM patients. Hyperinsulinemia may be associated with elevated plasma levels of VLDL cholesterol and triglyceride and decreased levels of HDL cholesterol [105]. Also there seems to be a link between hyperinsulinemia and hypertension [106, 107]. Three prospective population-based studies have shown that in non-diabetics elevated fasting and/or postprandial plasma insulin levels are associated with an increased risk of coronary heart disease independent of other risk factors, including blood glucose levels [108, 109, 110].

The suggestive evidence that hyperinsulinemia may play a role in the development of atherosclerosis in diabetic patients indicate that it could be beneficial, especially for the NIDDM patient, to design a therapeutic approach, based on the minimization of hyperinsulinemia. This is best achieved by reduction in obesity and by exercise. Weight loss reduces circulating insulin levels and improves glucose uptake by the peripheral tissue. Exercise increases the number of insulin receptors and results in a decrease in circulating insulin. A secondary advantage of exercise is an increase in the plasma levels of HDL cholesterol. Various types of oral hypoglycemic agents theoretically have differing abilities to stimulate insulin secretion and/or to improve insulin sensitivity. It is still being debated whether exogenous insulin therapy should be initiated early in NIDDM patients. This topic has recently been reviewed [111]. Since our knowledge is far from complete, strict therapeutical guidelines for the use of single oral hypoglycemic agents and for optimal use of exogenous insulin for the reduction of peripheral hyperinsulinemia cannot yet be outlined.

References

[1] Ganda OP, Williamson JR, Soeldner JS et al. Muscle Capillary Basement Membrane Width and Its Relationship to Diabetes Mellitus in Monozygotic Twins. Diabetes 1983; 32: 549–556.

[2] Steffes MW, Sutherland DER, Goetz FC et al. Studies of Kidney and muscle biopsy specimens from identical twins discordant for type I Diabetes Mellitus. N Engl J Med 1985; 312: 1282–1287.

[3] Feingold, KR, Lee TH, Chung MY et al. Muscle Capillary Basement Membrane Width in Patients with Vacor-induced Diabetes Mellitus. J Clin Invest 1986; 78: 102–107.

[4] Sosenko JM, Miettinen OS, Williamson JR et al. Muscle Capillary Basement-Membrane Thickness and Long-Term Glycemia in Type I Diabetes Mellitus. N Engl J Med 1984; 311: 694–698.

[5] Raskin P, Pietri AO, Unger R et al. The effect of diabetic control on the width of skeletal-muscle capillary basement membrane in patients with Type I diabetes mellitus. N Engl J Med 1983; 309: 1546–1550.

[6] Camerini-Davalos RA, Velasco C, Glasser M et al. Drug-induced reversal of early diabetic microangiopathy. N Engl J Med 1983; 309: 1551–1556.

[7] Mauer SM, Steffes MW, Connett J et al. The Development of Lesions in the Glomerular Basement Membrane and Mesangium After Transplantation of Normal Kidneys to Diabetic Patients. Diabetes 1983; 32: 948–952.

[8] Bohman S-O, Tydén G, Wilczek H et al. Prevention of Kidney Graft Diabetic Nephropathy by Pancreas Transplantation in Man. Diabetes 1985; 34: 306–308.

[9] Bilous RW, Mauer SM, Sutherland DER et al. Glomerular Structure and Function Following Successful Pancreas Transplantation (PTx) for Insulin-Dependent Diabetes Mellitus (IDDM). Diabetes 1987; 36 (suppl 2): 43A.

[10] Abouna GM, Kremer GD, Daddah SK et al. Reversal of diabetic nephropathy in human cadaveric kidneys after transplantation into non-diabetic recipients. Lancet 1983; 1274–1276.

[11] Weber B, Burger W, Hartmann R et al. Risk factors for the development of retinopathy in children and adolescents with Type 1 (insulin-dependent) diabetes mellitus. Diabetologia 1986; 29: 23–29.

[12] Doft BH, Kingsley LA, Orchard TJ et al. The Association Between Long-term Diabetic Control and Early Retinopathy. Ophthalmology 1984; 91: 763–769.

[13] Dahl-Jørgensen K, Brinchmann-Hansen O, Hanssen KF et al. Effect of near-normoglycemia for two years on progression of early diabetic retinopathy and neuropathy; the Oslo study. Br Med J 1986; 293: 1195–1199.

[14] Brinchmann-Hansen O, Dahl-Jørgensen K, Hanssen KF et al. Diabetic Retinopathy through 41 months with multiple injections, insulin pumps and conventional therapy. Arch Ophthalmol (Submitted for publication).

[15] Kohner EM, Lawson PM, Ghosh G et al. Assessment of Fluorescein Angiograms. Diabetes 1985; 34 (suppl 3): 56–60.

[16] The Kroc Collaborative Study Group. The Kroc Study Patients at Two Years: A Report on Further Retinal Changes. Diabetes 1985; 34 (suppl 1): 39A.

[17] Engerman R, Bloodworth Jr JMB, Nelson S. Relationship of Microvascular Disease in Diabetes to Metabolic Control. Diabetes 1977; 26: 760–769.

[18] Knatterud GL, Klimt CR, Levin ME et al. Effects of Hypoglycemic Agents on Vascular Complications in Patients With Adult-Onset Diabetes. JAMA 1978; 240: 37–42.

[19] Howard-Williams J, Hillson RM, Bron A et al. Retinopathy is associated with higher glycaemia in maturity-onset type diabetes. Diabetologia 1984; 27: 198–202.

[20] Hockaday TDR, Pandher KS, Bron A et al. Progression of Established Retinopathy Is Unrelated to Glycosylated Hemoglobin in Non-Insulin-Dependent Diabetes. Transplantation Proceedings 1986; 18 (6): 1574–1575.

[21] Nathan DM, Singer DE, Godine JE et al. Retinopathy in Older Type II Diabetics. Association With Glucose Control. Diabetes 1986; 35: 797–801.

[22] Lauritzen T, Frost-Larsen K, Larsen H-W et al. Two-Year Experience with Continuous Subcutaneous Insulin Infusion in Relation to Retinopathy and Neuropathy. Diabetes 1985; 34 (suppl 3): 74–79.

[23] Beck-Nielsen H, Richelsen B, Mogensen CE et al. Effect of Insulin Pump Treatment for One Year on Renal Function and Retinal Morphology in Patients with IDDM. Diabetes Care 1985; 8: 585–589.

[24] Rosenstock J, Friberg T, Raskin P. Effect of Glycemic Control on Microvascular Complications in Patients with Type I Diabetes Mellitus. Am J Med 1986; 81: 1012–1018.

[25] Italian National Research Council (CNR) Study. One year report. Metabolic control and diabetic retinopathy. Diabetologia 1986; 29: 111 (A).

[26] Lauritzen T, Larsen H-W, Frost-Larsen K et al. Effect of 1 year of near-normal blood glucose levels on retinopathy in insulin-dependent diabetics. Lancet 1983; 200–204.

[27] Helve E, Laatikainen L, Merenmies L et al. Continuous insulin infusion therapy and retinopathy in patients with type I diabetes. Acta Endocrinol 1987; 115 (3): 313–319.

[28] Krolewski AS, Warram JH, Rand LI et al. Risk of Proliferative Diabetic Retinopathy in Juvenile-Onset Type I Diabetes: a 40-yr Follow-up Study. Diabetes Care 1986; 9 (5): 443–452.

[29] Dornan T, Mann JI, Turner R. Factors protective against retinopathy in insulin-dependent diabetics free of retinopathy for 30 years. Br Med J 1982; 285: 1073–1077.

[30] Kofoed-Enevoldsen A, Jensen T, Borch-Johnsen K et al. Incidence of Retinopathy in Type I (insulin-dependent) Diabetes: Association with Clinical Nephropathy. Journal of Diabetic Complications 1987; 1: 96–99.

[31] Rand LI, Krolewski AS, Aiello LM et al. Multiple Factors in the Prediction of Risk of Proliferative Diabetic Retinopathy. N Engl J Med 1985; 313: 1433–1438.

[32] Klein R, Klein BEK, Moss SE et al. The Wisconsin Epidemiologic Study of Diabetes Retinopathy. II Prevalence and Risk of Diabetic Retinopathy When Age at Diagnosis Is Less Than 30 Years. Arch Ophthalmol 1984; 102: 520–526.

[33] Ramsay RC, Goetz FC, Sutherland DER et al. Progression of diabetic retinopathy after pancreas transplantation for insulin-dependent diabetes mellitus. N Engl J Med 1988; 318: 208–214.

[34] Graf RJ, Halter JB, Pfeifer MA et al. Glycemic control and nerve conduction abnormalities in noninsulin dependent diabetic subjects. Ann Intern Med 1981; 94: 307–311.
[35] Boulton AJM, Worth RC, Drury J et al. Genetic and metabolic studies in diabetic neuropathy. Diabetologia 1984: 26: 15–19.
[36] Porte Jr D. The Role of Metabolic Control in the Onset and Development of Diabetic Neuropathy. In: Andreani D, Crepaldi G, Di Mario U et al, eds. Diabetic Complications: Early Diagnosis and Treatment. John Wiley & Sons Ltd, 1987; 123–131.
[37] Dahl-Jørgensen K, Ganes T, Hanssen KF et al. Effects of two years of strict blood glucose control on peripheral nerve function in insulin dependent diabetes mellitus. The Oslo Study. Acta Neurol 1987 (Submitted for publication).
[38] Service FJ, Rizz RA, Daube JR et al. Near normoglycemia improved nerve conduction and vibration sensation in diabetic neuropathy. Diabetologia 1985; 28: 722–727.
[39] Ziegler D, Cicmir I, Mayer P et al. Somatic and autonomic nerve function during the first year after diagnosis of type 1 (insulin-dependent) diabetes. Diabetes Research 1988; 8 (In press).
[40] Holman RR, Mayon-White V, Orde-Pecker C et al. Prevention of deterioration of renal and sensory-nerve function by more intensive management of insulin-dependent diabetic patients. Lancet 1983; 204–208.
[41] Young RJ, Macintyre CCA, Martyn CN et al. Progression of subclinical polyneuropathy in young patients with Type 1 (insulin-dependent) diabetes: associations with glycaemic control and microangiopathy (microvascular complications). Diabetologia 1986; 29: 156–161.
[42] The St. Thomas's Diabetic Study Group. Failure of improved glycaemic control to reverse diabetic autonomic neuropathy. Diabetic Med 1986; 3: 330–334.
[43] Solders G, Wilczek H, Gunnarsson R. Effects of Combined Pancreatic and Renal Transplantation on Diabetic Neuropathy: A Two-year Follow-up Study. Lancet 1987; II: 1232–1235.
[44] Hanssen KF, Dahl-Jørgensen K, Lauritzen T et al. Diabetic control and microvascular complications: the near- normoglycaemic experience. Diabetologia 1986; 29: 677–684.
[45] Parving H-H, Noer I, Deckert T et al. The Effect of Metabolic Regulation on Microvascular Permeability to Small and Large Molecules in Short-Term Juvenile Diabetics. Diabetologia 1976; 12: 161–166.
[46] Sami N, Feldt-Rasmussen B, Deckert T. Microalbuminuria in Insulin-dependent Diabetes: Prevalence and Practical Consequences. Journal of Diabetic Complications 1987; 1: 76–80.
[47] Deckert T, Feldt-Rasmussen B, Djurup R et al. Glomerular size and charge selectivity in insulin-dependent diabetes mellitus. Kidney International 1988; 33: 100–106.
[48] Bending JJ, Viberti GC, Bilous RW et al. Eight-Month Correction of Hyperglycemia in Insulin-dependent Diabetes Mellitus Is Associated with a Significant and Sustained Reduction of Urinary Albumin Excretion Rates in Patients with Microalbuminuria. Diabetes 1985; 34 (suppl 3): 69–73.
[49] Mogensen CE, Beck-Nielsen H, Richelsen B et al. Long-term intervention studies: insulin pump treatment in normoalbuminuric diabetics aand antihypertensive treatment in incipient nephropathy. Five year follow-up studies, effect on GFR, blood pressure and urinary albumin excretion ratio. Proceedings of the International Symposium "Diabetic Complications "87", Rome, 29–31 October 1987.
[50] Dahl-Jørgensen K, Hanssen KF, Kierulf P et al. Reduction of urinary albumin excretion after 4 years of continuous subcutaneous insulin infusion in insulin-dependent diabetes mellitus. Acta Endocrinol 1988; 117: 19–25.
[51] Wiseman M, Viberti G, Mackintosh D et al. Glycaemia, arterial pressure and microalbuminuria in Type 1 (insulin-dependent) diabetes mellitus. Diabetologia 1984; 26: 401–405.
[52] Nørgaard K, Storm B, Graae M et al. Microalbuminuria and retinal changes in children with type 1 (insulin-dependent) diabetes mellitus are related to long-term poor metabolic control. Diabetic Medicine. (In press).

[53] Deckert T, Feldt-Rasmussen B, Borch-Johnsen K et al. Glycaemic control and Microvascular Complications in Type I Diabetic Patients. Pediat adolesc Endocr 1987; 17: 186–196.

[54] Schulz, B, Zander E, Mester J. Progession of Diabetic Nephropathy in Insulin-Independent Diabetes Mellitus in Relation to Metabolic Control and Blood Pressure. Transplantation Proceedings 1986; 18: 6, 1665.

[55] Bending, JJ, Pickup JC, Viberti GC et al. Glycaemic control in diabetic nephropathy. Br Med J 1984; 288: 1187–1191.

[56] Krolewski AS, Warram JH, Christlieb AR et al. The Changing Natural History of Nephropathy in Type I Diabetes. Am J Med 1985; 78: 785–793.

[57] Borch-Johnsen K, Nissen H, Salling N et al. The Natural History of Insulin-Dependent Diabetes in Denmark: 2. Long-term survival – who and why. Diabetic Medicine 1987; 4: 211–216.

[58] Borch-Johnsen K, Kreiner S, Deckert T. Diabetic nephropathy – susceptible to care? Diabetes Res 1986; 3: 397–400.

[59] Hasslacher Ch, Stech W, Wahl P et al. Blood pressure and metabolic control as risk factors for nephropathy in Type 1 (insulin-dependent) diabetes. Diabetologia 1985; 28: 6–11.

[60] Feldt-Rasmussen B, Mathiesen ER, Deckert T. Effect of two years of strict metabolic control on progression of incipient nephropathy in insulin-dependent diabetes. Lancet 1986; 1300–1304.

[61] Feldt-Rasmussen B, Mogensen CE, Christensen CK et al. Blood glucose control and diabetic microangiopathy. N Engl J Med 1984; 311: 1577–1578.

[62] Deckert T, Lauritzen T, Parving H-H et al. Effect of Two Years of Strict Metabolic Control on Kidney Function in Long-Term Insulin-Dependent Diabetics. Diabet Nephrop 1983; 2: 6–10.

[63] Deckert T, Feldt-Rasmussen B, Borch-Johnsen K et al. Proteinuria, an Indicator of Malignan Angiopathy. In: Andreani D, Crepaldi G, Di Mario U et al, eds. Diabetic Complications: Early Daignosis and Treatment. John Wiley & Sons Ltd, 1987; 257–261.

[64] Deckert T, Poulsen JE. Diabetic Nephropathy. Fault or Destiny? Diabetologia 1981; 21: 178–183.

[65] Parving H-H, Andersen AR, Smidt UM et al. Effect of antihypertensive treatment on kidney function in diabetic nephropathy. Br Med J 1987; 294: 1443–1447.

[66] Viberti GC, Bilous RW, Mackintosh D et al. Long term correction of hyperglycaemia and progression of renal failure in insulin dependent diabetes. Br Med J 1983; 286: 598–602.

[67] Ciavarella A, Vannini P, Flammini M et al. Effect of long-term near-normoglycemia on the progression of diabetic nephropathy. Diabete & Metabolisme 1985; 11: 3–8.

[68] Christiansen JS, Parving H-H. The effect of short-term strict metabolic control on albuminuria in insulin-dependent diabetics with normal kidney function and diabetic nephropathy. Diab Nephropathy 1984; 3: 127–129.

[69] Nyberg G, Blohmé G, Nordén G. Impact of metabolic control in progression of clinical diabetic nephropathy. Diabetologia 1987; 30: 82–86.

[70] Jarrett RJ. The epidemiology of coronary heart disease and related factors in the context of diabetes mellitus and impaired glucose tolerance. In: Jarrett RJ, ed. Diabetes and heart disease. Amsterdam–New York–Oxford: Elsevier, 1984; 1–23.

[71] Borch-Johnsen K, Kreiner S. Proteinuria: value as predictor of cardiovascular mortality in insulin dependent diabetes mellitus. Br Med J 1987; 294: 1651–1654.

[72] Rytter L, Troelsen S, Beck-Nielsen H. Prevalence and mortality of acute myocardial infarction in patients with diabetes. Diabetes Care 1985; 8: 230–234.

[73] The expert panel. Report of the national cholesterol education program expert panel on detection, evaluation, and treatment of high blood cholesterol in adults. Arch Intern Med 1988; 148: 36–69.

[74] Study group of the European Atherosclerosis Society. Strategies for the prevention of coronary heart disease: a policy statement of the European Atherosclerosis Society. Eur Heart J 1987; 8: 77–78.

[75] Castelli WP, Garrison RJ, Wilson PWF et al. Incidence of coronary heart disease and lipoprotein cholesterol levels: The Framingham Study. J Am Med Assoc 1986; 256: 2835–2838.

[76] Castelli WP. The triglyceride issue: a view from Framingham. Am Heart J 1986; 112: 432–437.

[77] Cambien F, Jacqueson A, Richard JL et al. Is the level of serum triglyceride a significant predictor of coronary death in nomorcholesterolaemic subjects? The Paris Prospective Study. Am J Epidemiol 1986; 124: 624–632.

[78] Dunn FL, Pietri A, Raskin P. Plasma lipid and lipoprotein levels with continuous subcutaneous insulin infusion in type I diabetes mellitus. Ann Intern Med 1981; 95: 426–431.

[79] Witztum JK, Majoney EM, Branks MJ et al. Nonenzymatic glycosylation of low density lipoprotein alters its biological activity. Diabetes 1982; 31: 283–291.

[80] Schonfeld G, Birge C, Miller P et al. Apoprotein B levels and altered lipoprotein composition in diabetes. Diabetes 1974; 23: 827–834.

[81] Weidman P, Gerber A, Mordasini R. Effects of antihypertensive treatment on serum lipoprotein. Hypertension 1983; 5 (suppl III): III-120–III-131.

[82] Das AK, Chandrasegaran S, Ramarkrishnan S, Chandrasekar S, Ghosh MN. Serum high density lipid-cholesterol, triglyceride and cholesterol in young Indian diabetics. Med Sci Res 1987; 15: 401–402.

[83] Jensen T, Stender S, Deckert T. Abnormalities in plasma concentrations of lipoproteins and fibrinogen in Type I (insulin-dependent) diabetic patients with increased urinary albumin excretion. Diabetologia 1988; 31: 142–145.

[84] Friedewald WT, Levy RI, Fredrickson DS. Estimation of the concentration of low-density lipoprotein cholesterol in plasma, without the use of the preparative ultracentrifuge. Clin Chem 1972; 18: 499–502.

[85] Mattsom FH, Grundy SM. Comparison of effects of dietary staturated, monosaturated and polyunsaturated fatty acids on plasma lipids and lipoproteins in man. J Lipid Res 1985; 26: 194–202.

[86] Lopes-Virella MF, Colwell JA. Pharmacological treatment of lipid disorders in diabetes mellitus. Diabetes/Metabol Rev 1987; 3: 691–722.

[87] Frick MH, Elo O, Haapa K et al. Helsinki Heart Study: Primary prevention trial with gemfibrozil in middleaged men with dyslipidenia. N Engl J Med 1987; 317: 1237–1245.

[88] Lipid Research Clinics Program. The Lipid Research Clinics Coronary Primary Prevention Trial Results. I. Reduction in incidence of coronary heart disease. J Am Med Assoc 1984; 251: 351–364.

[89] Blankenhorn DH, Nessim SA, Johnson RL et al. Beneficial effects of combined colestipol-niacin therapy on coronary atherosclerosis and coronary venous bypass grafts. J Am Med Assoc 1987; 257: 3233–3240.

[90] Banga JD, Sixma JJ. Diabetes mellitus, vascular disease and thrombosis. Clinics in Haematology 1986; 15: 465–492.

[91] Ostermann H, van de Loo J. Factors of the hemostatic system in diabetic patients. A survey of controlled studies. Haemostatis 1986; 16: 386–416.

[92] Allesandrini P, McRae J, Feman S et al. Thromboxane biosynthesis and platelet function in Type I diabetes mellitus. N Engl J Med 1988; 319: 208–212.

[93] Haines AP, Sanders TAB, Imeson JD et al. Effects of a fish oil supplement on platelet function, haemostatic variables and albuminuria in insulin-dependent diabetics. Thromb Res 1986; 43: 643–655.

[94] Beitz J, Schinke E, Liebang U et al. Influence of a cod liver oil diet in healthy and insulin-dependent diabetic volunteers on fatty acid pattern, inhibition of prostacyclin formation by low density lipoprotein (LDL) and platelet thromboxane. Klin Wochenschr 1986; 64: 793–799.

[95] Bang HO, Dyerberg J, Hjørne N. The composition of food consumed by Greenland Eskimos. Acta Med Scand 1976; 200: 69–73.

[96] Kohner E. Pathogenic mechanisms in the development of diabetic retinopathy. In: Andreani D, Crepaldi G, Di Mario U, Pozza G, eds. Diabetic complications: Early Diagnosis and Treatment. John Wiley & Sons Ltd, 1987; 55–63.
[97] Meade TW, Mellows S, Brozovic M et al. Haemostatic function in ischaemic heart disease. Principal results of the Northwick Park Heart Study. Lancet 1986; II: 533–537.
[98] Kannel WB, Wolf OA, Castelli WP et al. Fibrinogen and risk of cardiovascular disease. JAMA 1987; 258: 1183–1186.
[99] Jones RL, Peterson CM. The fluid phase of coagulation and the accelerated atherosclerosis of diabetes mellitus. Diabetes 1981; 30: 33–38.
[100] The working group on hypertension in diabetes. Statement on hypertension in diabetes mellitus: final report. Arch Intern Med 1987; 147: 830–842.
[101] Parving H-H, Andersen AR, Smidt UM et al. Effect of antihypertensive treatment on kidney function in diabetic nephropathy. Br Med J 1987; 294: 1443–1447.
[102] Valdorf-Hansen F, Jensen T, Borch-Johnsen et al. Cardiovascular risk factors in type I (insulin-dependent) diabetic patients with and without proteinuria. Acta Med Scand 1987; 222: 439–444.
[103] MRC trial of treatment of mild hypertension: Principal results. Medical Research Council Working Party. Br Med J (Clin Res) 1985; 291: 97–104.
[104] Stout RW. Insulin and atheroma – an update. Lancet 1987; I: 1077–1079.
[105] Uusitupa M, Sittonen O, Voutilained A et al. Serum lipids and lipoproteins in newly diagnosed non-insulin-dependent (type II) diabetic patients with special reference to factors influencing HDL-cholesterol and triglyceride levels. Diabetes Care 1986; 9: 17–22.
[106] DeFronzo RA. The effect of insulin on renal sodium metabolism. Diabetologia 1981; 21: 165–171.
[107] Singer P, Godicke W, Woigkt S. et al. Post prandial hyperinsulinemia in patients with mild essential hypertension. Hypertension 1985; 7: 182–186.
[108] Pyörälä K, Savolainen E, Kaukola S. et al. Plasma insulin as coronary heart disease risk factor: relationship to other risk factors and predictive value during 9 1/2-year follow-up of the Helsinki Policemen Study population. Acta Med Scand 1985; suppl 701: 38–52.
[109] Welborn TA, Wearne K. Coronary heart disease incidence and cardiovascular mortality in Busselton with reference to glucose and insulin concentration. Diabetes Care 1979; 2: 154–160.
[110] Eschwege E, Ducimetiere P, Thibult N et al. Coronary heart disease mortality in relation with diabetes, blood glucose and plasma insulin levels. The Paris prospective study, ten years later. Horm Metab Res 1985; 15 (suppl): 41–45.
[111] Stolar MW. Atherosclerosis in diabetes: the role of hyperinsulinemia. Metabolism 1988; 37 (suppl 1): 1–9.

Subject index